BREAST CARE

A Clinical Guidebook for Women's
Primary Health Care Providers

Springer

New York
Berlin
Heidelberg
Barcelona
Hong Kong
London
Milan
Paris
Singapore
Tokyo

William H. Hindle, M.D. Editor

Professor of Clinical Obstetrics and Gynecology
University of Southern California School of Medicine; and
Director, Breast Diagnostic Center
Women's and Children's Hospital
LAC + USC Medical Center
Los Angeles, California

BREAST CARE

A Clinical Guidebook for Women's Primary Health Care Providers

With a Foreword by Vicki Seltzer, M.D.

With 178 Illustrations, 16 in Color

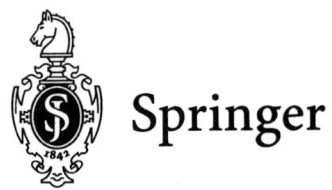

Springer

William H. Hindle, M.D.
Professor of Clinical Obstetrics and Gynecology
University of Southern California School of Medicine; and
Director, Breast Diagnostic Center
Women's and Children's Hospital
LAC + USC Medical Center
Los Angeles, CA 90033
USA

Library of Congress Cataloging-in-Publication Data
Breast care : a clinical guidebook for women's primary health care
    providers / [edited by] William H. Hindle.
        p.   cm.
    Includes index.
    ISBN 0-387-98348-1 (hardcover : alk. paper)
    1. Breast—Diseases. 2. Breast—Cancer. 3. Breast—Care and
hygiene. 4. Women's health services. 5. Women—Health and hygiene.
I. Hindle, William H.
    [DNLM: 1. Breast Diseases—diagnosis. 2. Breast Diseases—
therapy. 3. Primary Health Care. 4. Women's Health.   WP 840 B827
1998]
RG4993.B74   1998
618.1'9—dc21

97-49307

Printed on acid-free paper.

Production managed by Terry Kornak; manufacturing supervised by Joe Quatela.
Typeset by Best-set Typesetters, Hong Kong.
Printed and bound by Maple-Vail Book Manufacturing Group, York, PA.
Printed in the United States of America.

9 8 7 6 5 4 3 2 1

ISBN 0-387-98348-1 Springer-Verlag New York Berlin Heidelberg   SPIN 10645878

DEDICATION

With profound respect and admiration this book is dedicated to Daniel R. Mishell Jr., M.D., Lyle G. McNeile Professor and Chairman, Department of Obstetrics and Gynecology, University of Southern California School of Medicine, Los Angeles, California. Without Dr. Mishell, the Breast Diagnostic Center of Women's and Children's Hospital would not have come into being or flourished as it has. Dr. Mishell was the visionary and pioneering force behind the establishment and expansion of the Breast Diagnostic Center as a comprehensive breast service for the dual purpose of educating our obstetrics and gynecology resident physicians and providing breast care for women attending Women's and Children's Hospital. In addition, Dr. Mishell's continuing enthusiasm has sustained the creation and growth of all the breast services within the Department of Obstetrics and Gynecology. The experience gained from providing these services and from their relations to support services within the Los Angeles County and University of Southern California (LAC + USC) Medical Center form the basis of this book. Dr. Mishell has been a dear personal friend since our "early days" during the late 1950s when we were together in the Harbor (Harbor General Hospital/University of California at Los Angeles) combined obstetrics and gynecology residency training program. Above all, Dr. Mishell is a relentlessly productive medical educator who inspires all of us to teach "from the data."

W.H.H.

FOREWORD

Breast cancer is the most common cancer in women. There are more than 180,000 new cases a year diagnosed in the United States, and approximately 46,000 deaths. Although we certainly have not yet had the same degree of success in reducing breast cancer mortality as we have had in reducing cervical cancer mortality, progress is being made. Due to aggressive attempts by the Ob-Gyn community to educate women about the risks of breast cancer, and to make certain that women are being screened, there has been a reduction in the incidence of tumors larger than three centimeters, and an increase in the detection of small and in situ lesions. In addition, mortality from breast cancer in the United States finally appears to be beginning to decline.

Although one of the main responsibilities of the medical community with regard to breast disease is to do whatever is possible to reduce mortality from breast cancer, another important responsibility is to diagnose and treat nonmalignant breast problems. A common reason for women to seek health care is for breast complaints that are benign, but are troubling to the patient. It is very important for the physician to be able to rule out the presence of cancer, and then treat the problem.

Obstetrician-gynecologists have been at the forefront in helping women with breast problems. For decades they have been educating women about breast disease, fostering early detection of breast cancer, and treating benign breast problems. Dr. William Hindle has been one of the leaders in educating obstetrician-gynecologists about breast disease, having worked extensively both in training medical school students and resident physicians, and in providing continuing education courses for professionals already in practice.

In this book, Dr. Hindle covers all of the most relevant issues that a physician must understand in order to diagnose and treat breast problems. It is an important contribution to our continuing effort to provide the best possible health care for women.

Vicki Seltzer, M.D.
President (1997–8), American College of Obstetricians & Gynecologists

PREFACE

Historically, except for the surgical treatment of breast cancer, widespread and comprehensive medical education and pertinent research on breast disorders has been lacking. However, in the last 30 years the magnitude of the symptoms and disorders of the female breast, particularly breast cancer, have inspired a multitude of "breast books" both for the "lay public" and health care professionals. Many of these are expensive medical tomes packed with facts and figures from the medical literature but which are essentially irrelevant to the needs of primary health care providers. Furthermore, most of the data provided by the continuing medical information explosion is now available from medline and other computerized networks and software services.

How then are those with heretofore little formal instruction and experience in breast care to prepare themselves for their roles as HMO gatekeepers and front line managed care providers for women with breast concerns and problems?

This book attempts to set forth in a clear, concise, pragmatic, and well-illustrated format the nine-year experience of the Breast Diagnostic Center (BDC) of Women's and Children's Hospital, LAC + USC Medical Center, Los Angeles, California (1988–1997) along with the experience of those consultants in the various specialties to whom our patients are referred.

Included are a few chapters by authors of national reputation outside of the University of Southern California who have been invited to present their experience and particular expertise, which is not otherwise locally available.

Dr. David Grimes is a notable example of the appropriateness of such inclusion. His contribution (Chapter 2) on the importance of applying evidence-based medicine to breast care is positioned at the beginning of this book to emphasize the fundamental importance of having accurate data as the basis for clinical management. This approach exhorts the primary health care provider to stay current with the medical literature and the advances in breast care that are founded on scientific data in order to assure continuing quality medical care for the patient.

Dr. James Hall has unique and extensive experience as an obstetrician/gynecologist providing complete breast care, including surgical treatment of breast cancer, to his patients in rural north-central Indiana. His comprehensive approach and personal data presented in Chapter 38 should serve as an inspiration to others who may have the opportunity of providing comprehensive care in a private rural setting.

Dr. Audrey Arona (Chapters 13, 15, and 33) has taken her training at the BDC into private practice where she has successfully applied the principles and techniques she learned to a competitive clinical setting. Obtaining hospital surgical privileges for performing open surgical biopsy (OSBx) was initially a "struggle" but eventually she earned the acceptance and cooperation of the oncologic surgeons and pathologists with whom she works. Dr. Arona found that the OSBx training during her residency was more than satisfactory technical preparation. In fact, pathologists and other surgical personnel have commented that her technical skills and surgical specimens are more appropriate than those of some surgical specialists.

As a practitioner of family medicine, Dr. Suzanne Taylor contributes in Chapter 39 her compassionate adaptation of the general BDC principles to the breast care of her female patients in a rural setting located far from extensive support services or specialty consultants. As a primary care physician, Dr. Taylor stresses patient-doctor rapport and the close monitoring of continuity of care particularly during the diagnosis and treatment of breast cancer.

Finally, in Chapter 41, Dr. David Plotkin presents his unique insight and perspective into the natural history and biologic behavior of breast cancer based on his personal experience of more than 40 years of medical oncology observation.

As this book is intended as a practical guide for the evaluation and management of women's breast problems by primary care providers, the material presented is based on the experience of the various authors and they have not been required to give citations and references. However, by individual preference, some authors have included citations. In addition, certain key references that are fundamentally germane and pertinent are footnoted.

This book presents a practical and effective clinical approach to the specific patient population and health care setting at the BDC. The reader should freely adapt the material, procedures, techniques, and protocols given in this book to his or her local situation. The principles described herein are universally applicable. Each geographic location, physical setting, patient population, and practice situation will dictate some variation in the application of these principles. However—this is how WE do it!

William H. Hindle, M.D.
Los Angeles, California

ACKNOWLEDGMENTS

I wish to acknowledge the personal inspiration and professional contribution I have received from the following individuals: Drs. Bruce H. Drukker, John H. Isaacs, and Douglas J. Marchant, obstetrician/gynecologist pioneers in the study and surgery of the female breast (Dr. Marchant particularly who, in addition to being a prolific author and frequent lecturer on breast disease, has been at the forefront of recent developments in surgical diagnosis and treatment of breast cancer; Dr. Keith Russell for his untiring efforts to have care of the breast included as an integral part of obstetrics and gynecology; Drs. Ralph Hale, Purvis Martin, and Herman Rhu for their friendship and assistance with my involvement in the American College of Obstetricians and Gynecologists; Dr. C. Donald Christian for his energy and tenacity in moving the American Board of Obstetrics and Gynecology to hold a Conference on Breast Disease—An Initiative for Curriculum Development in Residency Education in 1986; Dr. Philip J. DiSaia for his courageous public stance and pioneering clinical work on the use of estrogen replacement therapy for estrogen-deficient women who have been treated for breast cancer; and Dr. Leo D. Lagasse for his compassionate counsel and enthusiastic support during my transition from private practice to academic medicine.

Dr. Laszlo Tabar deserves special mention for his dedication to the mammographic detection of breast lesions, particularly nonpalpable breast cancer, and his landmark two-county Swedish study that validated the efficacy of screening mammography in lowering the mortality from breast cancer. Dr. Tabar is a devoted student of breast disease and one of the most stimulating and enthusiastic teachers I have had the privilege to know. His contributions to the technical aspects of mammography and the interpretation of mammograms are profound.

Dr. Gary L. Dunnington is responsible for bringing the breast service of the Department of Surgery, Los Angeles County and University of Southern California (LAC + USC) Medical Center into the twenty-first century with firm preference for fine-needle aspiration cytologic diagnosis of palpable breast masses and breast-conserving therapy for invasive breast cancer. He served as founding director and inspirational team leader of the USC/Norris Breast Center, gathering into cooperative harmony all the diverse personalities and professional talents involved in the diagnosis, treatment, and research of breast cancer within the University of Southern California School of Medicine.

Drs. Raquel Arias and Susana Gonzalez have contributed their special energies and enthusiasm to the BDC. Dr. Arias has unmatched clinical intensity and vitality, which are infectious and stimulating to the resident physicians and their patients. An apt student of breast disorders, Dr. Arias is the favorite teacher of the resident physicians and their premier female professional role model. Dr. Gonzalez exhibits a calm compassion and confidence that are reassuring to patients and all associated with her. She has particular talents for patient care and is guided by uncompromising principles. Dr. Gonzalez is a quick learner and a warmly welcomed speaker.

The readability and correctness of language in this book is due to the scrutiny, persistence, and insistence of Nolie S. Howard who has read and critiqued every written word and sentence. She has tenaciously ferreted out redundancies and areas where technical and specialty jargon could be converted to clearly understandable terms. Her dedicated assistance is profoundly appreciated by the editor, the various authors, and, I am certain, the readers of this book.

Peggy Firth, our medical illustrator, merits special recognition for her line drawings that so clearly illustrate the pertinent anatomy, surgery, and clinical procedures. Peggy has a unique talent for visualizing exactly what the authors intended and then producing the appropriate explicit and informative line drawings.

Laura Gillan, Editor, Medicine, for the New York office of Springer-Verlag, has from the beginning supplied unflaggingly cheerful enthusiasm and a constantly positive approach regarding the origin and creation of this book. Without her apt attention and joyous support, this work would not have progressed to publication.

Finally, I wish to acknowledge my colleague, Dr. Robert Israel, who from the beginning expressed keen interest in breast cancer and the creation of the Breast Diagnostic Center. His encouragement and friendship have been a constant source of support and are deeply appreciated. I am especially grateful for his willingness to share the services of his secretary with me during the past many years. Michelle Ramsey is that shared individual and I wish to recognize her loyal and effective secretarial support and assistance. She is the gatekeeper of the fax and e-mail communications that have been essential to the creation of this book.

William H. Hindle, M.D.
Los Angeles, California

CONTENTS

CONTRIBUTORS

Raquel D. Arias, M.D., Associate Professor, Clinical Obstetrics and Gynecology, University of Southern California School of Medicine; Associate Director, Breast Diagnostic Center, Women's and Children's Hospital, LAC+USC Medical Center, Los Angeles, California

Audrey J. Arona, M.D., Department of Obstetrics and Gynecology, University of Southern California School of Medicine, Los Angeles, California; Private Practice, Los Gatos, California

R. James Brenner, M.D., J.D., Clinical Professor of Radiology, University of California, Los Angeles, School of Medicine, Los Angeles, California; Director of Breast Imaging, Joyce Eisenberg Keefer Breast Center, John Wayne Cancer Institute, St. Johns Hospital and Health Center, Santa Monica, California

Susan E. Downey, M.D., F.A.C.S., Associate Professor, Clinical Surgery—Plastic; University of Southern California School of Medicine, Los Angeles, California

Gary L. Dunnington, M.D., Professor and Chairman of General Surgery, Director, Breast Center, Southern Illinois University, Springfield, Illinois

Juan C. Felix, M.D., Associate Professor, Pathology and Obstetrics and Gynecology, University of Southern California School of Medicine; Director, Pathology, Women's and Children's Hospital, Los Angeles, California

Barbara Florentine, M.D., Assistant Professor, Clinical Pathology, University of Southern California School of Medicine, Los Angeles, California

Silvia C. Formenti, M.D., Associate Professor, Radiation Oncology, University of Southern California School of Medicine; USC/Kenneth Norris Jr. Comprehensive Cancer Center, Los Angeles, California

Steven D. Frankel, M.D., Assistant Clinical Professor, Department of Radiology, University of California at San Francisco; Chief of Breast Imaging, San Francisco General Hospital, San Francisco, California

Susana G. Gonzalez, M.D., Assistant Professor, Clinical Obstetrics and Gynecology and Family Medicine, University of Southern California School of Medicine; Assistant Director, Breast Diagnostic Center, Women's and Children's Hospital, LAC+USC Medical Center, Los Angeles, California

T. Murphy Goodwin, M.D., Associate Professor, Obstetrics and Gynecology; Co-Director of the Division of Maternal-Fetal Medicine, University of Southern California School of Medicine; Director, Maternal-Fetal Medicine, The Hospital of The Good Samaritan, Los Angeles, California

David A. Grimes, M.D., Vice President of Biomedical Affairs, Family Health International, Research Triangle Park, North Carolina; Clinical Professor, Department of Obstetrics and Gynecology, University of North Carolina School of Medicine, Chapel Hill, North Carolina

James A. Hall, M.D., Women's Health Center of Logansport, Logansport, Indiana; Associate Clinical Professor, Department of Obstetrics and Gynecology, Indiana University, Indianapolis, Indiana

William H. Hindle, M.D., Professor, Clinical Obstetrics and Gynecology, University of Southern California School of Medicine; Director, Breast Diagnostic Center, Women's and Children's Hospital, LAC+USC Medical Center, Los Angeles, California

Patricia Kelly, Ph.D., Medical Geneticist, Catholic Healthcare West, San Francisco, California

William H. Kern, M.D., Emeritus Clinical Professor, Pathology, University of Southern California School of Medicine; Past President, American Society of Cytopathology, Recipient, Papanicolaou Award, 1987

Carol P. Marcusen, L.C.S.W., M.S.W., B.C.D., Director, Social Services Department, USC/Kenneth Norris Jr. Cancer Center and Hospital, Los Angeles, California

Daniel R. Mishell Jr., M.D., The Lyle G. McNeile Professor and Chairman, Department of Obstetrics and Gynecology, University of Southern California School of Medicine, Los Angeles, California

Yuri Parisky, M.D., Associate Professor of Radiology, University of Southern California School of Medicine, Los Angeles, California

Richard J. Paulson, M.D., Professor, Obstetrics and Gynecology; Chief, Division of Reproductive Endocrinology and Infertility, University of Southern California School of Medicine, Los Angeles, California

John G. Pearce, M.B.Ch.B., M.S.R.R., M.B.A., B.C.F.E., B.C.F.M., Professor, Radiology and Surgery, University of Southern California School of Medicine; Director, University of Southern California Mammography Services, Los Angeles, California

David Plotkin, M.D, Clinical Professor, Medicine—Oncology, University of Southern California School of Medicine; Director, Memorial Cancer Research Foundation of Southern California, Los Angeles, California

Diana E. Ramos, M.D., Department of Obstetrics and Gynecology, University of Southern California School of Medicine, Los Angeles, California

Barbara Rabinowitz, PhD, MSW, RN, Vice President for Oncology, Saint Barnabas Health Care System, Livingston, New Jersey

Eric L. Rosen, M.D., Department of Radiology, Breast Imaging Section, University of California at San Francisco, San Francisco, California

Subir Roy, M.D., Professor, Obstetrics and Gynecology, University of Southern California School of Medicine, Los Angeles, California

Christy A. Russell, M.D., Associate Professor of Clinical Medicine, Oncology, University of Southern California School of Medicine; USC/Kenneth Norris Jr. Comprehensive Cancer Center, Los Angeles, California

Katherine Schlaerth, M.D, Clinical Associate Professor of Family Medicine and Pediatrics, University of Southern California School of Medicine, Los Angeles, California

Vicki Seltzer, M.D., Professor, Obstetrics & Gynecology and Women's Health, Albert Einstein College of Medicine, New York, New York; Chairman, Obstetrics and Gynecology, Long Island Jewish Medical Center; President, American College of Obstetricians and Gynecologists (1997–1998)

Randy Sherman, M.D., Professor and Chief, Division of Plastic and Reconstructive Surgery, University of Southern California School of Medicine, Los Angeles, California

Edward A. Sickles, M.D., Professor of Radiology, Chief, Breast Imaging Section, University of California at San Francisco, San Francisco, California

Kristin A. Skinner, M.D., Assistant Professor, Surgery, University of Southern California School of Medicine, Division of Tumor & Endocrine Surgery, USC/ Kenneth Norris Jr. Comprehensive Cancer Center, Los Angeles, California

Maida Taylor, M.D., M.P.H., Associate Clinical Professor, Department of Reproductive Sciences, Obstetrics and Gynecology, University of California at San Francisco, San Francisco, California

Suzanne M. Taylor, M.D., Clinical Assistant Professor, Department of Family Medicine and Comprehensive Care, LSU Medical Center, Shreveport, Louisiana; Medical Director, David Wade Correctional Center/Forcht Wade Correctional Center, Louisiana Department of Public Safety and Corrections

Angela Demman Treinen, R.N., M.N., O.C.N., Oncology Clinical Nurse Specialist, USC/Norris Breast Center, USC/Kenneth Norris Jr. Comprehensive Cancer Center, Los Angeles, California

Arnold Walder, M.D., M.S., Ph.D., Clinical Professor of Surgery, University of Texas School of Medicine, San Antonio, Texas

1 BREAST DISEASE FOR PRIMARY HEALTH CARE PROVIDERS FOR WOMEN: AN OVERVIEW

William H. Hindle

The media, in all its forms, has found a ready market for "news" about breast cancer and other breast disorders. The topic of breast cancer is everywhere: in all the women's magzines, on the front pages of the news-papers, and on the nightly news and talk shows. Stories abound of surgical disfigurement and treatments that cause loss of hair and vomiting. Most women and their families know of someone who either has the disease or who has died of it. Myths and misinformation persist.

Historically the health care system in the United States, with its method of episodic delivery and diverse multipractitioner workforce, has been ill-equipped to meet the needs of women with breast problems or to answer their concerns in a compassionate and comprehensive way. In the past, training and experience in breast care have been lacking in health care education, and there is no medical specialty trained to provide comprehensive breast evaluation and treatment.

In recent years the scene has begun to change. Women's advocacy groups have motivated women to seek answers and to become involved in decisions regarding their own health issues; more and more medical schools are establishing programs that emphasize instruction and experience in breast disease and care; and the various health institutions are creating breast health centers, such as the one that inspired this book, offering comprehensive care and treatment for women who have breast problems. Meanwhile, understanding of the biologic behavior and natural history of breast disorders, effective diagnostic techniques, and efficient treatments have all advanced during the last 25 years.

The expansion of managed medical care has pushed primary health care pro-viders into the "front line" as preliminary evaluators and then as gatekeepers to further specialized treatment. This situation provides an opportunity for the primary health care practitioner, often the obstetrician/gynecologist, to take the lead in providing diagnosis and management of female breast problems.

HISTORICAL PERSPECTIVE

At the turn of the century Dr. Halsted, at John Hopkins Hospital in Baltimore, pioneered the effective surgical management of what today is considered rela-tively advanced breast cancer. Before Dr. Halsted's surgical innovations, breast cancer was accompanied by a local ulcerated, fungating spread that became intolerable to the woman so afflicted and to everyone near her: the diagnosis was considered a repugnant death sentence.

For its time, the Halsted radical mastectomy (HRM) achieved miraculous results. Five-year local control was obtained in more than 90% of his cases, and the 5-year survival rate was greater than 40%. Such successful results were previously unknown no matter what treatments were tried. During the late 1940s Dr. Patty in England, followed during the mid-1960s by Dr. Auchincloss in the United States (and others, e.g., Drs. Baker, Handily, Madden, Robins, and Turner), published breast cancer surgery results with preservation of the pectoralis muscle and limitation of the axillary dissection to levels I and II lymph node areas. This change in the HRM became known as the modified radical mastectomy (MRM). The MRM allowed breast reconstruction and lessened the deformity of the anterior chest wall while improving the viability of the overlying skin. It took more than 10 years for the MRM to become the standard of surgical care for breast cancer in the United States. Then, Dr. Bernard Fisher at the University of Pittsburgh and others (Drs. Blicher-Toft, Clark, Freeman, Harris, Hayward, Lichter, Sarrazin, VanDongen, and Veronsi) published their work proving the equal effectiveness of breast-conserving therapy (BCT). Finally, the landmark National Surgical Adjuvant Breast and Bowel Project (NSABP) randomized prospective clinical trials validated both the transition to MRM from the Halsted method and the equivalent success of BCT.

Meanwhile, over the last few decades, mammography has evolved into an effective breast imaging technique, with minimal radiation risk, for mammographic diagnosis of palpable breast lesions and breast cancer screening of asymptomatic women. Much of the current knowledge about the natural history of breast cancer has been gleaned from serial mammograms obtained during population-based clinical trials. During this same time, effective and tolerable adjuvant therapy with multidrug chemotherapy and hormonal therapy (e.g., tamoxifen) was developed for the treatment of metastatic breast cancer; radiation therapy (RT) progressed through technical advances to become an effective, tolerable breast cancer therapy; and breast reconstruction with various prostheses or autologous tissue flaps became commonplace.

Until recently, other breast disorders, such as pain (mastalgia), fibrocystic changes, fibroadenomas, and nipple discharge, received meager medical attention and study. This lack of clinical focus and research is now changing.

ESTIMATED BREAST CANCER STATISTICS

Invasive breast cancer is the second most common cancer of women (following malignant skin lesions). It was estimated that 180,200 women in the United States would be diagnosed with invasive breast cancer (Table 1.1) in 1997. In addition to the 180,200 invasive breast cancers, more than 36,000 women would be diagnosed with in situ breast cancer. Breast cancer deaths for 1997 were estimated at 43,900, a number second only to lung cancer deaths in women. This level of invasive

Table 1.1. Invasive breast cancer: 1997

30% of all diagnosed cancer in women

17% of all cancer deaths in women

180,200 new cases

43,900 deaths

Source: ACS,[1] with permission.

Table 1.2. Invasive gynecologic cancer: 1997

Type	Incidence (new cases)	Mortality (deaths)	Percent[a] (mortality/incidence)
Breast	180,200	43,900	24
Cervix uteri	14,500	4,800	33
Corpus uteri	34,900	6,000	17
Ovary	26,800	14,200	53
Vulva	3,300	800	24
Vagina/others	2,300	700	30

Source: ACS,[1] with permission.

[a] Percents (mortality/incidence) were added by the author.

breast cancer mortality is almost twice the total number of all gynecologic pelvic cancers combined (Table 1.2). The estimated incidence of female breast cancer reported by the American Cancer Society has been increasing 1–2% a year for more than 40 years but has shown a downward trend over the past few years and may be stabilizing. Hopefully, this trend will continue and not prove to be a temporary aberration.

The yearly incidence of invasive breast cancer in the general female population of the United States is 1:1000 for ages 30–39, 2:1000 for ages 40–49, and 3:1000 for ages 50–59. Unfortunately, the breast cancer mortality rate has remained essentially the same for more than 50 years (Fig. 1.1) despite improved treatments that have allowed many women with breast cancer to live longer than before. There appears to be a downward trend over the past few years in the estimated breast cancer mortality in the United States. The current estimated median survival after diagnosis and treatment of invasive breast cancer in the United States is more than 10 years.

The number of living women in the United States who have been treated for invasive breast cancer is approaching 2 million. This number represents about 40% of the estimated female survivors of all types of cancer (1995 data). Most of these women are under continuous medical surveillance; many, particularly those who were postmenopausal at the time of diagnosis, are on tamoxifen adjuvant therapy.

The odds of having invasive breast cancer diagnosed by 5-year age groups based on the Surveillance, Epidemiology, and End Results of the National Cancer Institute (SEER—NCI) cancer statistics of 1973–1992 data for women in the United States are listed in Table 1.3. They range from 1:19,608 at age 25 to 1:9 at age 85. The "lifetime" odds of 1:8 are twice the calculated odds back in 1940. The calcu-

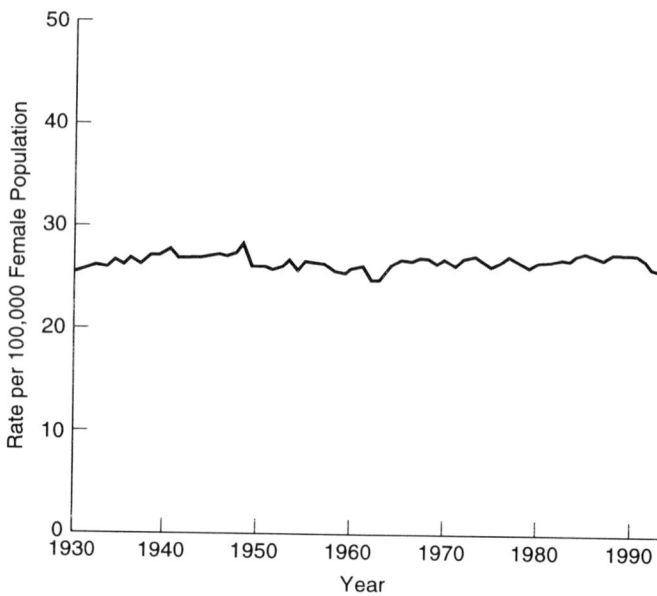

Figure 1.1.   Death rate for invasive breast cancer in U.S. women 1930–1993. Age-adjusted rate per 100,000 women in the United States. (After Parker et al.,[1] with permission.)

Table 1.3. Breast cancer: odds of occurrence by decades of age

By age (years)	Odds
25	1:19,608
35	1:622
45	1:93
55	1:33
65	1:17
75	1:11
85	1:9
Ever	1:8

Sources: SEER—NCI and Marshall,[3] with permission.

lated cumulative lifetime probability of being diagnosed with invasive breast cancer based on the same SEER data ranges from 0.03% for ages 25–29 to 12.6% for women over 95 (Table 1.4). The optimistic view is that women in the United States who live to be over age 95 have an 87.4% probability of *not* being diagnosed with invasive breast cancer. Furthermore, using the 1997 estimates of the ratio of breast cancer mortality to incidence (43,900:180,200 or 1.0:4.1) the lifetime probability of dying of breast cancer would be less than 3.1%, the good news being that the lifetime probability of not dying of breast cancer is more than 96.9%.

Table 1.4. Cumulative lifetime probability of a woman's being diagnosed with invasive breast cancer

Age (years)	Percent probability
25–29	0.03
30–39	0.16–0.45
40–49	1.1–1.9
50–59	3.0–4.2
60–69	5.7–7.3
70–79	8.9–10.4
80–89	11.5–12.1
95+	12.6

Source: After Feuer,[4] with permission.
The probabilities are based on SEER data 1973–1992.

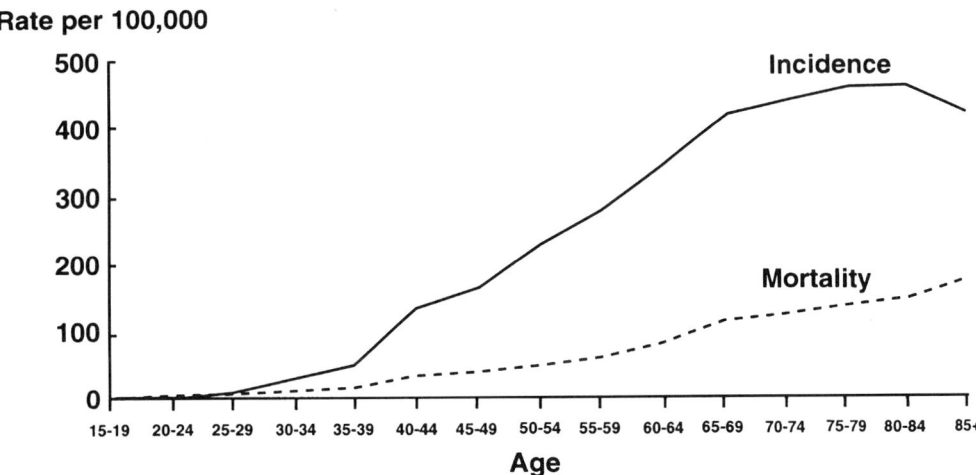

Figure 1.2. Age-related incidence and mortality for invasive breast cancer in U.S. women. (From Harris,[2] with permission.)

Invasive breast cancer has the capacity to lie clinically dormant after the initial diagnosis and treatment for 5, 10, 20, even 30 years before recurrence and metastasis become apparent. Thus it is not accurate to describe a woman treated for invasive breast cancer as "cured," as the disease may manifest again at any time during her life. Metastatic breast cancer is most commonly clinically apparent within 3 years of the initial diagnosis of invasive breast cancer.

Geographic location, age, and ethnic background are important variables in breast cancer statistics. Primary health care providers need to know the demographics of the particular patient population for which they are caring. The incidence of breast cancer, as well as benign breast disorders, varies with age. The incidence and mortality rates for breast cancer plotted for 5-year age intervals are depicted in Figure 1.2. Beginning at about age 25 the incidence of invasive

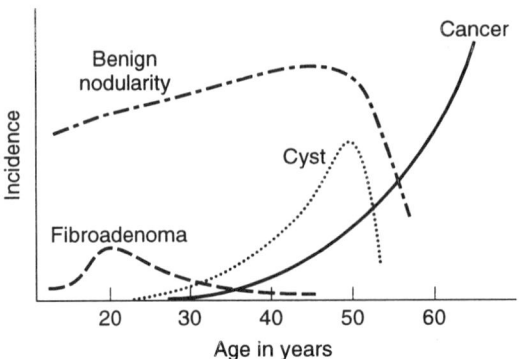

Figure 1.3. Incidence of common breast lesions as a function of age. (After Mansel and Bundred,[5] with permission.)

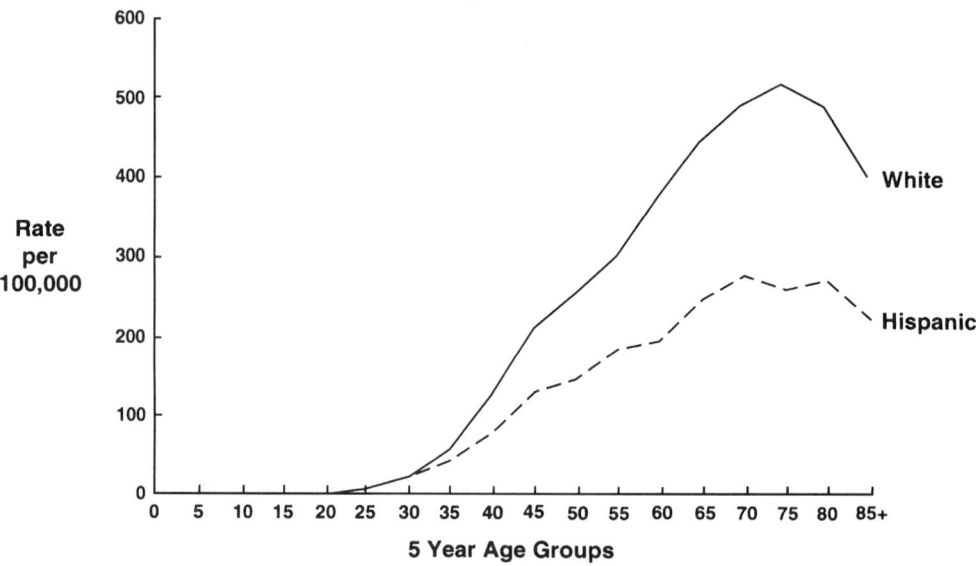

Figure 1.4. Incidence of invasive breast cancer per 100,000 women, White and Hispanic, in California as a function of age. (From Morris,[6] with permission.)

breast cancer increases with advancing age. The dip after age 84 may be artifactual, as statistics beyond this age are often not reliable. Age-related curves for benign masses and cancer are depicted in Figure 1.3. The California data for the incidence of breast cancer by age are depicted in Figure 1.4 for the White and Hispanic populations and in Figure 1.5 for the White, Black, and Asian/other populations.

Table 1.5 lists the incidence for various racial/ethnic groups living in the United States based on SEER data for 1988–1992. The highest rate (for Whites,

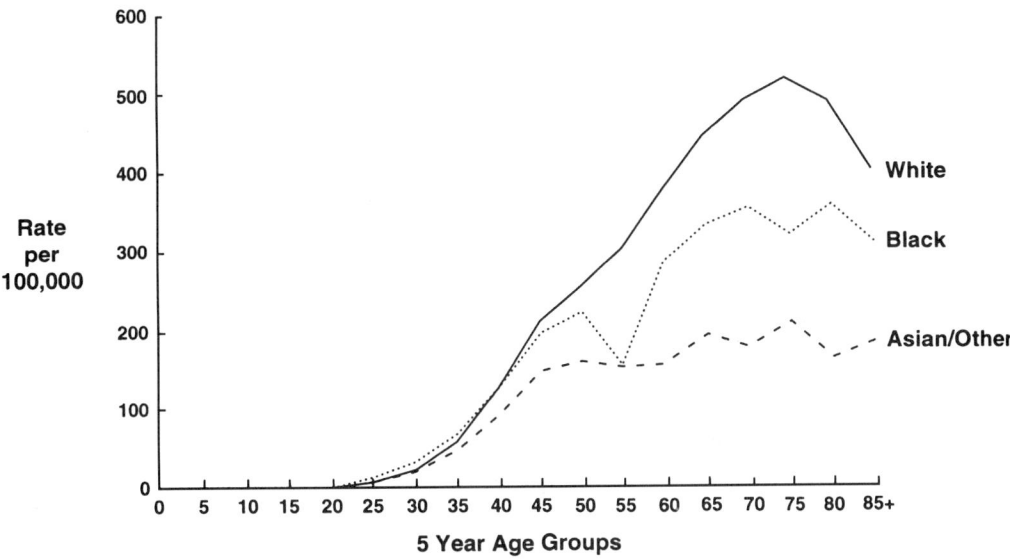

Figure 1.5. Incidence of invasive breast cancer per 100,000 women, White, Black, and Asian/Other, in California as a function of age. (From Morris,[6] with permission.)

Table 1.5. Incidence of invasive breast cancer by ethnic group

Ethnic group (living in U.S.)	Incidence (per 100,000)
White	111.8
Hawaiian	105.6
African American	95.4
Japanese	82.3
Alaskan Native	78.9
Filipino	73.1
Hispanic	69.8
Chinese	55.0
Vietnamese	37.5
American Indian	31.6
Korean	28.5

Source: SEER—NIH.[7]
Rate per 100,000 women age-adjusted to 1970 U.S. standards.

at 111.8/100,000 women) is nearly four times that of the lowest (for Koreans, at 28.5/100,000). The rate among African-Americans is reported at 95.4/100,000 and for Hispanics at 69.8/100,000. Thus there is wide variation in the incidence of invasive breast cancer in the United States among women of different ethnic/racial backgrounds.

BREAST-ORIENTED HISTORY

The essential breast-oriented items of the patient's medical history are listed in Table 1.6. Initial inquiries should focus on the patient's presenting complaint. The patient's anxiety about the possibility of breast cancer can be lessened by beginning with a focused physical examination of the area in question. Thereafter the clinically meaningful breast-oriented history can be obtained in a more relaxed atmosphere and other pertinent history obtained.

Precise questions about the presenting complaint should lead to a clear clinical impression and assessment of the intrinsic breast pathology. The patient's age is relevant to her potential risk of breast cancer and generally correlates with the probability of a mass being fibrocystic changes, a fibroadenoma, a cyst, or cancer (Fig. 1.3). The date of her last menstrual period should identify the possibility of pregnancy or the occurrence of menopause.

A personal history of breast cancer carries a fivefold increased risk of breast cancer occurring in the other breast. History of a first-degree relative (mother or sister) with diagnosed breast cancer increases the relative risk of breast cancer to about threefold. Furthermore, the exact diagnosis of any surgery (and exact type of surgery performed) is critical information. Breast surgery can result in changes noted at the physical examination and on subsequent mammograms.

Specific inquiry as to prior fine-needle aspiration (indications and findings) is essential. Recent trauma to the breast can be associated with pain, ecchymosis, or Mondor's disease (thrombophlebitis of the superficial veins of the breast). Past trauma can produce evidence of fat necrosis on mammography.

The dates and results of prior mammograms are essential, and the films should be obtained for review if there is a possibility of breast cancer. Exogenous hormone therapy (oral contraceptive therapy, estrogen replacement therapy, or hormone replacement therapy) can increase the mammographic density in some women and can be associated with breast pain, although it does not alter the clinically meaningful relative risk of breast cancer. Other current nonhormonal medications can be related to breast pain or nipple discharge. A sample form for taking the patient's breast-oriented history (Fig. A.1) lists additional questions.

Table 1.6. Clinically meaningful breast-oriented history

Chief complaint
Age
Last menstrual period
Personal history of breast cancer
History of mother or sister with breast cancer
Breast surgery
Breast trauma
Last mammogram (date and result)
Currently taking oral contraceptive therapy, estrogen replacement therapy, hormone
    replacement therapy

BREAST EXAMINATION

The most important breast procedure performed by primary care providers is a complete clinical breast examination (CBE). It should be carried out annually and at any time a woman presents with a breast complaint or concern. The CBE should follow a systematic routine. An effective, thorough CBE is described and illustrated in a step-by-step approach in Chapter 4.

SCREENING MAMMOGRAPHY

By definition, screening mammography is a periodic imaging evaluation for asymptomatic women (i.e., women without breast complaints or clinically meaningful CBE findings). Multiple prospective randomized clinical trials have demonstrated that only population-based screening mammography has the ability to lower the mortality from breast cancer by detecting invasive breast cancer before it is large enough to be palpated. Mammography is accurate, effective, and efficient for this purpose.

When to Begin Screening Mammography

Although each woman's health situation should be individually evaluated, in general all women should begin annual screening mammography at age 40. Why not begin sooner? The incidence of breast cancer begins to rise at about age 25 and increases steadily thereafter (Fig. 1.2). Although it may be indicated on an individual case basis, population screening before age 40 is not cost-effective because of the low incidence of breast cancer before age 40.

Although there are considerable clinical screening data that interval cancers grow more rapidly in the 40- to 49-year age group, the debate over a national health care policy continues regarding the indication for and value of screening mammography for those under age 50. Cost is a major issue, as it is estimated that there are more than 20 million women in the 40- to 50-year age group in the United States. The various population-based clinical trials for the 40- to 49-year age group (Fig. 1.6) demonstrate a trend toward decreased mortality; and when the results of these trials are combined, the reduction in breast cancer death is statistically significant. However, if the Canadian trial (not population-based) data are included, the statistical significance is lost.

Some women with a family history of breast cancer should begin screening mammography earlier. For example, a woman with a family history of breast (or ovarian) cancer in three successive generations, suggestive of an autosomal dominant pattern, should begin annual screening mammography 10 years before the age at which her mother was diagnosed with breast cancer (i.e., if the mother was diagnosed at age 43, the daughter should begin annual screening mammography at age 33). Thereafter mammography and CBEs should be repeated annually. In addition, a woman with such a family history would benefit from consultation with a breast specialist.

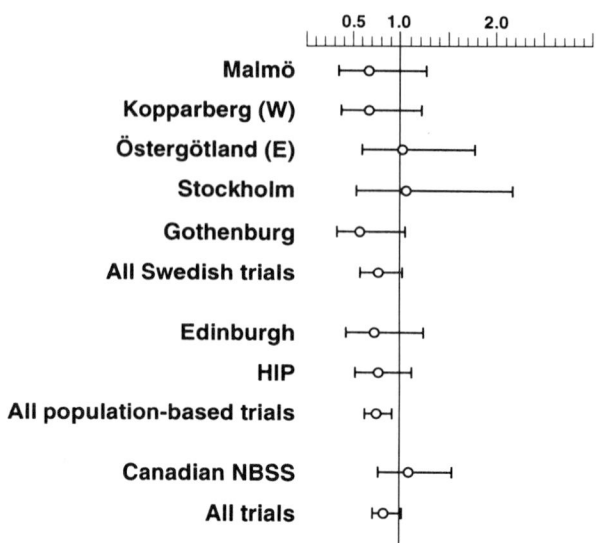

Figure 1.6. Relative risk (RR) of invasive breast cancer from English-language published clinical trials of screening mammography for women aged 40 to 49. Circles indicate the mean; lines indicate the confidence intervals (CI). Only the total for "all population-based trials" CI result does not cross the vertical line at 1.0 RR and is therefore statistically significant. It demonstrates a reduction in breast cancer mortality for the screened group versus the nonscreened (control) group. (From Organizing Committee and Collaborators,[8] with permission.)

The primary health care provider is responsible for obtaining a breast-oriented history and performing CBE when referring a woman for screening mammography. This clinical information should be included on the mammography request (requisition or referral form). Furnishing two sets of prior mammogram films (e.g., the prior year and another year before that) allows the mammographer to search for slow, subtle changes that may not otherwise become apparent.

Screening Mammogram Report

The screening mammogram report should conclude with a mammographic impression utilizing the BI-RADS terminology (lexicon) including the assessment category.[9] It should be followed by a specific recommendation (e.g., "recommend annual mammography"). If further mammography is recommended, such as spot compression or magnification views, the patient should be instructed to return to the mammographer for completion of the imaging evaluation. The primary health care provider has a prominent role in advising the patient, explaining the procedures and indications, answering questions she may have, and tracking her to be certain that the recommendations are carried out (or if not, documenting that fact and the reason for it in the medical record).

See Chapter 5 for a complete discussion of screening mammography.

DIAGNOSTIC MAMMOGRAPHY

Diagnostic mammography, by definition, is performed when a woman has a breast complaint (e.g., a perceived mass, localized pain, or a clinically meaningful abnormal CBE finding). Diagnostic mammography is a medical consultation, and the clinician should provide the breast-oriented history and CBE findings to the mammographer, including the exact location of the lesion (e.g., "a mass in the upper outer quadrant of the right breast") and if fine-needle aspiration has been performed.

After the breast imaging evaluation has been completed, a specific plan of action should be agreed on by the mammographer, the clinician, and the patient (e.g., referral to a breast surgeon for biopsy, short interval follow-up mammography in 6 months, or follow-up with annual mammography and CBE).

Of keen interest to primary care providers is the probability of cancer estimated for each of the BI-RADS categories.

0%—Category 2 (benign finding)
1%—Category 3 (probably benign finding); short-interval follow-up suggested
25%—Category 4 (suspicious abnormality); biopsy should be considered
>98%—Category 5 (highly suggestive of malignancy)

ULTRASONOGRAPHY

When the mammographic findings are uncertain, it is becoming standard practice to proceed with a focused ultrasound evaluation of the area in question. In the experience of Los Angeles County and University of Southern California (LAC + USC) Medical Center, when mammographic indeterminate densities are perceived the probability of malignancy as the final diagnosis is about 15%.

Ultrasound examination of the breast requires specific equipment (e.g., a 7.5-mHz linear array, close field, hand-held transducer) and is an intensely operator-dependent imaging procedure. Optimum interpretation necessitates that the mammographer perform or at least be present throughout the breast ultrasound examination. Ultrasonography is a dynamic "on-line" procedure that, for the breast, is focused on a specific clinical area of concern. Ultrasound imaging of the breast is an accepted, effective technique for differentiating a cyst from a solid mass, particularly a nonpalpable mass: mammography does not do this reliably. There are established criteria for characterizing the various breast lesions by ultrasound imaging. Ultrasonography is not appropriate for breast cancer screening. For further discussion of ultrasound imaging, refer to Chapter 7.

FINE-NEEDLE ASPIRATION

Fine-needle aspiration (FNA) is an essential component of the diagnostic triad (CBE, FNA, mammography) for evaluating a palpable breast mass (Table 1.7). It is a convenient, accurate, efficient, cost-effective procedure. FNA technique is

KEY PRACTICE POINTS
MASS: A persistent palpable dominant breast mass must be definitively diagnosed without delay.

Table 1.7. Breast diagnostic triad[a]

Clinical breast examination

Fine-needle aspiration

Mammography

[a] Also called triple assessment, triple diagnosis, triple test.

readily learned and can be performed in the office setting with medical supplies and equipment that are already available in the primary care office or clinic. FNA technique is described and illustrated in Chapter 8.

BREAST COMPLAINTS

Almost all women presenting to a primary health care provider with a breast complaint have a powerful fear, of which they may or may not be aware, of breast cancer. Although it may not be appropriate to extract an expression or acknowledgment of this fear from the patient, her primary health care provider should be sensitive to the profound emotion associated with the breast and especially with the fear of breast cancer. Compassion, understanding, and patience are called for when a woman presents with a breast complaint.

The most common presenting breast complaint is a perceived mass, followed by breast pain, an abnormal mammogram, and nipple discharge.

Breast Mass

A persistent palpable breast mass is appropriately evaluated by the diagnostic triad (CBE, FNA, mammography). If there is concurrence of results from the three procedures, the diagnosis can be relied on with confidence, and an appropriate clinical plan of action (follow-up or treatment) can be pursued. Unless there is clinical suspicion of breast cancer, the mammographic component of the diagnostic triad is omitted for women under age 30. However, when FNA reveals cancer, diagnostic mammography should be performed regardless of age to map the lesion and to look for any abnormalities in the remainder of the breast or in the other breast. FNA should be performed on every palpable dominant breast mass even if excision is planned because knowing whether the mass is cancer or a benign lesion can determine the surgical technique to be used (see Chapter 14).

If the primary care provider has not been trained, is not experienced in performing FNA, or has doubt as to the presence of a breast mass or the appropriate treatment, the patient should be referred to a breast specialist. Again, the patient should be followed during the evaluation and treatment process and thereafter.

Breast Pain

The breast-oriented history (Table 1.6) and subsequent questions pertinent to the complaint of breast pain should direct the examiner to the clinical diagnosis (see Chapter 15). It is imperative to ascertain if the pain is associated with a mass. If a mass is present, a timely diagnosis is paramount. Complete CBE should be performed on all women presenting with the complaint of breast pain; and for women 30 or older, mammography should be performed to detect a nonpalpable lesion.

Abnormal Mammogram

When a woman presents as a result of an abnormal mammogram (see Chapter 6), the clinician obtains a breast-oriented history and performs a CBE. If no mass is palpated, the patient is referred to a mammographer for evaluation of her films (and comparison to her prior mammograms, if available), to obtain another mammographic impression, and for imaging recommendations, such as additional mammographic views or referral for biopsy. Requesting a second mammographic interpretation is a common, appropriate clinical practice.

The evaluation of nonpalpable lesions and ordering of the ultimate definitive diagnostic test, usually tissue histology, is within the purview of the mammographer. If tissue confirmation is not to be requested, the mammographer should be 90% certain that the lesion is benign and the patient should be closely followed thereafter. If there is a mammographic suspicion of malignancy, a timely definitive diagnosis, usually by tissue histology, is mandatory.

The primary care provider should follow the patient undergoing imaging evaluation until a definite conclusion is reached. Many patients, and not infrequently their relatives, seek information and answers to their questions from the patient's primary care provider. Furthermore, the primary care provider should continue to follow the patient with annual CBEs and mammography after the imaging evaluation is completed and the indicated therapy carried out.

Nipple Discharge

As with breast pain, the breast-oriented history and subsequent questions pertinent to the complaint of nipple discharge (see Chapter 16) should give clues to the clinical diagnosis. The clinical impression is then confirmed (or otherwise) by CBE. If there is no palpable mass, evaluation of pathologic nipple discharge proceeds with imaging studies, usually galactography. If an intraluminal lesion is identified, surgical excision of the involved area can lead to the definitive histologic diagnosis.

It is important to know if the reported nipple discharge is coming from the duct opening(s) on the top of the nipple or from other areas in the nipple–areolar complex (e.g., near the periphery of the areola). Abrasion, *Candida* (*Monilia*) infection, eczema, excoriation, dermatitis, intradermal inclusion cyst (infected or not infected), Montgomery's tubercles (physiologic secretion or infection), Paget's disease, sebaceous gland (physiologic secretions or infection), a subareolar fistula, and traumatic changes can be experienced and described by the patient as "nipple discharge."

BREAST CANCER

Therapeutic Discussion

When a breast cancer has been diagnosed, a structured interdisciplinary treatment planning conference (usually available in a multidisciplinary comprehensive breast cancer center) can expose the patient to the variety of opinions by specialists (Table 1.8) involved in cancer therapy (see Chapter 21). It is imperative that all the oncologic specialists be trained, experienced, and actively involved in the comprehensive evaluation and management of women with breast cancer.

The patient may not wish to participate directly in the treatment planning conference, but she and her selected relatives should have that opportunity whenever possible. Most patients prefer a person-to-person conference in a relaxed, comfortable private setting. Oncologic counseling with a review of all the options, given in an empathetic, compassionate manner, enables the patient to evaluate the

Table 1.8. Comprehensive treatment team

Patient
Spouse/significant other
Family/near relatives

Primary care physician
Cytopathologist
Mammographer
Medical oncologist
Oncologic (genetic) counselor
Oncologic nurse
Oncologic surgeon
Pathologist
Physiotherapist
Plastic surgeon
Psychologist or psychiatrist
Psychosocial therapist
Radiation oncologist
Social worker

Successfully treated breast cancer patients
Breast cancer support group

current accurate information about her particular case. Then, over time (there is no medical rush), she can assess her own risk tolerance and life style and make an informed choice about a specific individualized treatment plan.

It is estimated that more than 75% of women diagnosed with invasive breast cancer are eligible for breast-conserving therapy (BCT): lumpectomy, axillary lymph node dissection, and anterior chest wall irradiation. BCT is now the "preferred therapy for stage I and II breast cancer," according to the National Institutes of Health.[10]

When her therapy is completed, the cancer patient should be followed closely (seen twice a year for at least 3 years) and then annually for the rest of her life. Tragically, with invasive breast cancer there is the long-term risk of recurrence locally, systemically (metastatic), or both. Long-term follow-up requires a supportive, compassionate approach by the woman's primary health care provider, who should be readily available to respond to her questions and concerns.

Interpretation of Published Literature

Survival, without clinical evidence of recurrent cancer, is the ultimate criterion of successful cancer treatment. Ideally, overall survival figures should be stratified to differentiate between those breast cancer patients who are alive and those who died (1) from breast cancer or (2) from other causes. There ought to be multiple studies done by a variety of institutions utilizing uniform techniques to confirm (with appropriate statistical analysis) the treatment results. Unfortunately, many published studies give only short-term (5-year survival or less) disease-free survival figures. Prolonged survival should be documented by more than 20 years of follow-up. Even if there is no clinical evidence of recurrent cancer (so-called disease-free survival), subsequent recurrent cancer and metastases may occur. Furthermore, no clinical trial or published study can predict the outcome for an individual patient. The data apply to groups of patients with similar clinical characteristics (age, type of cancer, stage of cancer) and uniform application of therapy.

The search by epidemiologists for "statistically significant" risk factors for breast cancer has yielded a multitude of published mathematic correlations, most of which are at low levels of relative risk: for example, $RR < 2$, which is a "weak association" without evidence of causality and which, for clinical purposes, is likely a chance correlation.

When evaluating population-based screening mammography and similar clinical trials, one should be aware of exactly what the figures represent and how the groups were selected and maintained. For example, in the Swedish screening mammography clinical trials, the data are kept epidemiologically pure based on the initial designation. For example, women in the study group offered screening mammography may refuse it, yet their clinical information remains in the study group data. Likewise, women in the control group (not offered screening mammography) may have mammography outside the study, and their data remain in the control group. As a result, the final difference between the study group and the control group probably represents a minimum calculation of the clinical outcome (difference in the overall breast cancer mortality in the two groups). Thus the effect of the intervention (in this example population-based screening mammography) is likely underestimated.

Goal in Clinical Practice

The goal in primary care clinical practice is to discover, diagnose, and treat a breast cancer before it has grown to a palpable size. With current methods of treatment, nonpalpable (e.g., <1 cm) breast cancer has better than 90% 10-year disease-free survival. In population-based studies, screening mammography has been proved to be effective for detecting nonpalpable breast cancer. More than a 35% reduction in breast cancer mortality has been reported in some screening mammography studies. However, even in these favorable reports, the implication is that the other 65% of breast cancer patients who underwent screening mammography died of their disease. Thus screening mammography is an imperfect method for "early detection" of breast cancer, but it is currently the only effective population-based method we have. Again, there is no guarantee for an individual woman.

Nonmalignant Breast Disorders

Benign breast lesions and symptoms can be appropriately evaluated, and most can be treated and followed, by primary care providers. Referral consultation with a breast specialist should be obtained when the evaluation or treatment of a breast problem is beyond the scope of the training and experience of the primary care provider. The primary care provider should be responsible for doing annual CBEs and ordering screening mammography for all women age 40 and over.

Breast Surveillance

After a treatment plan for a breast disorder has been recommended for the patient, her case should be followed by her primary care provider. If the woman has breast cancer, a formal systematic patient tracking system should be in place to ensure that the patient is followed and supervised as outlined by the oncologists who treated her. With rare exceptions, the minimum follow-up includes annual CBE and mammography. In addition, a woman with a breast disorder of any type should be instructed in breast self-examination (BSE) and told to return for CBE and reevaluation if she notices any distinct change in her breasts.

Effect of Steroid Hormone Therapy on Breast Evaluation

The breast complaints or findings of women on oral contraceptive therapy, estrogen replacement therapy, or hormone replacement therapy should be evaluated in the same timely and thorough manner as for women who are not on steroid hormone therapy. In some women, estrogen therapy in any form can affect CBE and mammograms, particularly the mammographic density. If the estrogen therapy is judged to be interfering with the interpretation of either the CBE or the mammogram, the estrogen therapy should be discontinued (for more than a month) and the procedure repeated.

EFFECT OF PREGNANCY OR LACTATION ON BREAST EVALUATION

The breast complaints or findings of women who are pregnant or lactating should be evaluated in the same timely and thorough manner as for women who are not pregnant or lactating. The increased size, engorgement, and tenderness of the breast during pregnancy and lactation decreases the accuracy of CBE and mammography, and so screening mammography should be deferred during this time. If diagnostic mammography is indicated for a clinical suspicion of breast cancer, mammography can be performed immediately after draining the breast if the woman is lactating, or with the fetus protected by a lead shield during pregnancy. It is imperative that the mammographer (and the cytopathologist when an FNA is performed) be informed that the woman is pregnant. With modifications in the sequencing (timing) of treatments, breast cancer therapy can be the same for a pregnant woman as for a nonpregnant woman. However, the patient's fully informed consent is mandatory, as most of the risks of breast cancer therapy to the unborn fetus are unknown, and an adverse effect may not be clinically apparent until the child grows to adulthood.

See Chapters 33, 34, and 35 for further details on pregnancy and lactation.

GENETIC COUNSELING AND TESTING

The knowledge that she has a relative who has breast cancer or who has died of it can make a woman anxious and heighten her concern about a breast problem. Concern about a history of a relative's breast cancer may motivate a woman to

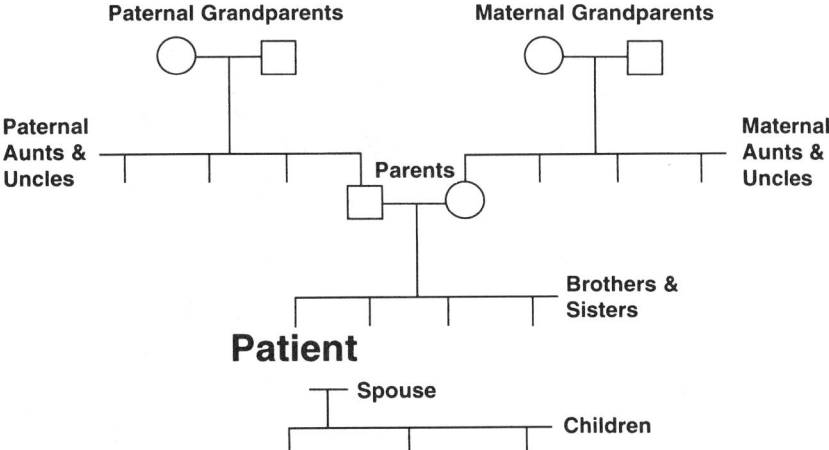

Figure 1.7. Sample pedigree that can be used to evaluate the applicability of *BRCA1* and *BRCA2* testing for a woman with invasive breast cancer by plotting her relatives who were ever diagnosed with breast, ovarian, colon, or prostate cancer.

seek medical advice and breast evaluation. As genetic testing becomes commercially available (e.g., for the genes BRCA1 and BRCA2), primary health care providers should be prepared to give preliminary advice: in-depth genetic counseling requires special training and expertise. The topic is discussed in Chapter 28.

A complete family pedigree noting the occurrence of breast cancer, ovarian cancer, colon cancer, and prostate cancer should be obtained. Ideally, the diagnosis and cancer-specific mortality should be verified. A four-generation family pedigree is diagrammed in Figure 1.7. If there appears to be an autosomal dominant inherited pattern of breast cancer, the patient diagnosed with breast cancer should be offered specialized genetic counseling and genetic testing (e.g., for BRCA1). If she decides to have genetic testing, she (and probably her immediate family) should be counseled further when the test results are obtained.

Medicolegal Considerations

A persistent dominant breast mass must be definitively diagnosed. If a woman of reproductive age has an indistinct mass, it is appropriate to reexamine the breast in a month or two at another time in her menstrual cycle (e.g., shortly after her menstruation has stopped). Several jurisdictions have held that a persistent palpable dominant breast mass should be diagnosed, or be in the active process thereof, within 4 months of the initial presentation of symptoms or physical findings to her health care provider.

Legally, all care must be "reasonable" and according to the current standards of care. With any breast lesion or complaint, particularly a mass, a specific plan of action and follow-up should be recorded in the patient's medical record. Scheduled return appointments should be documented in the medical records or in permanent appointment files in the health care provider's office.

All women with breast findings or symptoms should be instructed to examine their breasts on a monthly basis (see Chapter 4) and to return promptly if there is any progression of symptoms (e.g., should a vague mass-like lesion become distinct or increase in size). When a health care provider orders a mammogram, he or she is responsible for getting the results and reporting them to the patient. If a patient persists in not keeping her mammography appointment, she should be notified by mail that she is due to have a mammogram performed, with a copy of the letter kept in her medical record.

If a practitioner is in doubt as to how to proceed with a breast complaint, he or she should refer the patient to a breast specialist. The practitioner then shares responsibility for obtaining the consultation and for ascertaining that the patient keeps her appointment and follows the recommendations of the consultant. For example, if the consultant says, "Oh that's nothing, just forget it," the referring clinician should reevaluate the patient or obtain a second opinion.

Second (or even third and fourth) opinions are common in the medical care of the breast, as everyone does not always agree on the specific diagnosis, the extent of the disease, or the most appropriate management. Primary health care providers should be comfortable with the practice of obtaining additional opinions, particularly as to the diagnosis and treatment of breast cancer. See Chapter 36 for more extensive discussion of this topic.

References

1. Parker SL, Tong T, Bolden S, et al. Cancer statistics, 1997. CA Cancer J Clin 1997;47:14
2. Harris R, Leinninger L. Clinical strategies for breast cancer screening: weighing and using the evidence. Ann Intern Med 1995;122:539
3. Marshall E. Search for a killer: focus shifts from fat to hormones. Science 1993;259:618
4. Feuer EJ, Wun LM, Boring CC, et al. The lifetime risk of developing breast cancer. J Natl Cancer Inst 1993;85:892
5. Mansel RE, Bundred NJ. Color Atlas of Breast Disease. London, Mosby-Wolfe, 1995
6. Morris CR, Wright WE, eds. Breast Cancer in California. Sacramento CA, California Department of Health Services 1996
7. Miller, BA, Kolonel LN, Bernstein, et al. Racial/ethnic patterns of cancer in the United States 1988–1992, (NIH: Pub. No. 96-4104). Bethesda, Md. National Cancer Institute, 1996
8. Organizing Committee and Collaborators. Breast cancer screening with mammography in women aged 40–49 years. Int J Cancer 1996;68:693
9. American College of Radiology (ACR). Breast imaging reporting and data system (BI-RADS™), 2nd ed. Reston, VA, American College of Radiology, 1995
10. NIH Consensus Conference. Treatment of early-stage breast cancer. JAMA 1991;265:391

Recommended Reading

Ahmed A. Diagnostic Breast Pathology. New York, Churchill-Livingstone, 1992

Bland KI, Copeland EM III (eds). The Breast: Comprehensive Management of Benign and Malignant Diseases. Philadelphia, Saunders, 1991

De Paredes ES. Atlas of Film-Screen Mammography (2nd ed). Baltimore, Williams & Wilkins, 1992

Harris JR, Hellman S, Henderson IC, Kinne DW (eds). Breast Disease (3rd ed). New York, Lippincott, 1996

Hindle WH (ed). Breast Disease for Gynecologists. East Norwalk, CT, Appleton & Lange, 1990

Hughes LE, Mansel RE, Webster DJT. Benign Disorders and Diseases of the Breast. Philadelphia, Baillière, 1989

Kopans DB. Breast Imaging. Philadelphia, Lippincott, 1989

Masood S. Cytopathology of the Breast. Chicago, ASCP (American Society of Clinical Pathologists), Press, 1996

Page DL, Anderson TJ. Diagnostic Histopathology of the Breast. New York, Churchill-Livingstone, 1987

Smallwood JA, Taylor I (eds). Benign Breast Disease. Baltimore, Urban & Schwarzenberg, 1990

Tabar L, Dean PB. Teaching Atlas of Mammography (2nd ed). New York, Thieme, 1985

For Patients

Love SM, Lindsey K. Dr. Susan Love's Breast Book (2nd ed). New York, Addison-Wesley, 1995

2 APPLICATION OF EVIDENCE-BASED MEDICINE TO THE CARE OF THE BREAST

David A. Grimes

Evidence-based medicine has direct relevance to the care of the breast. Breast diseases, both benign and malignant, are a major public health problem in the United States; and they are sexist, being largely limited to women. Because of the sexual importance of the breast in contemporary society, the controversy over detection and treatment of breast cancer has been strident and divisive.

What primary care providers—and their patients—need today are not impassioned pleas from scientific authorities or lay activists. What is needed is a dispassionate evaluation of the data at hand. It is here that evidence-based medicine can help. In this chapter, I define evidence-based medicine, describe its two components, review several major study designs, explain an evaluation system for evidence, and discuss measures of association in clinical studies.

WHAT IS EVIDENCE-BASED MEDICINE?

Evidence-based medicine is the systematic application of the best available evidence to clinical problems, with the clinician serving as the ultimate filter. Some critics charge, "But this is how medicine has always been practiced." Although it may have been the goal, medicine has consistently fallen short of the mark. For several millennia, authority, not science, has dictated the practice of medicine. We have looked to respected leaders in fields of practice and research for guidance. However, no individual can have a comprehensive knowledge of the scientific literature.

"Experts" are often dangerously out of touch with the scientific literature. In a classic study of the advice of medical authorities, Antman et al.[1] performed cumulative meta-analyses of randomized controlled trials of myocardial infarction treatments. They determined in what year the scientific evidence for benefit of a given treatment reached statistical significance. They then compared these results with the recommendations found in review articles and textbook chapters published over the same years by cardiology experts. Thrombolytic therapy was a prototype: more than a decade elapsed between demonstration of its benefit and its recommendation by most authorities. The clinical implications are clear: thousands died needlessly over this interval. The experts' lack of systematic access to knowledge about treatments was indirectly lethal.

The same problem prevails in obstetrics. By 1990 randomized controlled trials had established that administration of glucocorticoids to women at risk of delivering prematurely saves babies' lives and reduces morbidity. Nevertheless, by 1994 only an estimated 18% of women with a fetus at risk were receiving this life-saving therapy. Again, delay in adoption of effective treatment cost thousands of lives and squandered precious medical resources. Evidence-based medicine can save us (and our patients) from our good intentions.

Two Essential Components of Evidence-Based Medicine

Evidence-based medicine blends the best available evidence with the clinical acumen of the clinician. Each is indispensable. For example, if one practices scientific medicine without skill or compassion, few patients voluntarily seek such care. On the other hand, if one practices compassionate, attentive care that is not scientific, one's practice quickly becomes stale—and potentially dangerous.

What constitutes the "best available evidence"? Randomized controlled trials stand at the pinnacle of the scientific hierarchy. Medicine has learned a painful lesson in recent decades: observational studies (most of the published literature) routinely exaggerate the benefit of new treatments or tests, reflecting the inherent biases in such research. Hence, randomized, controlled trials carry the most weight in evidence-based medicine. Often, however, observational studies are the only (and thus the best) evidence available.

The clinician must always filter the scientific evidence. Without the clinician's judgment, skill, and experience, the evidence can tyrannize the patient. Evidence-based medicine does not lead to cookbook medicine; the clinician always plays the pivotal role in applying the evidence. For example, a study might be valid (that is, it measures accurately what it sets out to measure) but completely irrelevant to a given patient. An example is the RADIUS trial, which evaluated the benefit of routine ultrasonography during pregnancy in low-risk women. The study found no benefit overall in low-risk women, but this finding may not pertain to other groups of women at higher risk. Often the evidence is insufficient to dictate a course of action. In these vast "gray zones" of clinical practice, clinicians should give patient preferences great weight.

Types of Clinical Studies

All clinical studies fall into two broad categories: observational and experimental. Observational studies, the more frequent, involve the passive observation of clinical practice as it occurs in the community. Within observational studies, another dichotomy exists: descriptive studies and analytic studies.

Descriptive studies are the simplest type of observational study. The case report is the "least publishable unit." An example would be a report of a new technique for fine-needle aspiration used for one patient. When more than one case appears in a report, the aggregate is called a "case-series report." An example of such is a report of 100 consecutive fine-needle aspirations in a newly established breast clinic.

Descriptive studies are often the first foray into new medical territory, such as toxic shock syndrome. They serve several purposes, including trend analysis and health care planning. Most importantly, descriptive studies can generate hypotheses that can then be tested in more rigorous studies. For example, case reports of benign hepatocellular adenomas among women taking high-dose oral contraceptives led to a more sophisticated study that confirmed the hunch of a causal link. Importantly, descriptive studies lack control or comparison groups and thus cannot test hypotheses or judge causal associations.

Analytic studies are the other type of observational study. As the name implies, these studies have comparison groups and thus enable testing of hypotheses. For example, do oral contraceptive users have a reduced risk of benign breast disease compared with women not using birth control pills?

Two general types of analytic study exist: cohort and case-control studies. The word "cohort" comes from Roman military terminology: a cohort was one-tenth of a legion of soldiers, or 300–600 men. Hence a cohort study can be considered a group of persons "marching forward" in time from exposure (e.g., oral contraceptives) to outcome (e.g., benign breast disease).

Case-control studies are the other type of analytic study. Most clinicians (and many editors) remain confused about case-control studies, which relates to the "backward" nature of this kind of research. Unlike a cohort study, which moves forward in time, a case-control study works backward. Indeed, Alvin Feinstein of Yale, nicknamed case-control studies "trohoc" studies ("cohort" spelled backward). Here an investigator starts with an outcome (e.g., breast cancer) and looks back in time for exposures of interest (e.g., late age at first childbirth).

Given their confusing nature, why perform case-control studies at all? This type of research is useful for studying outcomes that are rare or that take many years to develop. Breast cancer is a prototype. Following cohorts of women forward for decades to look for cases of breast cancer can be logistically difficult or prohibitively expensive. Stated alternatively, case-control studies can be efficient in terms of time and resources.

Case-control studies are often easy to do. Regrettably, they are also easy to do poorly. The literature is strewn with poorly performed case-control studies. Selection bias is the nemesis of these studies. Difficulties choosing an appropriate comparison group are often to blame.

The prototype of the experimental study is the randomized controlled trial. In an observational study the investigator merely observes; in a randomized controlled trial the investigator intervenes by assigning exposures. An example is the community trials of mammography screening for breast cancer. The investigator determines which group undergoes the screening test.

Randomized trials have several unique features. Randomization is the only known way to avoid selection bias. It also balances confounding factors, both known and unsuspected, between treatment groups. Finally, predetermined definitions of outcomes (sometimes complemented by blinding of treatments) minimize information bias. Because of this lack of bias, randomized controlled trials offer the best prospect for identifying small but important differences between treatments or tests.

Randomized controlled trials have important limitations as well. Because only volunteers take part in such trials, the results may not be capable of extrapolation to others (lack of external validity). In general, volunteers for trials are healthier and more health-oriented than are those who do not volunteer. Human experimentation carries important ethical concerns. For example, randomized trials cannot be used to study known harmful exposures such as cigarette smoking or bacteria. In addition, the design and conduct of randomized controlled trials can be cumbersome and costly. As with cohort studies, they are not practical for studying rare events or those that take years to develop.

CLASSIFICATION SYSTEM FOR CLINICAL EVIDENCE

The U.S. Preventive Services Task Force (and its Canadian counterpart) have popularized a taxonomy for clinical research (Table 2.1). Level I evidence is the most credible and level III the least. Level III evidence consists of descriptive studies without control (comparison) groups, such as case reports and case-series reports. Also included in this category are opinions of experts and committees. The latter, often termed a "Delphi panel," has also been dubbed the "BOGSAT" approach, a wry acronym for "bunch of old guys sitting around a table." This reflects the limited scientific value of conventional clinical wisdom.

Level II evidence includes analytic studies of three types. Level II-3 evidence is that obtained from multiple time series with and without the intervention. Likewise, dramatic results of uncontrolled natural experiments can be regarded as level II-3 evidence. An example is the marked decline in mortality due to tuberculosis after the introduction of streptomycin in the United States.

Table 2.1. Quality of evidence

I. Evidence obtained from at least one properly randomized controlled trial.

II-1. Evidence obtained from well designed controlled trials without randomization.

II-2. Evidence obtained from well designed cohort or case-control analytic studies, preferably from more than one center or research group.

II-3. Evidence obtained from multiple time series with or without intervention. Dramatic results in uncontrolled experiments (such as the results of introducing penicillin treatment during the 1940s) could also be regarded as this type of evidence.

III. Opinions of respected authorities, based on clinical experience; descriptive studies and case reports; or reports of expert committees.

Source: US Preventive Services Task Force,[2] with permission.

Level II-2 evidence encompasses both cohort and case-control studies. Level II-1 evidence includes well designed trials without randomization. An example is a trial of prophylactic antibiotics for surgery. Patients are assigned to the two treatments during alternating months: in January all patients get antibiotic A, in February antibiotic B, in March antibiotic A, and so forth.

Finally, at the pinnacle of the scientific hierarchy is level I evidence, indicating one or more properly randomized controlled trials. The U.S. Preventive Services Task Force notes "properly randomized" trials, but a better index of quality might be "properly done randomized trials." As recently shown by Schulz et al.,[3] other elements of randomized trials may be more important for avoiding bias than proper randomization. Indeed, failure to conceal the allocation sequence from clinicians and prospective participants can exaggerate treatment effects by 30–40%. Hence it is imperative that those who enroll participants (and the participants themselves) be kept unaware of the upcoming assignment to avoid selection bias.

STRENGTH OF RECOMMENDATIONS

Based on the quality of evidence described above, clinicians can judge how strong a clinical recommendation can be. The scale used by the U.S. Preventive Services Task Force has five classes (Table 2.2). A direct correlation does not exist between the quality of evidence and strength of recommendation. Although randomized controlled trials often support an "A" recommendation (e.g., mammography screening for women aged 50–69 years), even well done trials may lead to inconclusive results (e.g., mammography screening for women younger than 50 years) (Table 2.3).

Table 2.2. Strength of recommendations

A. There is good evidence to support the recommendation that the condition be specifically considered during a periodic health examination.

B. There is fair evidence to support the recommendation that the condition be specifically considered during a periodic health examination.

C. There is insufficient evidence to recommend for or against the inclusion of the condition during a periodic health examination, but recommendations may be made on other grounds.

D. There is fair evidence to support the recommendation that the condition be excluded from consideration during a periodic health examination.

E. There is good evidence to support the recommendation that the condition be excluded from consideration during a periodic health examination.

Source: US Preventive Service Task Force,[2] with permission.

Table 2.3. US preventive services task force recommendations for breast cancer screening

Intervention/age (years)	Level of evidence[a]	Strength of recommendation[b]
Routine mammogram every 1–2 years with or without annual clinical breast examination		
40–49	I	C
50–69	I, II-2	A
70–74	I, II-3	C
≥75	III	C
Annual clinical breast examination without periodic mammograms		
40–49	III	C
50–59	I	C
≥60	III	C
Routine breast self-examination	I, II-2, III	C

Source: U.S. Preventive Services Task Force,[2] with permission.
[a] See Table 2.1.
[b] See Table 2.2.

MEASURING ASSOCIATIONS IN STUDIES

Breast disease studies often present incidence rates which reflect the likelihood of developing disease during a given interval, such as a year. The numerator includes those with the outcome of interest (e.g., breast cancer), and the denominator contains all those at risk of the outcome. Rates usually appear as numbers to the base 10, such as per 100, 1000, or 100,000 persons.

Age-specific rates offer additional information. For example, the annual incidence of breast cancer among U.S. women increases from 127/100,000 at age 40–44 years to 450/100,000 women at age 70–74 years.

In a classic Marx brothers movie, one of the brothers asks Groucho, "Say, Groucho, howsa' you' wife?" Groucho replies, "Compared to what?" Although unacceptably sexist for modern times, Groucho's response several decades ago framed the clinical question for contemporary readers. No study should be evaluated in a vacuum; clinicians must view the findings in context. For example, what is the risk of breast cancer among women exposed to oral contraceptives compared to women not exposed to oral contraceptives?

Relative risks address Groucho's question. A relative risk is a ratio of rates. A synonym for relative risk is "risk ratio." One divides the rate for the exposed group (e.g., women who have used oral contraceptives) by the rate for the unexposed group (those who have not). If the rates are equal, the ratio (relative risk) is 1.0, implying no effect of oral contraceptives on the risk of breast cancer.

Relative risks above 1.0 indicate an increased risk of disease associated with the exposure. For example, nulliparity is associated with an increased risk of breast cancer. Here the relative risk associated with nulliparity would be higher than 1.0, with parous women serving as the referent group. Conversely, relative risks below 1.0 imply a protective effect: use of oral contraceptives (OCs) lowers a woman's risk of benign breast disease. The relative risk associated with OC use would be less than 1.0, with women not using OCs serving as the referent group. Relative risks above and below 1.0 are reciprocally related. For example, a relative risk of 2.0 is equal in strength but opposite in direction to a relative risk of 0.5.

In any study using a sample, researchers obtain only an approximation of the true situation for the entire population. This guess, based on the particular sample studied, is termed a "point estimate." Point estimates tend to be imprecise in small studies due to statistical instability. Conversely, large studies have more statistical precision.

Authors can help readers understand the precision of their findings by reporting confidence intervals around rates, such as 95% confidence intervals. These figures can be found in statistical tables or calculated with commercially available software. For example, if 2 of 10 women given a new chemotherapy for breast cancer develop serious bone marrow toxicity, the incidence rate is 20%. However, the 95% confidence interval for the rate of 20% runs from 3% to 56%. If this study were repeated many times using the same number of participants, 95% of the time the true rate for the whole population would fall within this range. Because this interval is so wide, this hypothetical study of 10 women contributes little information. One knew in advance that the rate was between 0% and 100%; the estimate of 3–56% is not much more precise.

Researchers customarily present confidence intervals for relative risks as well. These intervals indicate the precision of the relative risk point estimates. Wide confidence intervals imply poor precision and vice versa. By definition, if the 95% confidence interval does not cross 1.0, the difference observed is statistically significant at the traditional $p < 0.05$.

In case-control studies, investigators cannot determine incidence rates. This problem stems from the fact that the denominator is unknown in this type of study. Hence researchers calculate "odds ratios." In situations where the disease or condition is rare (e.g., <5%), the odds ratio becomes a good substitute for relative risk. Indeed, authors commonly use these two terms interchangeably. Odds ratios also use confidence intervals to show precision. As with relative risk, if a 95% confidence interval around an odds ratio does not cross 1.0, the difference is statistically significant at $p < 0.05$.

Conclusions

Evidence-based medicine combines the best available evidence with the seasoned judgment of the clinician. It ensures that medical practice is up to date. More importantly, it prevents a clinician's practice from becoming obsolete in the future.

All clinical research can be categorized in a simple hierarchy of scientific rigor. Descriptive studies are most useful for generating hypotheses about causal associations. Analytic studies, such as cohort and case-control studies, can test hypotheses about cause and effect. However, selection bias, information bias, and confounding always act to bias observation research to some extent. Randomized controlled trials offer the best hope for finding real effects if they exist. Hence these trials receive the greatest weight in evidence-based medicine.

Cohort studies and randomized controlled trials should express their results using relative risks and confidence intervals. Case-control studies use odds ratios and confidence intervals.

The recommendations of the U.S. Preventive Services Task Force on screening for breast cancer are a prototype for the critical appraisal of the scientific literature. Important health policy questions, such as the advisability of mammography for women in their forties, should be resolved by scientific evidence, not by administrative fiat or political pressure.

References

1. Antman E, Lau J, Kupelnick B, Mosteller F, Chalmers TC. A comparison of results of meta-analyses of randomized control trials and recommendations of clinical experts. JAMA 1992;268:240–248

2. US Preventive Services Task Force. Guide to Clinical Preventive Services (2nd ed). Baltimore, Williams & Wilkins, 1995, pp 861, 862, 864

3. Schulz KF, Chalmers I, Hayes RJ, Altman DG. Empirical evidence of bias: dimensions of methodological quality associated with estimates of treatment effects in controlled trials. JAMA 1995;273:408–412

Recommended Rending

Evidence-Based Working Group. Evidence-based medicine: a new approach to teaching the practice of medicine. JAMA 1992;268:2420–2425

Ewigman BG, Crane JP, Frigoletto FD, et al. Effect of prenatal ultrasound screening on perinatal outcome: the RADIUS Study Group. N Engl J Med 1993;329:821–827

Nystrom L, Rutqvist LE, Wall S, et al. Breast cancer screening with mammography: overview of Swedish randomised trials. Lancet 1993;341:973–978

Sackett DL, Haynes RB, Guyatt GH, Tugwell P. Clinical Epidemiology: A Basic Science for Clinical Medicine (2nd ed). Boston, Little Brown, 1991

US Preventive Services Task Force. Guide to clinical preventive services (2nd ed). Baltimore, Williams & Wilkins, 1995

3 DEVELOPMENT AND GROWTH OF THE BREAST

William H. Hindle

EMBRYOLOGY

The breast ductal and glandular system develops in the embryo from ectoderm that buds and invaginates into the mesenchyme (Fig. 3.1). Canalization of the central lactiferous ducts occurs near term birth. Until puberty the male and female breasts are anatomically similar. The cells of the breast tissues contain the DNA, genes, and chromosomes that were genetically determined at conception.

Although variations in the onset and rate of female breast development and differences in the size, shape, and symmetry of mature breasts are common, congenital abnormalities are rare (Table 3.1). Congenital abnormalities can be classified as unilateral or bilateral and as hypoplasia or hyperplasia. In severe cases reconstructive plastic surgery is indicated, but it should be deferred until the breast tissue has completely matured (approximately age 18). If surgery is elected, the patient (family) should seek a plastic surgeon experienced in the uniquely specialized field of correcting breast developmental abnormalities.

The two most common developmental abnormalities are ectopic breast tissue (polymastia) and accessory or supernumerary nipples (polythelia). Both anomalies can occur on the embryonic milk line (Fig. 3.2). An accessory nipple is most commonly located below the breast or in the axilla and may appear bilaterally. The incidence of accessory nipples has been reported at 2–6%. Ectopic breast tissue is usually unilateral and located in the axilla. Neither lesion requires treatment unless the patient insists on surgical excision.

The stages of normal female breast development with approximate age ranges for each stage are listed in Table 3.2. The median age at which girls in the United States begin visible breast development is shortly before 10 years. The onset of physical breast development (thelarche) precedes the onset of menstruation (menarche) by about 3 years.

ENDOCRINOLOGY

When a girl reaches puberty, estrogen, progesterone, adrenal glucocorticoids, growth hormones, insulin, and prolactin (and probably other hormones not yet identified), in balanced proportions and acting in concert, bring about the glandu-

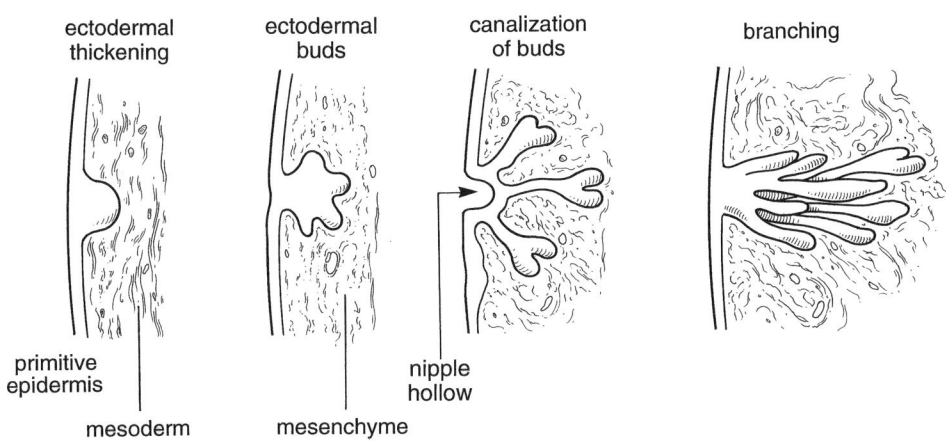

Figure 3.1. Early embryologic epithelial development of the human breast.

Table 3.1. Congenital and developmental breast abnormalities

Accessory axillary breast tissue: ectopic breast tissue, usually bilateral and often symptomatic with pregnancy

Amastia: absence of one or both breasts

Delayed thelarche: no breast development by age 15

Macromastia (gigantomastia): grossly enlarged breasts occurring with pregnancy or drug-induced

Juvenile hypertrophy: excessively enlarged breasts, usually bilateral

Poland syndrome: absence of the breasts, pectoralis muscles, and shoulder girdle; upper limb malformations

Polymastia: supernumerary breast

Polythelia: supernumerary nipples

Symmastia: midline confluence or webbing

Source: After Hindle and Pan,[1] with permission.

lar maturation of the breast and the functionality of the terminal duct lobular units (TDLUs). The primary effects of estrogen are (1) development of the stroma, (2) growth of the ducts, (3) deposition of the adipose tissue, 4) some lobular development, and (5) some alveolar development. Progesterone assists in these effects. The primarily progesterone effects are (1) lobular growth, (2) alveolar budding, and (3) alveolar secretory changes. Estrogen assists in these effects.

Milk secretion takes place in the glandular TDLUs of the mature breast. Lactation requires the coordinated actions of (1) cortisol, (2) growth hormone, (3) oxytocin, (4) parathyroid hormone, (5) placental lactogen, (6) prolactin, and (7) thyroxine. Paradoxically, high doses of estrogen and progesterone can suppress lactation.

The work on breast biopsy tissue by Ferguson, Anderson, and colleagues,[3,4] published in 1981 and 1982, remains one of the few breast endocrine studies on

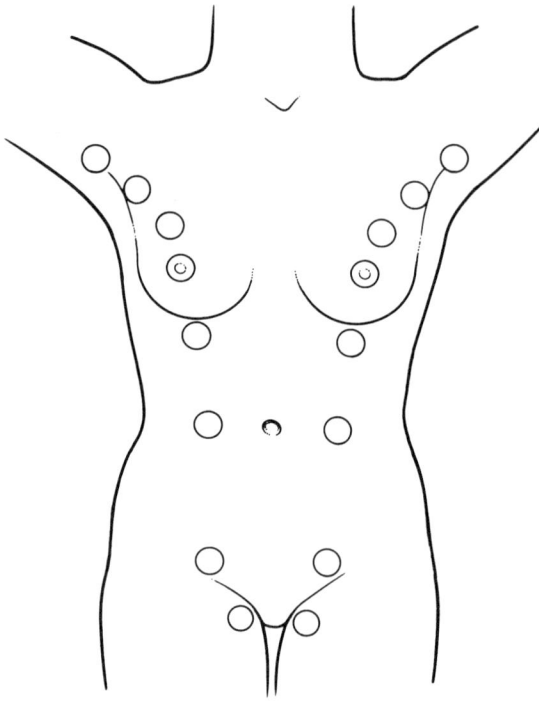

Figure 3.2. Sites of ectopic breast tissue and supernumerary nipples follow the embryologic milk line.

MILK LINES

Table 3.2. Stages of breast development at approximate age ranges

Age (years)	Stage	Development
9–10	I	Nipple elevation with no palpable glandular tissue and no pigmentation of the areola
10–12$\frac{1}{4}$	II	Palpable subareolar glandular tissue with projection of the nipple and breast as a single mound
11–13$\frac{1}{4}$	III	Nipple and breast remain a single mound; palpable glandular tissue increases; breast size and diameter enlarge; areola becomes pigmented
12–14$\frac{1}{4}$	IV	Nipple and areola rise above the breast, forming a second mound; areola enlarges; areolar pigmentation increases
13$\frac{1}{2}$–17	V	Breast shape becomes a smooth contour without projection of the areola and nipple

Source: After Tanner,[2] with permission.

human females (Figs. 3.3, 3.4). These studies demonstrated that the highest evidence of mitotic activity in female breast tissue occurs late during the luteal phase (shortly before the onset of menstruation), in contrast to the known increased mitotic activity that occurs during the follicular phase in the endometrium. The implication is that hormones (natural and synthetic—endogenous and exogenous)

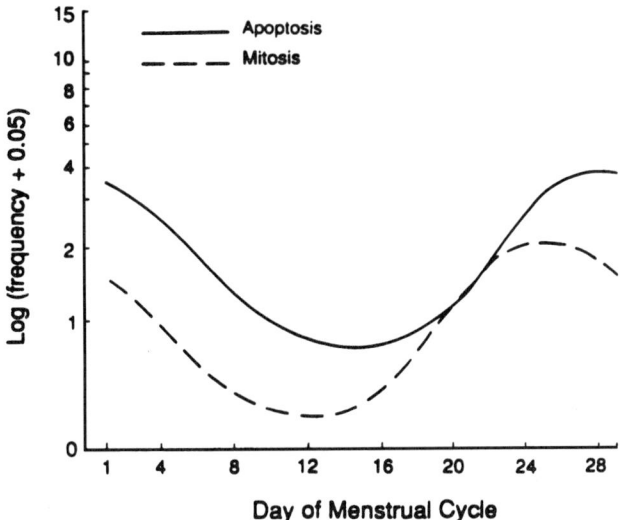

Figure 3.3. Variation of mitotic activity (cell replication) and apoptosis (programmed cellular death) in human female breast epithelium charted for each day of the menstrual cycle. The highest level of mitotic activity occurs during the late luteal (secretory) phase of the menstrual cycle. (From Ferguson and Anderson,[3] with permission.)

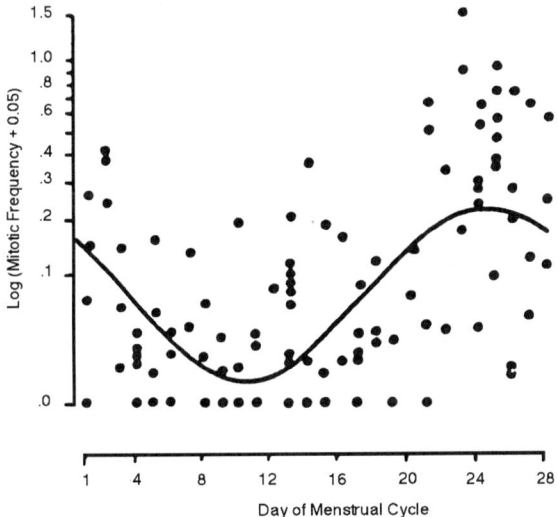

Figure 3.4. Log of the transformed values for the mitotic frequencies plotted against the day of the menstrual cycles, along with the fitted curve for the average sinusoidal variation. The highest mitotic activity occurs during the late luteal phase when progesterone is dominant (versus estrogen). (From Anderson et al.,[4] with permission.)

cannot be inferred to have the same effect, including known and potential benefits and dangers, on the breast epithelium that they have on the uterine endometrium. This point has important clinical considerations for counseling patients and prescribing estrogen, progesterone, and tamoxifen.

KEY PRACTICE POINTS

Breast epithelium: The maximum mitotic activity occurs during the late luteal phase, in contrast to the endometrial epithelium in which the maximum mitotic activity occurs during the follicular (proliferative) phase. The effect of progesterone dominant stimulation is distinctly different (seemingly opposite) in the breast epithelium compared to the endometrial epithelium.

PHYSIOLOGY

Lactation is the physiologic function of the female breast. The precipitous fall in serum progesterone level (with a similar fall, but lesser impact, of the estrogen level) and the decreased dopamine inhibition of prolactin (with stimulation by serotonin and other hormones) produces milk "let-down" after childbirth. The precise mechanisms and endocrinology of human milk production are complex and not well defined.

During the menstrual cycle there are observable cyclic histologic changes in the stroma, ductal lumen, and epithelium of the breast. Numerous studies have validated that during the reproductive years of a woman's life the ductal epithelium goes through monthly (approximately) cycles of proliferation and apoptosis (physiologic "planned" cellular death). In addition, there are cyclic fluctuations in vascularity and fluid retention. These physiologic cyclic changes are not uniform throughout the breast.

At menopause, physiologic estrogen withdrawal produces glandular and stromal atrophy. The atrophic changes are not uniform throughout the breast. The glandular atrophy begins in the distal portion of the TDLU and progresses "up" the lobules until eventually all that remains is the collecting ductal system with a few attached flattened atrophic lobules. There is a general correlation between the progressive atrophic breast changes and the decreasing mammographic density.

Estrogen receptors (ERs) occur in the ductal and lobular cells but not in the stroma. One study found that 7% of the breast epithelium was ER-positive. Generally, invasive breast cancers diagnosed during a woman's premenopausal years are ER-negative and during the postmenopausal years ER-positive. The progesterone receptors display a similar pattern but are more variable.

ANATOMY

Most of the mature breast is composed of adipose tissue, regardless of the size and shape of the breast or the weight and age of the woman. Furthermore, the process of fatty replacement of the glandular tissue of the breast begins during a woman's twenties and progresses with increasing age. Thus by age 70–80 women often have minimal amounts of ductal or glandular tissue remaining in their breasts. Nevertheless, the incidence of invasive carcinoma continues to increase with advancing age.

The ductal and glandular tissue of the breast is divided into individual lobes with no direct anatomic connection between them (Fig. 3.5). Each lobe empties into an individual lactiferous sinus with a collecting duct that has a separate opening on the top of the nipple. (The separate structure of each lobe accounts for the fact that nipple discharge from an intraductal papilloma appears only from a single opening on the nipple.) Inspection of the nipple during lactation reveals the 10–15 (or sometimes more) lobe openings on the nipple. Pathology of the lobes tends to originate in specific locations within the lobe (Fig. 3.6) and to be specific to the anatomy of that location (Fig. 3.7).

The term "tail of Spence" refers to the axillary extension of breast tissue over the pectoralis major muscle and into the axilla. The term "Montgomery's tubercles"

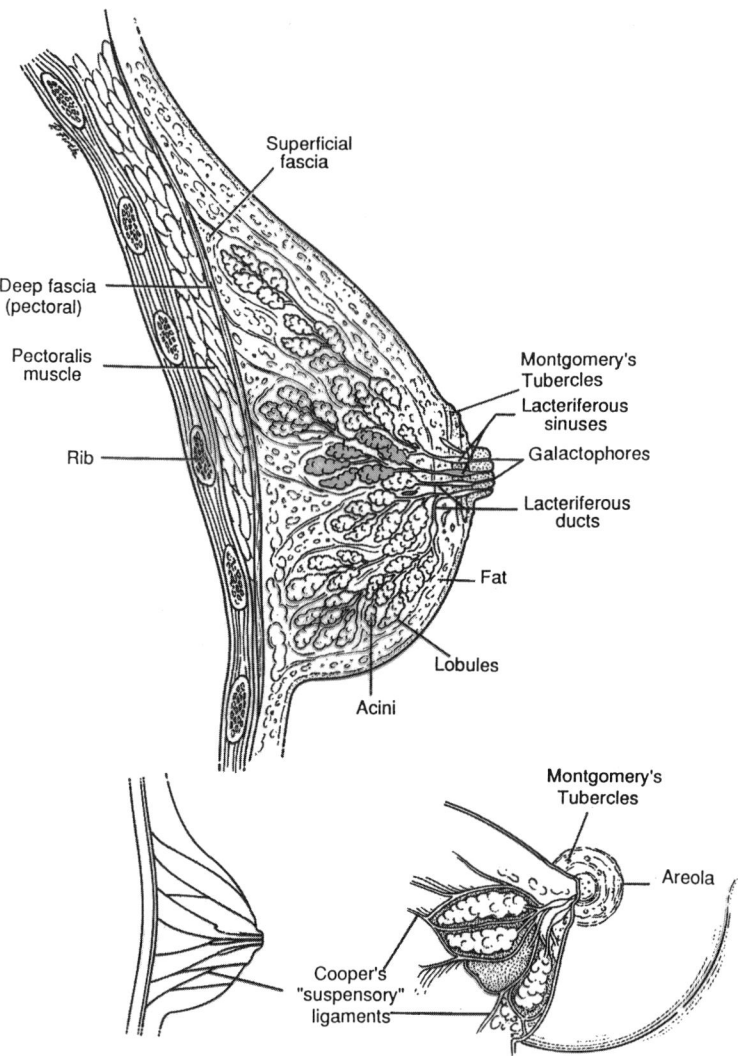

Figure 3.5. Anatomy of the human female breast showing separate lobes connected to the nipple by collecting ducts. (From Hindle,[5] with permission.)

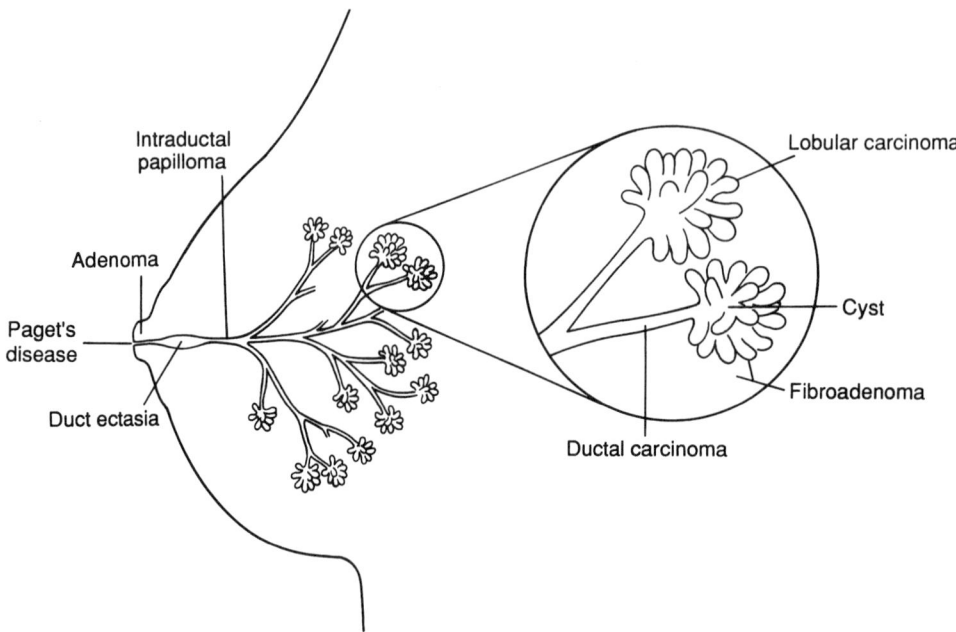

Figure 3.6. Common sites of pathology within a breast lobe.

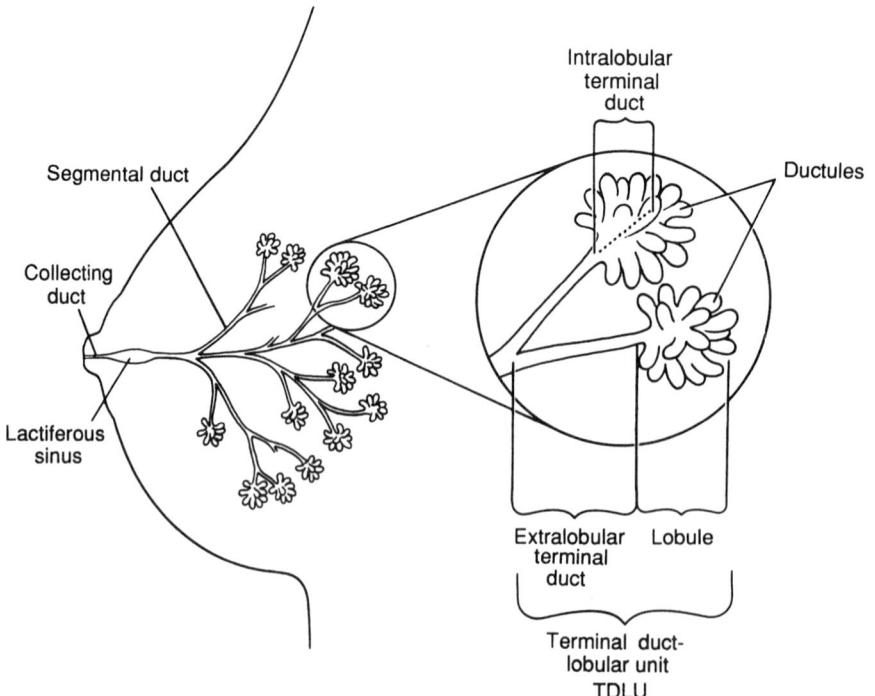

Figure 3.7. Anatomy of a breast lobe and terminal duct lobular unit. (From Hindle,[5] with permission.)

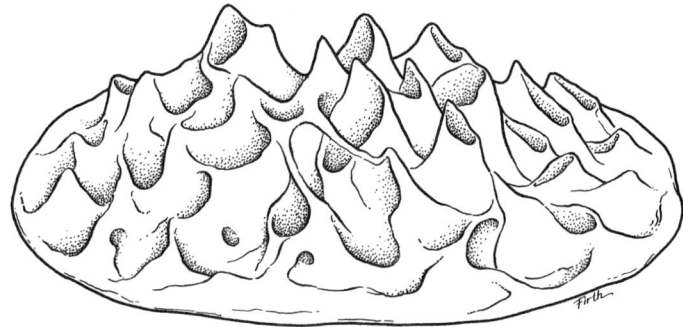

Figure 3.8. Random pattern of Cooper's ligaments of the breast.

(glands of Montgomery) refers to the elevated modified sebaceous glands, which are most prominent near the periphery of the areola. The glands may produce thick, creamy secretions or become infected.

Cooper's Ligaments

Sir Astley Cooper described the "ligaments" of the breast in 1845. They are thin, fibrous bands that run in a random pattern throughout the breast (Fig. 3.8) from the fascia on top (deep layer of the superficial pectoral fascia) of the pectoralis muscle to the superficial layer (of the superficial pectoral fascia), which joins Camper's superficial abdominal fascia below the dermis. Carcinoma invading the ligaments can shorten them, effectively contracting them, so that changes occur on the skin (dimpling, puckering, peau d'orange,* or nipple retraction) even though the primary cancer is deeper in the breast. Trauma to the breast can also damage the ligaments and result in similar contour and skin changes. Cooper's ligaments are the "loculations," or bands (septations), that surgeons break up when surgically opening and draining a large breast abscess.

Nerve Supply to the Breast

The anterior and middle branches of the second, third, fourth, and fifth intercostal nerves are the primary innervation of the skin over breast tissue. The supraclavicular branches of the cervical plexus supply the skin of the upper portion of the breast. The third, fourth, fifth, and sixth lateral cutaneous nerves supply the skin of the lateral aspects of the breast. The lateral cutaneous branches of the fourth intercostal thoracic nerve are the primary innervation of the nipple. The third and fifth intercostal nerves add to the innervation of the nipple–areolar complex.

Vascular Supply to the Breast

The arterial blood supply to the breast comes primarily from the anterior perforating branches of the internal mammary artery and the lateral thoracic artery. In addition, some of the blood supply comes from the lateral branches of the third,

---

*Although peau d'orange can result from edema related to congestive heart failure, dependency, or infection, classic peau d'orange is a clinical sign of inflammatory carcinoma.

fourth, and fifth intercostal arteries; the pectoral branch of the thoracoacromial artery; the suprascapular artery; and the thoracodorsal artery. Venous drainage of the breast is primarily by the internal thoracic vein, with additional drainage via the axillary vein and the second, third, and fourth intercostal veins.

Lymphatic Drainage and Lymph Nodes

The primary lymphatic drainage from the breast is into the axilla and the axillary lymph nodes (AxLNs). The internal mammary node chain drains the medial aspect of the breast. The rectus abdominis muscle sheath lymphatics (connecting via the epigastric plexus to the subdiaphragmatic lymphatics and to the intra-abdominal nodes) drain the inferior portion of the breast. Anatomy studies indicate that more than 90% of the lymphatic drainage of the breast goes to the axillae and less than 5% to the substernal internal mammary lymphatic channels. The lymphatic drainage of a cancer (e.g., the pattern of lymph node involvement) relates directly to the location of the cancer within the breast. Clinical research on axillary sentinel node dissection is confounded by the lymphatic drainage and the location of the primary cancer.

Meticulous autopsy and mastectomy studies reveal 30–60 lymph nodes in the axillary fat pad. However, a typical surgical pathology report of an axillary lymph node dissection (AxLND) or a modified radical mastectomy (MRM) states that 15–20 nodes have been identified and evaluated for evidence of involvement with cancer. The AxLNs are described in surgical anatomy as: level I, lateral to the insertion of the pectoralis minor muscle; level II, under the insertion of the pectoralis minor muscle; and level III, medial to the pectoralis minor muscle (Fig. 3.9). During an MRM or breast-conserving therapy (BCT), the AxLND removes levels I and II en bloc. A higher incidence of postoperative lymphedema of the arm results from removal of the level III nodes. The accepted incidence of "skip metastasis" (level III involvement despite none at level II) is about 1%.

Dissection of the AxLNs is an essential component of stage I and II cancer therapy for loco-regional control and categorical prognostic information. The latter assists in adjuvant therapy decisions and counseling the individual patient. Multiple studies have demonstrated that the AxLN involvement with cancer (presence and extent, i.e., number of nodes involved) correlates directly with the disease-specific mortality outcome. Figure 3.10 illustrates the correlation between AxLN involvement and disease-free survival after treatment of breast cancer. However, these numerically impressive data (and similar published data) relate to the prognosis for groups of breast cancer patients and may not apply to an individual patient.

MALIGNANT TRANSFORMATION AND CANCER GROWTH

It is generally accepted that most invasive ductal carcinomas begin in the ductules leading to the TDLUs or in the intralobular ductules. The process is usually malignant transformation (Fig. 3.11) from normal ductal epithelium to intraductal hyperplasia, to atypical intraductal hyperplasia, and then to ductal carcinoma in

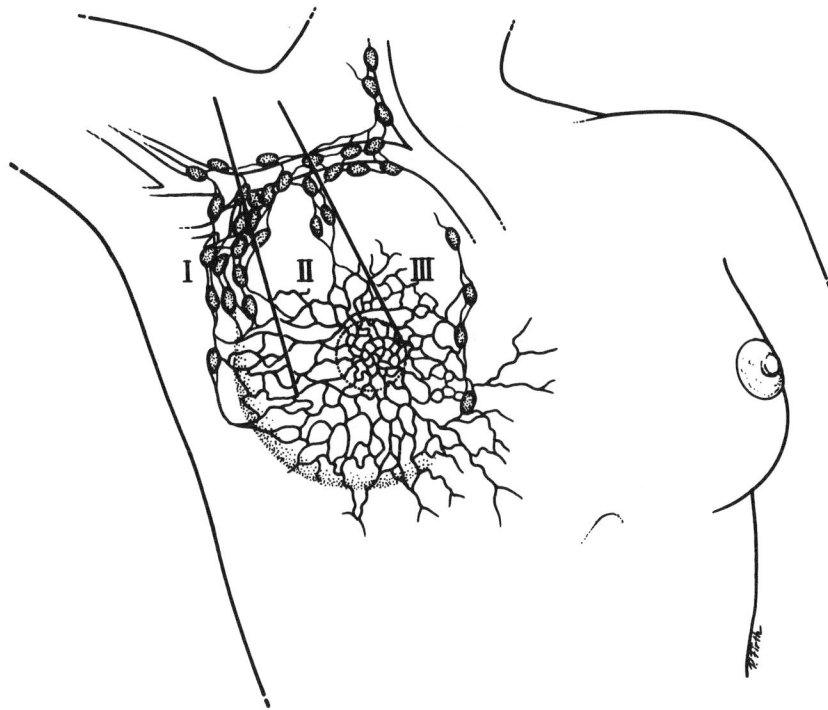

Figure 3.9. Levels I, II, and III of the axillary lymph nodes that drain the breast.

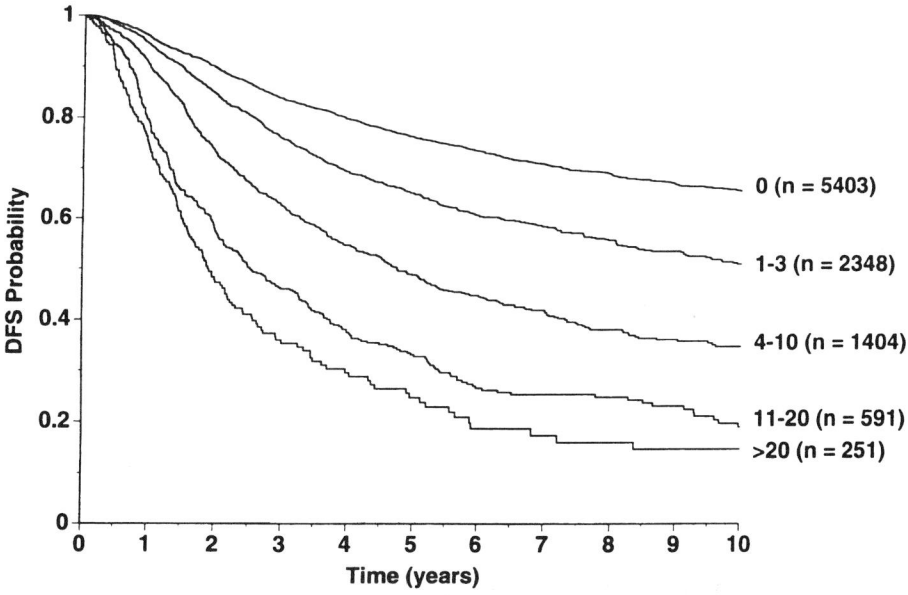

Figure 3.10. Correlation between the number of involved (with cancer) lymph nodes and disease-free survival over time. Data are from the San Antonio Data Base, with a median follow-up of 51 months. (After Clark,[6] with permission.)

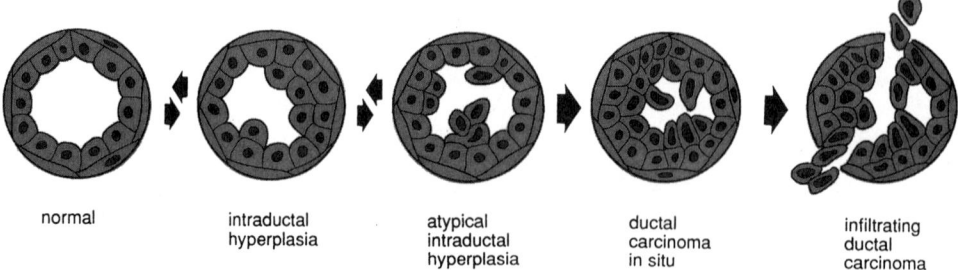

Figure 3.11. Potential progression of hyperplasia and atypia of the ductal epithelium to invasive carcinoma. All changes are spontaneously reversible up to (and possibly including) ductal carcinoma in situ. (After Kopans,[7] with permission.)

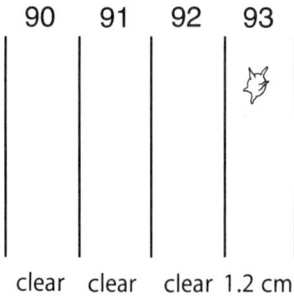

Figure 3.12. Serial annual mammograms showing the "sudden" appearance of a 1.2-cm mammographically malignant mass, implying uncharacteristically rapid growth of a cancer (short doubling time).

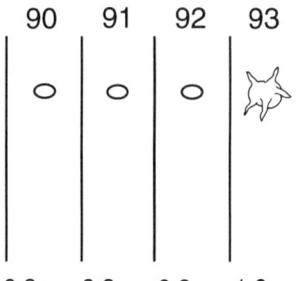

Figure 3.13. "Stable," benign-appearing 0.8-cm mass on serial annual mammograms suddenly appears as a 1.6-cm mammographically malignant lesion.

situ. There is evidence that malignant transformation of the ductal epithelium is spontaneously reversible up to and including carcinoma in situ. It is also clear that many of the changes in the ductal epithelium do not progress.

Furthermore, serial screening mammography studies have shown that ductal carcinoma can appear suddenly (interval cancer) in a size that usually takes several years to develop (Fig. 3.12) and that a "stable," benign-looking, nonpalpable mass can suddenly appear as a larger mammographically malignant mass (Fig. 3.13). Thus breast cancer clinical growth patterns are variable. Cancer doubling times, growth patterns, and biologic behavior are discussed in Chapter 41.

References

1. Hindle WH, Pan EY. Breast disorders in female adolescents. In Sanfilippo JS, Finkelstein JW, Styne DM (eds) Adolescent Medicine: State of the Art Reviews (vol 5). Philadelphia, Hanley & Belfus, 1994, pp 123–129

2. Tanner J. Growth at Adolescence. Oxford, Blackwell, 1962 (modified in Hindle and Pan[1])

3. Ferguson DJ, Anderson TJ. Morphological evaluation of cell turnover in relation to menstrual cycle in the "resting" human female breast. Br J Cancer 1981;44:177–181

4. Anderson TJ, Ferguson DJ, Rabb GM. Cell turnover in the "resting" human breast: influence of parity, contraceptive pill, age and laterality. Br J Cancer 1982;46:376–382

5. Hindle WH. Breast Disease. In Morrow CP, Curtin JP, Townsend DE (eds) Synopsis in Gynecologic Oncology (4th ed). New York, Churchill Livingstone, 1993

6. Clark MC. Prognostic and predictive factors. In: Harris JR, Lippman ME, Morrow M, et al (eds) Diseases of the Breast. Philadelphia, Lippincott-Raven, 1996

7. Kopans DB. Breast Imaging. Philadelphia, Lippincott, 1989, p 31

4   BREAST EXAMINATION

William H. Hindle

CLINICAL BREAST EXAMINATION

A simple, thorough clinical breast examination (CBE) is the most important diagnostic technique available to those primary health care providers called on to evaluate the female breast. Whether the examination is for a routine annual physical or for a specific breast complaint, CBE should be performed in the same systematic fashion. The results, including any abnormal findings beyond the limits of normal anatomic and physiologic variation, should be recorded in the patient's medical record.

The CBE should be performed in a pleasant relaxed atmosphere wherein the patient has complete privacy and is as comfortable as possible during the examination. The patient is instructed to remove all clothing from above the waist and is given an examination gown that opens at the front. The lighting should be equivalent to bright sunlight and should cast as few shadows as possible.

The CBE begins by inspection of the entire anterior chest with the patient sitting or standing (Fig. 4.1). Observe the breasts carefully for any variations, comparing the right to the left and to a prior examination if one has been previously performed by the examiner. Look for dimpling, discoloration, erythema, nodules, pitting, prominent vascularity, puckering, retraction, scars, ulceration; abnormal nipple position, nipple inversion or retraction; variations in breast size, shape, and contour; and any suggestion of an underlying mass. The woman then raises her arms above her head, and the same observations are made (Fig. 4.2). In this position more of the underside of the breast is visible, as are the axillary areas. The woman then presses firmly on her hips with her open hands, which tenses the pectoralis muscle underlying the breast (Fig. 4.3). An attachment from the pectoralis fascia to the skin can produce visible skin signs in this position. Next, the woman leans forward far enough so that the breasts hang free from the chest (Fig. 4.4). Nipple changes (e.g., position and "pointing," or direction) are apparent in this position. Most examiners prefer to conclude the standing or sitting inspection with palpation of both axillae (Fig. 4.5) and then the supraclavicular areas. Healthy lymph nodes are not palpable, but enlarged lymph nodes can be felt. Occasionally a mass is felt in the axillary area that is not consistent with a lymph node. If persistent, the axillary mass should be evaluated further. Frequently there are minor skin changes in the axilla, often related to shaving.

The most important phase of the CBE is palpation of the entire breast for the presence of a mass. This step is performed with the patient resting comfortably on her back (Fig. 4.6). A pillow under the head adds to her comfort during the examination. Many examiners prefer to place a pillow under the shoulder on the side being examined, which opens up the anterior chest wall area and allows the arm to relax and fall away from the chest; or she can place her arm comfortably over her head, which spreads out the tissue on the anterior chest and facilitates thorough palpation.

Palpation of the breast should cover the entire anterior chest wall (Fig. 4.7). The pads of the second, third, and fourth fingers are the most useful and most sensitive for breast palpation (Fig. 4.8). The fingers are gently rotated in concentric dime-sized circles (Fig. 4.9). This circular pattern is continued while applying varying degrees of pressure, mild to moderate to firm (Fig. 4.10), so that the entire depth of the breast is palpated, from the surface to the underlying ribs. The increasing pressure helps ensure that a small mass that is not attached to the skin or pectoralis fascia can be felt and not be pushed away by sudden movement. Moreover, the use of gently increasing pressure is more comfortable for the patient. The vertical strip pattern has been documented as the most effective pattern of palpation for detecting a breast mass (Fig. 4.11).

Subareolar Area

Special attention should be paid to the subareolar area. Palpation of the areola reveals normal findings different from the remainder of the breast. The usual diffuse nodularity palpated in the glandular breast of women of reproductive age is not present under the areola. Furthermore, if prominent, the collecting ducts can be felt as concentric cord-like structures. At the periphery of the areola there is often the impression of a circular "ridge" where the usual glandular tissue of the breast begins. Some women have prominent nodularity on this circular ridge. Occasionally, similar nodularity can be palpated along the inframammary fold.

The areola and its underlying tissue are more sensitive and can be tender to palpation compared to the rest of the breast; examination of this area should be gentle but thorough. About 15% of invasive carcinomas occur in the subareolar area.

Mastalgia

True diffuse pain within the breast can often be reproduced by firmly compressing the breast between the parallel surfaces of the palms held above and below the breast. This maneuver is reserved for women with a complaint of diffuse breast pain and is performed with the woman sitting or standing.

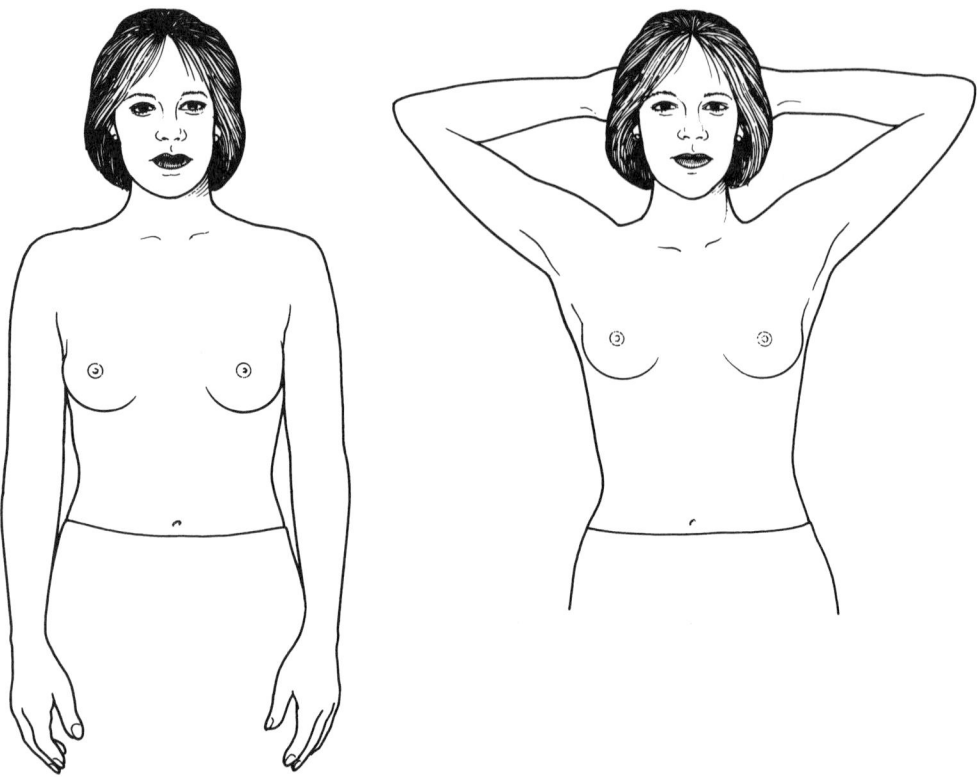

Figure 4.1. Inspection of the anterior chest with the patient standing (or sitting) at ease.

Figure 4.2. Inspection of the anterior chest with the patient's hands behind her head.

Nipple Discharge

If the woman has complained of nipple discharge, the top of the nipple should be inspected for the presence of discharge at the duct openings onto the nipple. Gentle but firm pressure is applied by the two index fingers simultaneously pressing downward and inward from the areolar skin margin to the base of the nipple in a clockwise pattern until the entire areola has been compressed (Fig. 4.12). This "milking" maneuver empties the collecting ducts below the nipple; and, if present, a discharge appears on the top of the nipple. Squeezing the nipple per se is not necessary and can be uncomfortable for the patient. If discharge is present, it is important to note whether it is bilateral or unilateral and from how many duct openings it appears. Pathologic nipple discharge related to neoplasms (e.g., intraductal papilloma or cancer) characteristically appears from a single duct opening on the nipple. Discharge associated with mammary duct ectasia (periductal mastitis) comes from multiple duct openings. If the discharge appears to be bloody, a dipstick for blood (e.g., a Hemastix or equivalent) confirms whether blood is present. Milky (physiologic) nipple discharge almost invariably can be expressed from multiple duct openings and is often bilateral.

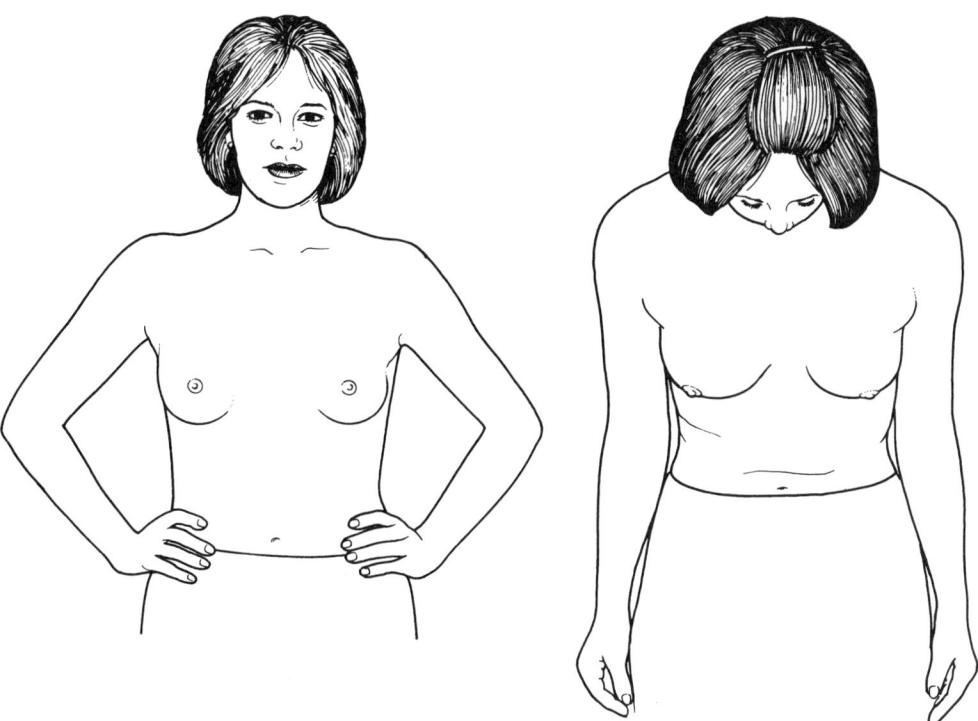

Figure 4.3. Inspection of the anterior chest with the patient pressing her hands on her hips.

Figure 4.4. Inspection of the breasts with the patient leaning forward.

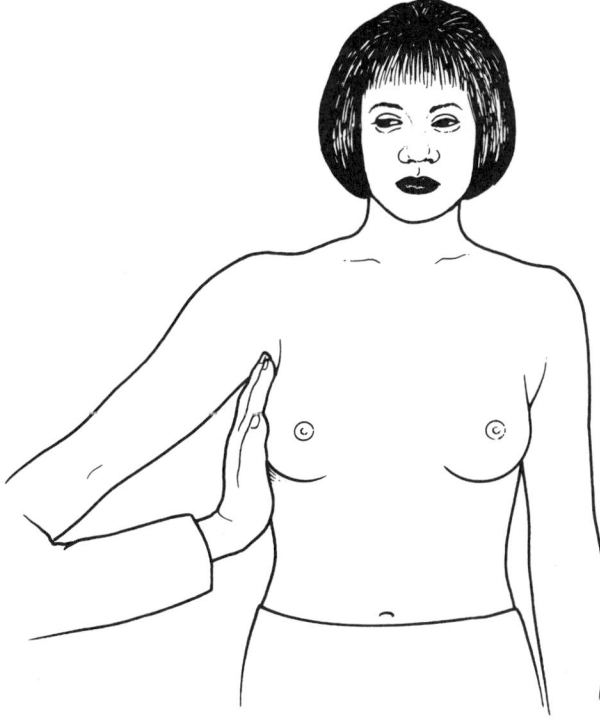

Figure 4.5. Palpation of the axillary area.

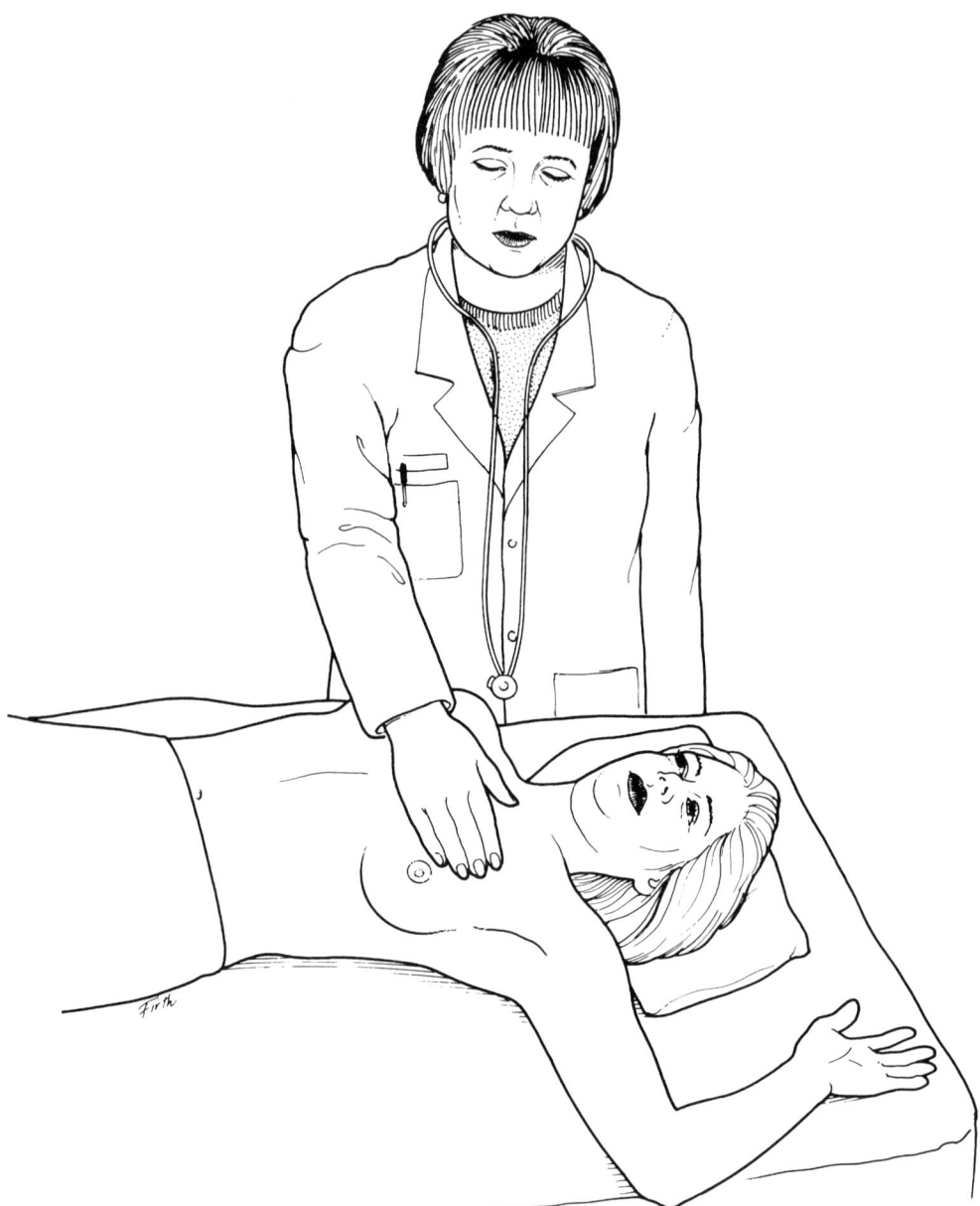

Figure 4.6. Proper position for palpation of the breast with the patient comfortably supine.

Pregnancy

Breast examination and evaluation are performed in the same manner when a woman is pregnant or lactating. Routine CBE should be performed and recorded on the first prenatal visit and repeated if the patient reports a problem during the pregnancy or lactation.

KEY PRACTICE POINTS

Breast examination: The paramount objective of the clinical breast examination is detection of a dominant breast mass.

Palpable dominant mass: A palpable dominant mass is defined as a readily felt, distinct, three-dimensional mass that is different in character from the remainder of that breast and from the other breast.

Routine breast examinations: Women should have annual clinical breast examinations and do regular breast self-examinations beginning at age 20.

Routine screening mammography: Women should have annual screening mammography beginning at age 40.

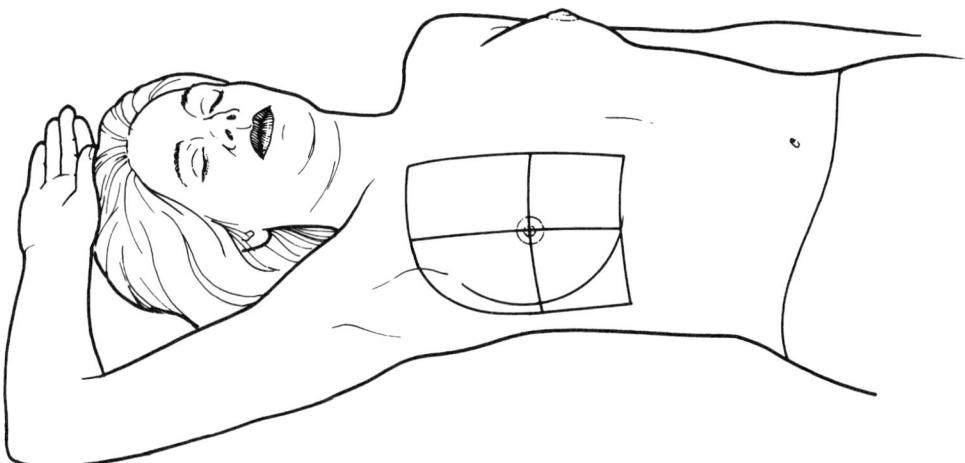

Figure 4.7. Outline of breast and surrounding area to be palpated systematically.

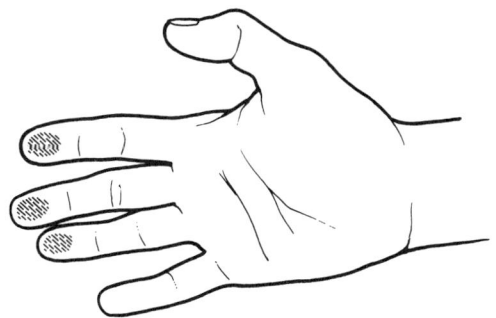

Figure 4.8. Pads of the second, third, and fourth fingers are the most sensitive for breast palpation.

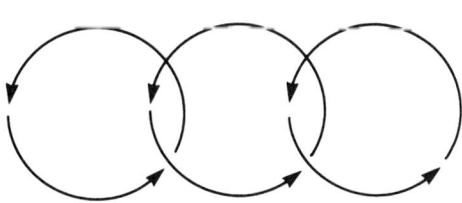

Figure 4.9. Pads of the fingers are rotated in concentric "dime-sized" circles for effective palpation of the breast.

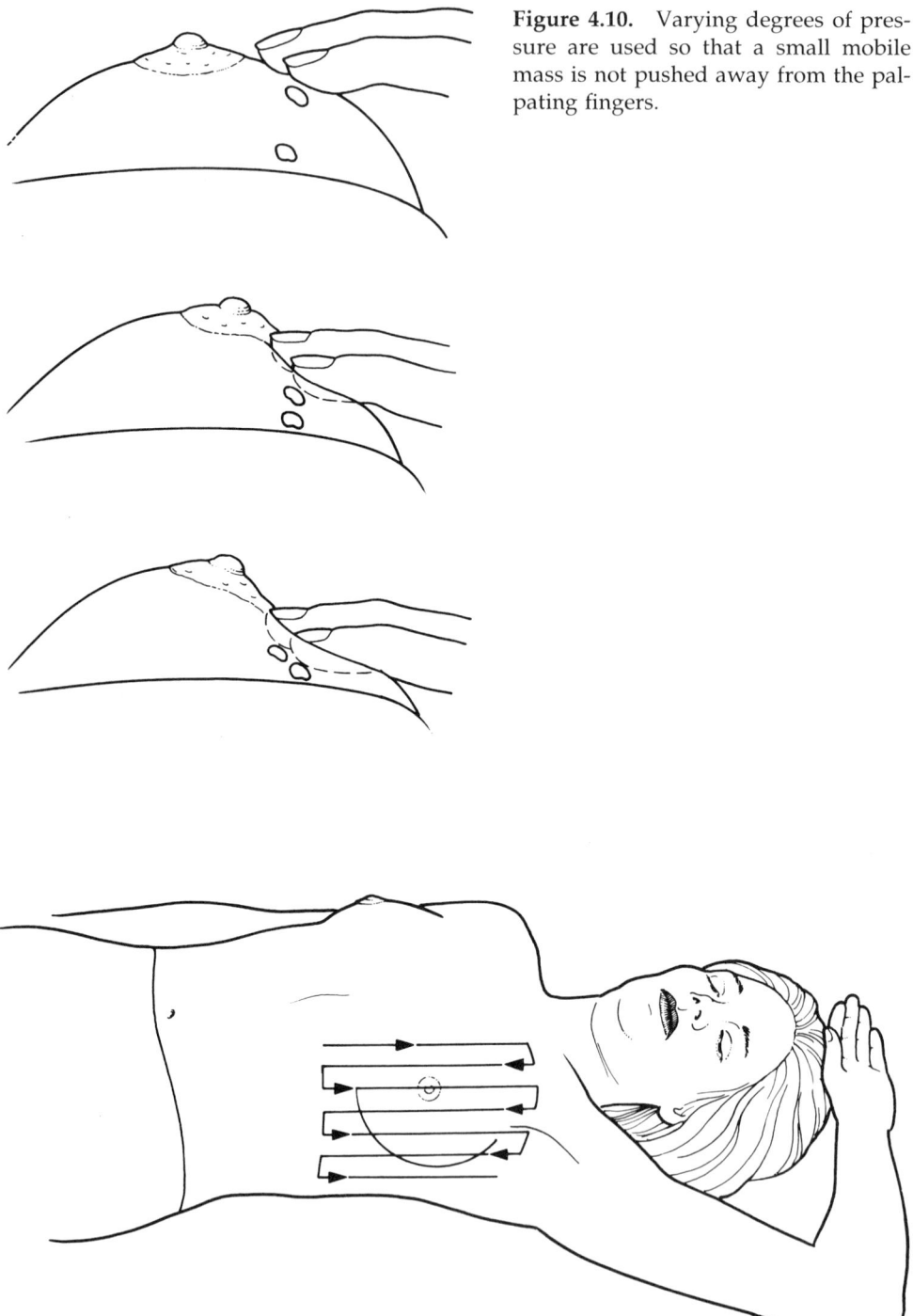

Figure 4.10. Varying degrees of pressure are used so that a small mobile mass is not pushed away from the palpating fingers.

Figure 4.11. A vertical strip pattern is most effective for systematic palpation of the breast.

Figure 4.12. Gentle massage of the areola in a systematic concentric radial pattern effectively "milks" the underlying ducts toward their openings on the nipple.

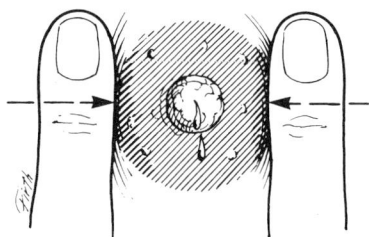

Breast Self-Examination

Breast self-examination (BSE) is optimally performed in the same methodical manner as the CBE using the contralateral hand to palpate each breast. A few days after the cessation of menstruation flow is usually the most comfortable time for a woman of reproductive age to examine her breasts. Women not having routine periods should choose a regular calendar date (e.g., the first day of the month) to do a BSE. Palpation of the axillary area is not an effective maneuver for BSE, nor is it necessary to squeeze or massage the nipples. Most women of reproductive age can elicit some nipple discharge; it is physiologic and not a cause for alarm or medical evaluation.

Effective instruction requires step-by-step demonstration of the BSE technique (Fig. 4.13). Compliance is encouraged by having the woman demonstrate back to her instructor what she has learned (Fig. 4.14). Further instruction and encouragement should be given if the patient's BSE is less detailed than described above. Optimally, BSE demonstration and reinforcement are performed at each annual examination.

Even though the typical breast mass is accidentally found by the patient herself, the BSE should not be "sold" as cancer prevention. There is no published documented evidence that routine BSE decreases the mortality from breast cancer, although several studies have shown a trend toward the detection of smaller masses (e.g., "earlier" cancer) when the mass is detected by a woman performing her routine monthly BSE. Beginning at age 20, all women should regularly examine their breasts so they are familiar with their own anatomy and can note any physiologic changes. Hopefully, this knowledge makes detection of a dominant mass or significant abnormality apparent before it becomes obvious by casual or coincidental palpation.

Recording Breast Examination Findings

Physical findings that are clinically pathologic should be documented in the patient's medical record. The description should be in clear concise "plain English" (e.g., firm, fixed, hard, indistinct, irregular, lobular, mobile, nodular, oblong, round, smooth, soft, tender, thickened, vague).

The exact location of any lesion should be noted (or drawn) utilizing the clock method of description (Fig. 4.15). Measurements are taken with the patient lying

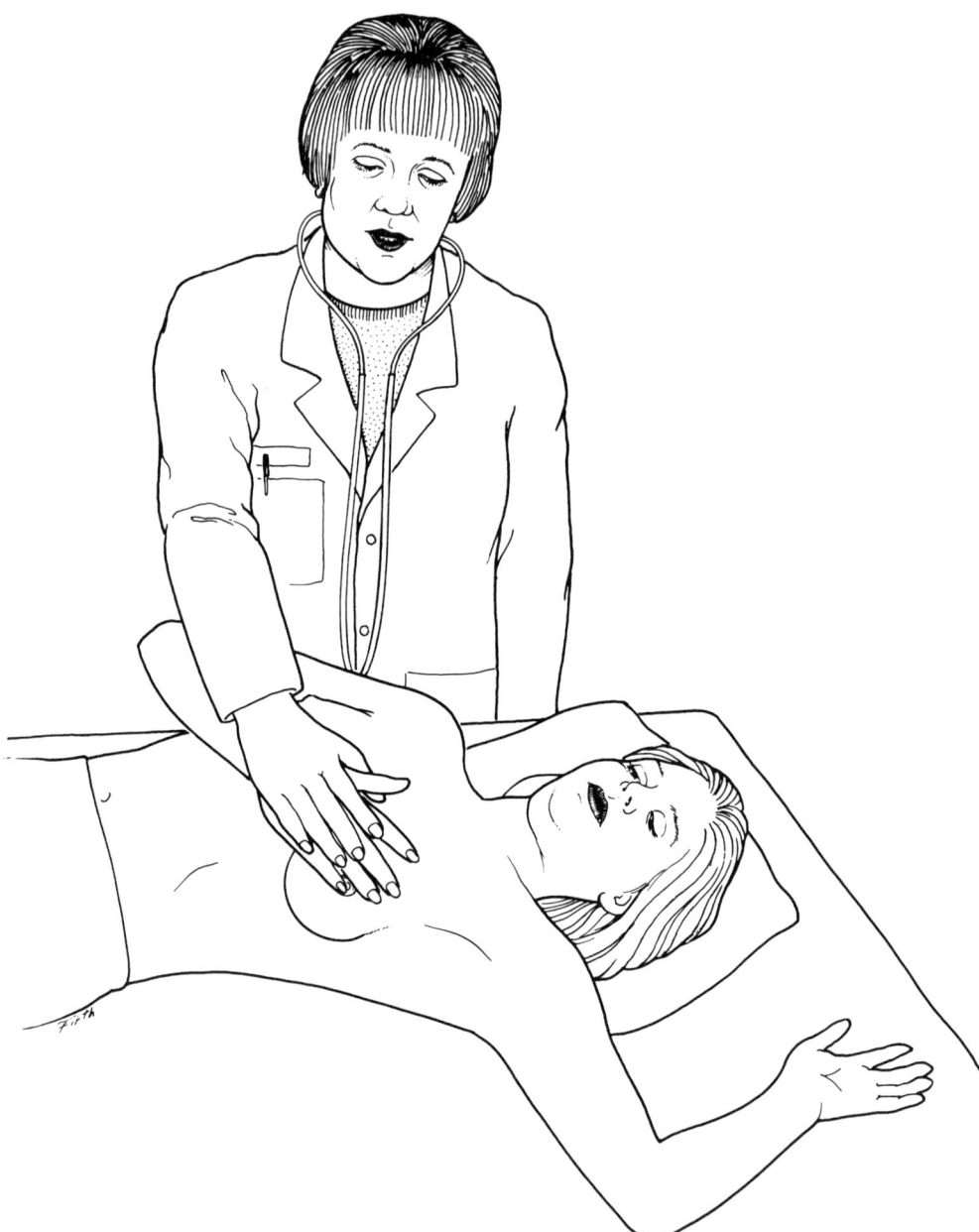

Figure 4.13.   Instructor demonstrates the breast self-examination technique to the patient.

supine. Actual dimensions (in centimeters) are ideal, or they may be estimated (and recorded as such) from palpation. It is essential that any recordings be labeled "right breast" or "left breast," as the case may be. Preprinted (Fig. 4.16), stamped (Fig. 4.17), or sketched breast diagrams are strongly encouraged because they require less writing, allow precise depiction of location, and are less liable to be misinterpreted. A word of caution is necessary: Drawing a circle or writing down measurements (e.g., 2 × 2 cm) are viewed in a courtroom as evidence that

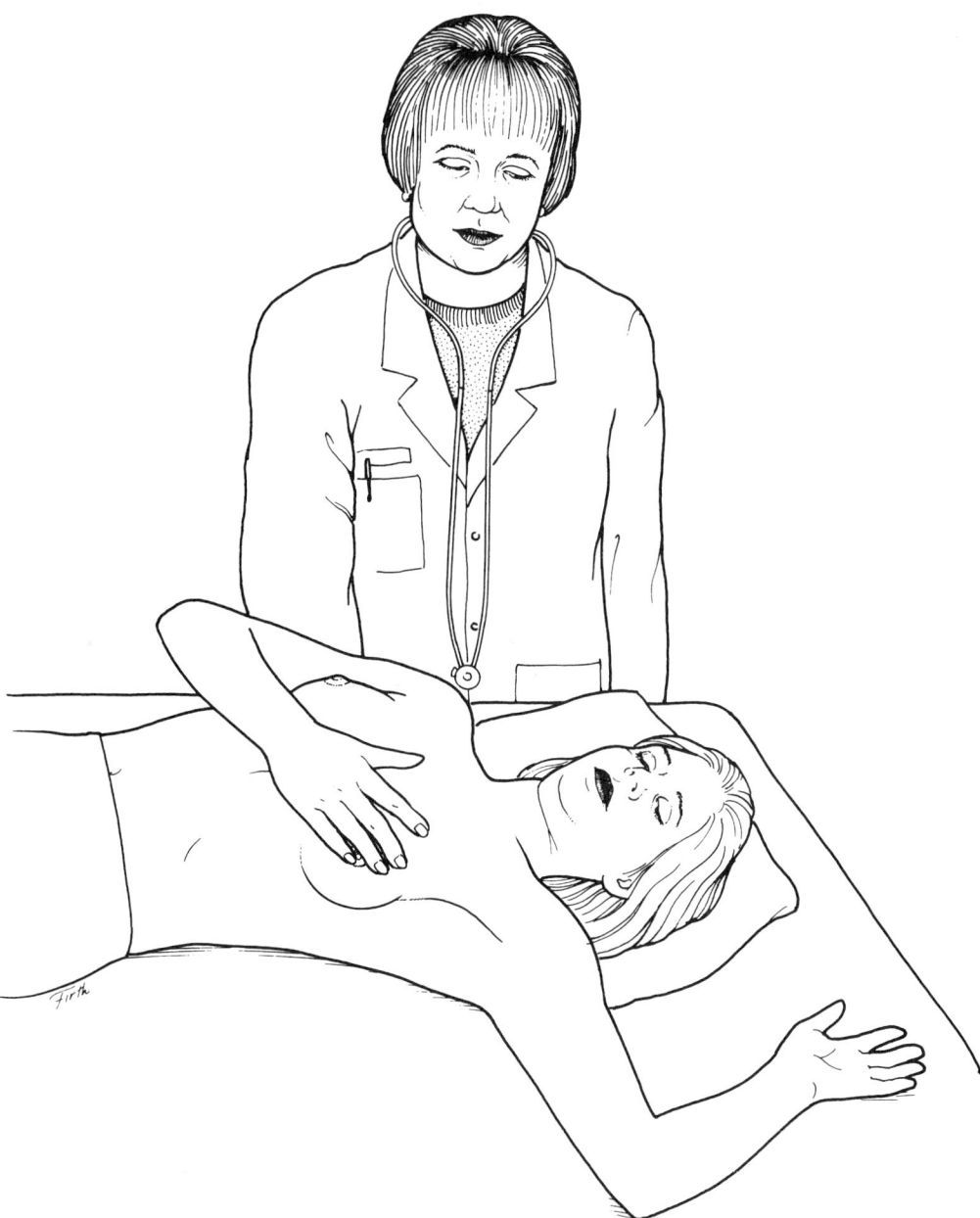

Figure 4.14. Instruction in breast self-examination is reinforced by having the patient demonstrate to her instructor what she has learned.

the examiner has found a dominant breast mass. If a localized area of vague diffuse nodularity or thickening is noted, it should be so described in the record or drawn with shaded lines or crosshatching, but *not as a circle* and *not* with precise dimensions. An example of an appropriate notation would be: "Left breast: diffuse nodularity in the upper outer quadrant. No dominant mass."

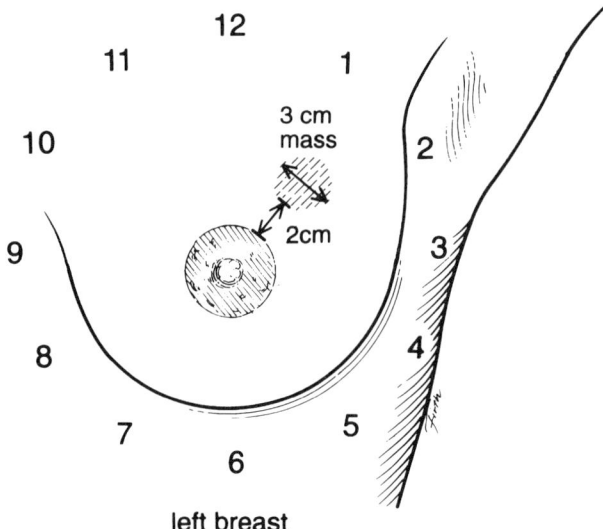

Figure 4.15. Precise location and measured size of a mass can be effectively described using a clock position. The mass in this illustration should be recorded as: "Left breast, dominant 3 cm mass at 1 o'clock position, 2 cm from the areola."

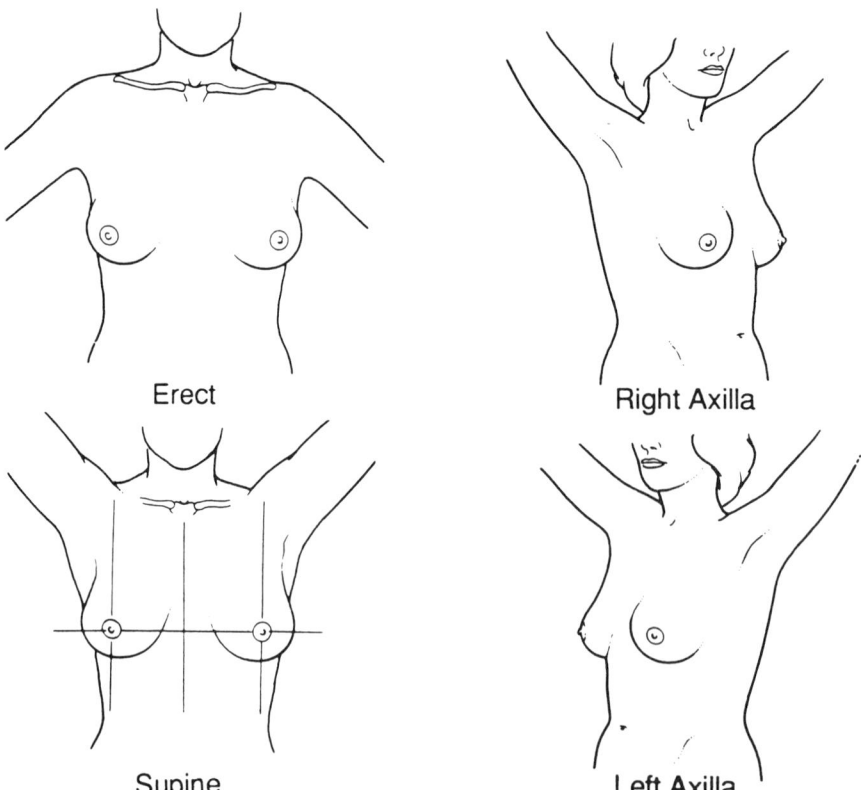

Figure 4.16. Example of a printed from used for recording the location of findings during CBE.

Figure 4.17. Diagram that can be "rubber-stamped" in the patient's chart for drawing the precise location of a physical finding.

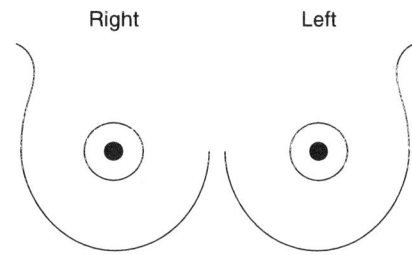

Right   Left

Some physicians fall into the habit of recording their physical findings with descriptions that are better reserved for final diagnoses (e.g., fibroadenoma and fibrocystic changes). These specific diagnostic terms can only be used after cytologic or histologic evaluation. If the physician must use such terms to characterize abnormal findings during examination, a qualifying phrase such as "consistent with" or "suggestive of" should be used in connection with the diagnostic term. Nevertheless, it is appropriate for the examiner to think in terms of specific histopathology when performing a breast examination. "What does this represent?" is an appropriate mental question when an abnormality is located.

When a clinically significant abnormality is recorded, the notation should be followed by a written plan of action (e.g., "recheck in 1 month" or "surgical consultation" or "schedule mammogram" or "patient to examine herself every week and return immediately if the lesion progresses"). Of course, a persistent palpable dominant breast demands timely diagnosis and should not simply be followed.

When a patient with a breast abnormality makes a return visit, the current status of the abnormality should be added to her medical record (e.g., cleared, larger, less prominent, no longer palpable, no longer tender, smaller, unchanged). If the lesion in question has not cleared or resolved, a new plan of action should be written.

CONCLUSIONS

Routine CBE should begin when a woman is 20 years of age and continue annually throughout her life. In addition, routine BSE should be encouraged after age 20. A complete CBE should be performed when a woman initially presents with a breast complaint or concern. It is prudent to have a patient palpate any abnormality the examiner detects in her breasts. This practice allows her to detect an anatomic or physiologic variation with her own periodic examinations and to demonstrate the area in question if she is sent for consultation. If ever the clinician has doubts as to the nature of the findings or proper management thereof, the patient should be referred to a breast specialist for consultation.

5   SCREENING MAMMOGRAPHY

Eric L. Rosen

Steven D. Frankel

Edward A. Sickles

The combination of mammography and clinical breast examination (CBE), performed at standard intervals, is currently the best way to provide breast cancer screening. Mammography employs x-rays to image the breast and requires specialized equipment, highly trained technologists, and specially trained physicians (almost always radiologists) to interpret the images. Mammography can be utilized either to detect unsuspected breast abnormalities (screening) or to evaluate known abnormalities (diagnosis). These two functions are most often performed separately because it allows screening examinations to be done in a more streamlined fashion and hence more rapidly and at lower cost.

Diagnostic mammography involves targeted x-ray images to evaluate an abnormality previously identified at either screening mammography or CBE. It is a tailored examination designed to determine if there is need for tissue diagnosis. Other imaging modalities such as ultrasonography and magnetic resonance imaging (MRI) are also utilized occasionally to provide additional information not available from mammography and CBE. Imaging procedures can be used to assist in the performance of minimally invasive biopsies of suspicious abnormalities or to localize nonpalpable abnormalities prior to surgical excision. An understanding of the various types of breast imaging examinations is crucial for proper clinical management of breast disease. It is also important to become familiar with specific mammographic abnormalities and their significance, as well as the terminology radiologists use to describe them.

WHY SCREEN WITH MAMMOGRAPHY?

Screening mammography has been shown to reduce the mortality from breast cancer by approximately 30% by detecting early and clinically occult breast cancer. Mammography is effective for detecting cancer, and studies show that the sensitivity (true-positive/true-positive + false-negative rate) of mammography is approximately 90% for detectable breast cancer (80–85% for all breast cancer). The other approximately 10% of detectable breast cancers are discovered by CBE. Therefore screening mammography should always be performed in conjunction with screening CBE to maximize the detection of breast cancer.

Mammography is less specific than sensitive, and therefore it is usually impossible to determine by imaging alone whether a mammographic abnormality truly represents cancer. Among every 1000 women who undergo screening mammography for the first time, approximately 70 demonstrate an abnormality that requires additional evaluation. Further evaluation with diagnostic mammography and ultrasonography results in a recommendation of biopsy for approximately 20 of the 70 women (the other 50 demonstrate characteristics typical for benign lesions). Subsequent biopsy reveals approximately seven cancers. If prior mammograms are available for comparison, the recall rate for additional imaging is reduced by at least 50%, as some of the less strikingly abnormal findings demonstrate stability when compared to the prior mammograms, indicating benignity. Comparison to prior mammograms is crucial to maximize the specificity of mammography and to reduce the number of false-positive examinations. To facilitate comparison, it is preferable to have women undergo mammography at the same facility each year. Alternatively, women should be encouraged to bring prior mammograms with them when undergoing subsequent screening.

WHO SHOULD UNDERGO SCREENING MAMMOGRAPHY?

Although the issue of who should have mammography is controversial, the American Cancer Society and many other national organizations currently recommend that routine mammographic screening begin at age 40. These guidelines state that women between 40 and 49 years of age should undergo routine mammography at 1- to 2-year intervals, and that women over age 50 should undergo annual mammography. Patients with a strong family history of breast cancer probably should begin annual screening before age 40, although no official standard has been set. Routine screening mammography is performed on few women younger than 30, principally because breast cancer is so rare in this age group but also because the younger breast is relatively more sensitive to radiation exposure.

The efficacy of screening women age 50 and older by routine mammography is well established, but there is controversy about the recommendations concerning women ages 40–49. Although full discussion of this topic is beyond the scope of this chapter, suffice it to say that almost all of the randomized controlled trials designed to evaluate the effectiveness of screening mammography were not designed with a sufficient number of patients in the younger age group to address this issue specifically. Nonetheless, two of the trials have produced statistically significant evidence of reduced breast cancer mortality among women ages 40–49 invited to undergo screening. The issue is further complicated because most of these studies differ substantially in their design and execution, making meta-analysis less reliable. Some meta-analyses of the studies have, however, demonstrated statistically significant mortality reductions among women ages 40–49, ranging from 18% to 23%. In addition, multiple studies have demonstrated that cancers detected by mammography in women ages 40–49 are similar in size and stage to those detected in older women, in whom the benefits of screening are established beyond dispute. These data suggest that mammography is capable of reducing breast cancer mortality in women ages 40–49 by detecting early cancer. Other studies strongly suggest that the proper screening interval for women ages 40–49 is every year, and it is likely that American Cancer Society guidelines will soon change to reflect these findings.

Do Women Under Age 50 Have Dense Breasts, Thereby Limiting the Sensitivity of Mammography?

The adult female breast is an involuting organ, and in general a woman's breasts lose some fibroglandular tissue over time and undergo fatty replacement. However, independent of age, the percentage of fibroglandular tissue in the breast is highly variable, and it is this underlying composition that determines the overall sensitivity of mammography. Mammograms of women with dense breasts do have a slightly lower sensitivity to cancer detection, but, it is likely that if a woman's breast tissue is dense before age 50, it will remain dense, even when she is 80. There is no magic age when all breasts become amenable to mammography. Instead, there is marked variability in the composition of breast tissue at all ages. The change in an individual's breast composition, to the extent that it occurs, is a gradual process.

Is There a Radiation Risk of Mammography?

Mammography utilizes ionizing radiation to image the breast, but the oncogenic risk associated with routine mammography is so small it is impossible to measure directly. Instead, estimates have been made by extrapolating data obtained from much higher radiation exposures, such as data from the Japanese atomic explosions and from women with tuberculosis undergoing routine chest fluoroscopy. These estimates suggest that the risk of inducing breast cancer from mammography is one cancer per one million examinations. This figure must be compared to the lifetime risk of developing breast cancer, which is currently $1:8$, and the evidence indicating that screening mammography reduces breast cancer mortality by about 30%. The radiation risk of mammography is negligible compared to the benefit it produces.

What Is a Screening Mammogram?

A screening mammography examination consists of four standard x-ray images, two of each breast, which are obtained from an asymptomatic woman at regular intervals. The examination, which typically takes 15–30 minutes to complete, is performed by a radiology technologist who has received special training in mammography. The patient remains standing as the technologist positions her breasts, one at a time, in the mammography unit. Once the breast is properly positioned, compression is applied to hold it in place, spread out the tissue, and minimize the amount of radiation needed to produce a proper image. The technologist then takes the image, releases the compression, and proceeds to the next exposure. When all four images have been taken, the technologist develops the films to ensure that the study is acceptable; if so, the patient is cleared to leave the imaging suite. The patient's films are then matched with those from her prior examinations, mounted on a viewing station, and interpreted by the radiologist.

WHAT ARE THE TWO STANDARD MAMMOGRAPHIC VIEWS?

In the United States routine screening mammography consists of two images of each breast: the mediolateral oblique (MLO) and the craniocaudal (CC) views. In both views the x-ray beam passes perpendicular to the plane of breast compression. The MLO view is obtained by compressing the breast in a plane parallel to the pectoralis muscle, usually 40–60 degrees from the horizontal plane. This view includes more breast tissue than any other view and is particularly useful for evaluating the upper outer breast. The craniocaudal view is obtained by compressing the breast in the horizontal plane. This view includes more medial tissue than the MLO view but less tissue in the upper and lateral breast. The routine use of two views maximizes inclusion of most of the breast tissue, improves the sensitivity and specificity of the examination, and permits most abnormalities to be localized to a particular quadrant in the breast.

IS COMPRESSION REALLY NEEDED?

Adequate breast compression is a prerequisite for high-quality mammography. The degree of breast compression is determined by the technologist at the time of the examination. Properly applied, breast compression is well tolerated by most women. Compression may be transiently uncomfortable but should not be painful; if pain is experienced, the patient should immediately alert the technologist, who reduces the degree of compression appropriately. High-quality mammograms are impossible without adequate compression because compression minimizes motion blurring, improves image contrast, spreads apart potentially confusing areas of otherwise overlapped tissue, and reduces radiation dose.

AT WHAT POINT IS THE MAMMOGRAM INTERPRETED BY A RADIOLOGIST?

Interpretation of the mammograms by the radiologist is timed variously from practice to practice. At our institution (University of California, San Francisco, Medical Center) screening examinations are interpreted in batches to maximize cancer detection efficiency and to minimize the cost of screening. Once a batch of examinations is completed, they are mounted on a film viewer that contains all the screening examinations performed that day.

Although the radiologist may not interpret a study immediately, all the screening examinations are read during one or two sessions within 24 hours of the examination. This practice allows us to interpret screening mammograms under optimal viewing conditions, uninterrupted, and without distraction from other examinations and other business.

How Are the Results of a Screening Examination Reported?

Screening mammography reports are typically standardized and are often computer-generated. Screening lends itself to this type of reporting in several ways. First, the use of standardized reports allows the radiologist to concentrate on interpreting the images, not on generating reports. Second, most screening mammograms are uncomplicated and normal, facilitating the use of standardized reports. Third, this approach allows tracking of patients, outcome analysis, and follow-up of abnormal examinations. Negative results are sent to the referring physician and to the patient. When an abnormality requiring further evaluation is detected, the physician is notified directly in addition to the written report. At our institution, patients with abnormal screening studies currently are not contacted by the radiology staff unless the referring physician requests us to do so. The regulations of the U.S. Mammography Quality Standards Act (MQSA) mandate that both normal and abnormal reports be sent to all patients.

Screening mammography reports should be short and concise and utilize standard terminology to eliminate ambiguous and meaningless terms. A normal or negative report comments on the density of the breasts, states that no mammographic features of malignancy are seen in either breast, and recommends when the patient's next screening examination should be performed. Any characteristically benign findings may (or may not) be described.

The density of the breasts is commented on because mammography is slightly less sensitive in women with dense breasts; for example, cancer may be obscured by overlying dense tissue. Overall breast density is typically reported as being fatty, mostly fatty (scattered fibroglandular densities), heterogeneously dense, or extremely dense.

An abnormal mammogram report describes the location and type of abnormality and indicates the need for any additional imaging studies to evaluate the finding. Typically abnormalities detected at screening require at least some additional imaging before a final recommendation can be made for management.

What Does a Normal Screening Mammography Report Mean?

Most women undergoing routine screening mammography have "normal" examination reports, which means that no features of malignancy were demonstrated on the current study. It is not a guarantee that the woman does not have cancer, as approximately 10% of detectable cancers are mammographically occult, and another 5–10% of cancers are undetectable and present clinically as interval cancers before the next screening examination. Each woman undergoing screening mammography should undergo a clinical breast examination (CBE). If a palpable abnormality is detected, a normal mammogram report does not negate the palpable finding nor does it indicate that the palpable finding is benign. Indeed, it places more responsibility on the clinician because the palpable finding may be mammographically occult, and thus its management should be based on the results of the physical examination. Any abnormality detected by CBE must be completely evaluated regardless of a normal or negative screening mammogram report. Furthermore, a woman with a palpable abnormality should not be sent for routine screening mammography; rather, the abnormality should be brought to the attention of the radiologist prior to imaging, and diagnostic (not screening) mammography should be performed instead.

WHAT IS THE SIGNIFICANCE OF AN ABNORMAL SCREENING MAMMOGRAM?

An abnormal screening mammogram simply indicates that an unexpected finding has been detected. Typically, additional imaging studies are required to determine if the abnormality is sufficiently suspicious for malignancy to justify tissue diagnosis. Approximately 70% of screening examinations interpreted as abnormal demonstrate findings characteristic of normal or probably benign entities on further evaluation. Only 30% of the abnormalities initially detected are suspicious for malignancy after additional evaluation, and biopsy is typically recommended for these women. Approximately 30% of these abnormalities represent cancer. Thus the abnormal screening report is not meant to be definitive but, rather, to identify patients who require additional imaging evaluation and to guide clinicians to the appropriate next step in the evaluation of a possible abnormality.

WHAT FINDINGS ARE DETECTED AT SCREENING MAMMOGRAPHY?

Screening mammography findings may be divided into three categories. First are findings that are characteristically benign according to their mammographic appearance, their demonstrated stability over time, or both. Patients with typically benign findings on their screening mammograms require no additional evaluation and are considered normal. They should undergo repeat mammography at regular intervals (usually yearly), depending on their age and breast cancer risk factors.

Second, a finding may be incompletely evaluated by the screening examination, and so the likelihood of benignity or malignancy cannot be determined. Most abnormalities detected at screening fall into this category. Typically, additional evaluations with diagnostic mammography or ultrasonography are requested to confirm that a true abnormality exists and to evaluate the finding more completely.

Third, a finding may be so characteristic of malignancy that no additional imaging evaluation is required, and biopsy is recommended on the basis of the screening images alone. This category is encountered relatively rarely because even findings suggestive of malignancy usually require further imaging evaluation to evaluate the extent of disease before biopsy is performed.

There are three major categories of abnormalities detected on screening mammograms: densities, masses, and calcifications. Each category is associated with a broad spectrum of entities, ranging from entirely benign to malignant. Other abnormalities, detected less commonly by mammography screening, reflect disruptions of normal breast structures: architectural distortion, nipple retraction, and skin thickening.

DENSITIES AND MASSES

An abnormal mammographic density is an area of increased opacity (whiteness) demonstrated on a single mammographic view. Most densities initially interpreted as abnormal on a screening mammogram represent superimposition of normal fibroglandular tissues. Superimposition and a true abnormality can usually be distinguished based on careful analysis of the two standard mammographic views, but additional images are required if the suspected area is not included on the complementary view or if there is dense fibroglandular tissue present that could obscure an underlying abnormality. This analysis is mandated to exclude the possibility that the density represents an underlying mass. A density that represents normal fibroglandular tissue demonstrates scalloped, concave-outward margins and possibly contains areas of interspersed fat. Densities that represent superimposition are normal and require no further evaluation.

A true mass is demonstrated on at least two different mammographic views; it typically has convex-outward borders and is denser (whiter) centrally than peripherally. Masses are frequently demonstrated on screening mammograms; and all solitary, dominant, and palpable masses should be further evaluated because of the possibility that they are malignant.

Not all densities are benign. Neodensities that appear on subsequent mammographic examinations usually are considered suspicious for malignancy, even if no true mass is demonstrated by additional imaging. Sometimes breast cancer, especially invasive lobular carcinoma, presents as a neodensity long before a true mass can be demonstrated. In fact, approximately 15% of neodensities are malignant, and each such new and focal mammographic finding (excepting superimposition) should undergo biopsy, even if the density looks like adjacent fibroglandular tissue. This same suspicion is not applied to the generalized, bilateral, diffuse increase in fibroglandular tissue seen in approximately 25% of women who are taking hormone replacement therapy.

In addition, not all densities can be easily characterized. Some demonstrate imaging features intermediate between those of densities and masses. These "focal asymmetric densities" are typically demonstrated on more than one mammographic view; they also have scalloped borders and may be denser peripherally than centrally. If a focal asymmetric density is new, enlarging, palpable, or associated with microcalcifications, architectural distortion, or skin and nipple changes, it is suspicious for malignancy and should undergo biopsy. Otherwise, a focal asymmetric density likely represents benign fibroglandular tissue and is so unlikely to represent cancer that, after further imaging evaluation has excluded a true mass, it should be followed with periodic mammographic surveillance to assess stability.

If a true mass is identified, it should be characterized by size, location, density, shape, and margins. In addition, temporal stability and solid versus cystic nature should be determined to allow recommendations for appropriate management. This diagnostic evaluation typically requires additional unilateral mammography and ultrasonography; at our institution it is performed after the referring physician has been contacted and consulted about the findings on the screening examination.

The size of a mass is not useful for determining a benign or malignant etiology but, rather, is a useful baseline for any future assessment. The size of a mass typically is indicated in at least two dimensions. Sometimes the mammographic size of a mass subsequently proved to be cancer is helpful when planning appropriate treatment.

Location is reported by the quadrant of the breast in which the lesion is located and by its approximate position on the clock-face. The location of a mass does not help predict its etiology, as both benign and malignant masses have the same distribution by quadrant; but the quadrant reflects the distribution of underlying fibroglandular tissue. The most frequent location of a mass is the upper outer breast (45%) followed by the retroareolar breast (25%), lower outer breast (15%), upper inner breast (10%), and lower inner breast (5%). Determining the location of a mass requires visualization on at least two views, preferably 90 degrees apart. If a mass is not seen on orthogonal (right angle) views, its location can be approximated by utilizing triangulation techniques and oblique views.

The density of a mass may be that of either fat or fibroglandular tissue. Completely fat-containing masses include lipomas, oil cysts (fat necrosis), and galactoceles. Partially fat-containing masses include hamartomas and intramammary lymph nodes. It is vital to identify fat-containing masses because they are benign and require no further evaluation. Masses composed of fibroglandular tissue can be subdivided into those that are relatively hypodense, isodense, or hyperdense compared to a similar volume of benign fibroglandular tissue. Malignant masses are often hyperdense compared to similar-size areas of fibroglandular tissue and thus may be more conspicuous. This increased density or whiteness of cancer as seen on mammograms is probably related to the relative noncompressibility of cancer compared to adjacent normal tissue, which results in a focal increase in x-ray attenuation. However, masses that are hypodense or isodense may represent malignancy, so a mass that has a density of fibroglandular tissue could represent a cancer.

Possible shapes of a mass include round, oval, lobular, and irregular. Masses that are round, oval, or lobular have a high likelihood of being benign. Masses with these shapes typically include cysts, fibroadenomas, and intramammary lymph nodes. Certain types of breast cancer occasionally present as round, oval, or lobular masses; and therefore these descriptors are not absolute indicators of benignity. An irregular mass is any mass not described by one of the other shapes; such masses are considered suspicious for malignancy.

The margin of a mass, the mammographic border between the mass and adjacent normal tissue, is useful for predicting benign versus malignant etiology. The terminology used to describe margins includes circumscribed, microlobulated, obscured, ill-defined, and spiculated. A mass with circumscribed margins has a well defined sharp border with adjacent tissue and is likely (>98%) benign. Masses with microlobulated margins demonstrate multiple 1- to 5-mm lobulations and are found to be malignant up to 50% of the time. The margins of a mass may be partially obscured if the mass is adjacent to dense fibroglandular tissue. If the margins of a mass are substantially obscured, overall mammographic assessment of the interface is not possible, and so this mass may be considered slightly suspicious for malignancy. Ill-defined and spiculated margins are inherently suspicious for malignancy and imply an infiltrative process. Figures 5.1 and 5.2

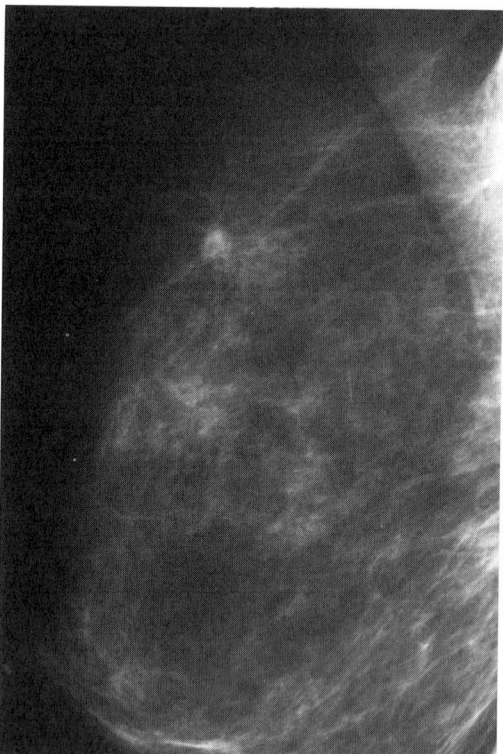

Figure 5.2. "Early" (small) invasive ductal carcinoma, MLO view, left breast (same lesion as in Figure 5.1). This spot compression magnification mammogram of the mass better illustrates the margins of this mass, which are clearly spiculated. Spot compression magnification mammograms provide improved resolution compared to standard mammographic images and are helpful for evaluating the margins of a mass and determining if there are associated microcalcifications that may not have been visible on the standard images.

Figure 5.1. "Early" (small) invasive ductal carcinoma, mediolateral oblique (MLO) view, left breast. This film demonstrates a typical clinically occult breast cancer detected on a screening mammogram. There is an irregular mass in the left upper breast that appears to have ill-defined, possibly spiculated, margins.

depict a typical speculated infiltrating ductal carcinoma. Spiculated margins are classic (although not pathognomonic) for cancer but are not commonly demonstrated among women undergoing regular screening, probably because routine screening allows detection of most malignant masses before they have developed spiculations.

The margins of a mass can be difficult to evaluate on screening mammograms unless the mass is completely or almost entirely surrounded by fat. Therefore spot-compression magnification mammography is performed on most masses to demonstrate the margins accurately. These high-resolution magnified images may also reveal any subtle microcalcifications associated with the mass.

Once a mass is identified, and additional imaging is performed to completely evaluate its shape and margins, the mass is assigned to one of three risk categories, each having different management. *Benign* masses have no risk of malignancy and require no further evaluation. Masses that can be confidently called benign are those that are fat-containing, have characteristic calcifications of a degenerating fibroadenoma, are proved to be simple cysts (see Ultrasonography, below), or demonstrate long-term (>2 years) mammographic stability if they otherwise would be categorized as "probably benign."

Probably benign masses carry such a low likelihood of malignancy (<2%) that they may safely be followed with periodic mammographic surveillance. A mass must fulfill strict imaging criteria before being classified as probably benign. This category is reserved for masses detected on initial mammograms (or previous films not available); they are round, oval, or lobular and have >75% circumscribed margins and no indistinct or spiculated margins. In addition, a probably benign mass must be nonpalpable and not associated with any secondary signs of malignancy (skin thickening or retraction, nipple retraction, suspicious microcalcifications, and architectural distortion). A spot-compression magnification view of a typical probably benign mass is illustrated in Figure 5.3. A new mass (not seen on prior mammograms) should not be classified as probably benign. A probably benign mass can be followed initially with a 6-month repeat unilateral mammogram and then, if stable, with bilateral mammography in 6 months followed by repeat mammography annually for a total follow-up of 2–3 years. Any change in a probably benign mass, except a decrease in size, should prompt biopsy.

Suspicious masses are biopsied to assess for malignancy. Features of suspicious masses include irregular shape, ill-defined or spiculated margins, skin or nipple retraction, associated architectural distortion, and certain types of calcification. Any enlarging mass that is not a simple cyst is suspicious for malignancy. It is important to identify patients who have had a prior biopsy, as postoperative scarring may mimic the mammographic features of malignancy. Obviously, one must correlate the location of the mammographic finding to the site of prior surgery to make sure they correspond. Approximately 30–50% of masses undergoing biopsy are malignant. Benign findings (masses and pseudomasses) frequently biopsied include fibroadenomas, complex cysts, papillomas, or entities such as fibrosis and sclerosing adenosis, which may simulate a mass.

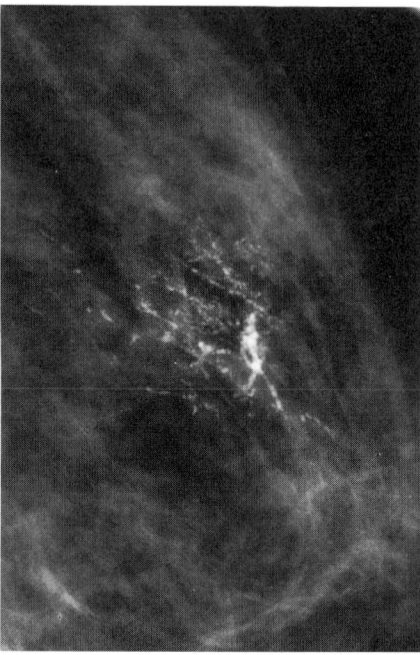

Figure 5.3. Probably benign mass. This spot compression magnification view demonstrates a lobular mass with mostly (>75%) circumscribed margins, except where obscured by adjacent fibroglandular tissue. A single coarse, benign-appearing calcification is associated with this mass, suggesting its solid nature. This mass was not palpable on clinical breast examination, and the patient had no prior mammograms. The imaging features of this mass predict a low probability of malignancy (<2%); therefore appropriate management would be short-term follow-up mammography in 6 months to assess stability. If the mass is unchanged at that time an additional 6-month follow-up mammography examination followed by yearly mammograms should be undertaken to establish the long-term stability of the mass. Any change in the mass should prompt biopsy to exclude malignancy.

Calcifications

Calcifications within the breasts are frequently seen on screening mammograms and may be indicators of benign or malignant processes. The mammographic demonstration of calcifications may be the earliest detectable indicator of a malignancy. Analysis of the size, shape, and distribution of breast calcifications can usually distinguish benign from malignant etiologies. Fortunately, most calcifications seen on screening mammograms are clearly benign and require no additional evaluation. In addition, malignant calcifications may also demonstrate characteristic features that, when present, are also easily identified and distinguished from their benign counterparts.

Because breast calcifications are the smallest structures identified on mammograms, fine-detail evaluation is often not possible on the screening examination and may require additional imaging utilizing high-resolution spot-compression magnification to define the calcific particles better. Frequently, these additional images demonstrate characteristic features of either benign or malignant calcifications not readily appreciated on standard screening images. Moreover, these high-resolution images can also be used to identify a subset of calcifications that, although not characteristically benign, are so unlikely to be malignant that they may safely be followed with periodic mammographic surveillance ("probably benign" calcifications). Calcifications that remain indeterminate after this additional workup are considered slightly suspicious for malignancy; and unless comparison studies demonstrate long-term stability, biopsy is recommended.

Vascular calcifications occur within the arterial walls and are typically seen as two parallel tracks of calcific particles. Early in this process when so little calcification is present that only one wall is calcified, the appearance may be ambiguous on standard images. In these cases spot-compression magnification mammography is usually sufficient to demonstrate the truly vascular nature of the suspect calcifications.

Skin calcifications occur in sebaceous glands and are typically polygonal in shape, lucent-centered, and frequently tightly clustered with other similar-appearing particles. These calcifications are typically located overlying the inferior and medial breast but also are found around the areola and the axilla. Skin calcifications may be demonstrated fortuitously to be within the skin on routine screening views but often require special tangential views to confirm their intradermal location. Some skin calcifications do not demonstrate the classic mammographic features, so any small cluster of calcifications seen near a skin surface should be evaluated with tangential views to exclude the possibility that they are skin calcifications and therefore benign.

Secretory calcifications result from a benign inflammatory process involving the ducts and periductal tissues. They represent calcifications of inspissated secretions in or adjacent to dilated benign ducts. The calcifications associated with this process are commonly rod-shaped, often with central lucency, and in a ductal or segmental distribution; they are usually bilateral in distribution. These calcifications are ordinarily so much larger than malignant calcifications, which are also ductal in location, that the two are rarely confused. Furthermore, benign secretory calcifications typically are oriented with their long axes pointing toward the nipple, whereas malignant calcifications demonstrate no such polarity.

Dystrophic calcifications result from prior trauma or surgery to the breast. These calcifications are usually large and coarse, and they may vary in size and shape. They may have central lucency. Typically, they are amorphous in shape and may be oriented in strands or sheets along the plane of injury or surgery. A particular type of dystrophic calcification forms within the wall of an oil cyst, resulting from fat necrosis, and appears as thin peripheral ("eggshell") calcifications outlining a fat-containing mass. Over time, the walls of the oil cyst may become completely calcified, and the appearance resembles that of a pearl.

Degenerating fibroadenomas may develop characteristic calcifications. Early calcification in a fibroadenoma is ordinarily at the periphery of the mass and is coarse and chunky. As this process progresses the calcifications become larger and occupy more of the mass until they display a characteristic "popcorn" appearance. Finally, the fibroadenoma may become completely calcified. Rarely, an atypical or early calcification within a fibroadenoma causes a diagnostic dilemma and is mistaken for malignancy, prompting biopsy.

Milk of calcium in tiny benign cysts is associated with benign proliferative processes in the breast. These calcifications typically occur in a scattered distribution involving both breasts. When they are unilateral and clustered, they may resemble malignant calcifications. Because milk of calcium sediments to the dependent portion of the cyst in which it is located, fluid-calcium levels are seen on lateral and oblique images as linear or curvilinear calcifications. Craniocaudal images, obtained at a right angle to the fluid-calcium levels, depict the calcifications as fuzzy, poorly defined smudges. This characteristic change in appearance on different mammographic views is typical of milk of calcium and is not seen with malignant calcifications. Spot-compression magnification mammograms in 90-degree lateral and craniocaudal projections may be required to establish the benign diagnosis of milk of calcium.

If calcifications are detected on screening mammograms and demonstrate the features of one of these benign types of calcifications or if the calcifications are not strikingly abnormal and demonstrate long-term stability, no further evaluation is required and the patient's calcifications are presumed to be benign. If the calcifications cannot be assigned to one of the characteristically benign categories, however, additional evaluation is required. This evaluation typically consists of spot-compression magnification mammograms in 90-degree lateral and craniocaudal projections. These mammograms provide magnified images with superior resolution and diminished noise compared to standard images and so better portray the number, distribution, and shapes of the calcific particles. Frequently these additional images reveal that the calcifications are indeed one of the benign types, thus requiring no additional evaluation.

Calcifications that fail to demonstrate features characteristic of benignity must be evaluated to determine the likelihood of malignancy and their exact location within the breast. Mammographic features suggestive of malignancy include small size (<5mm), pleomorphic shapes, and clustered distribution with linear or branching particles. Typical malignant microcalcifications are illustrated in Figures 5.4 and 5.5. These characteristically malignant calcifications usually represent calcification of necrotic debris within the lumens of neoplastic ducts, that is, ductal carcinoma in situ (DCIS). A mammographically significant cluster is usually considered to be at least 5–10 calcific particles within a volume of $1\,cm^3$. A cluster of calcifications that demonstrates these features must be regarded as suspicious for malignancy, and a biopsy should be performed. Biopsy requires determining the exact location and distribution of the suspicious cluster prior to biopsy and is usually accomplished by spot-compression magnification mammography to define the distribution and by orthogonal mammograms to determine the location.

Calcifications that are neither characteristically benign nor malignant, despite optimal visualization with spot-compression magnification mammography are indeterminate, and carry a 20–30% chance of malignancy. Sometimes it is possible to identify a subset within this category consisting of clustered calcifications that

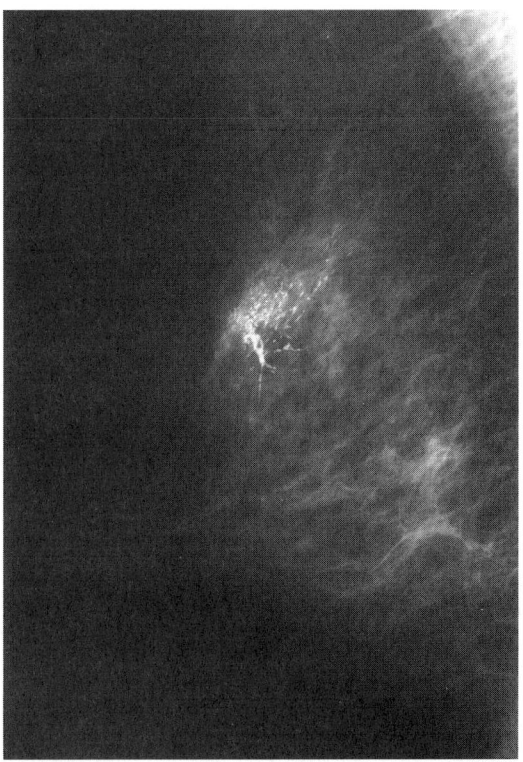

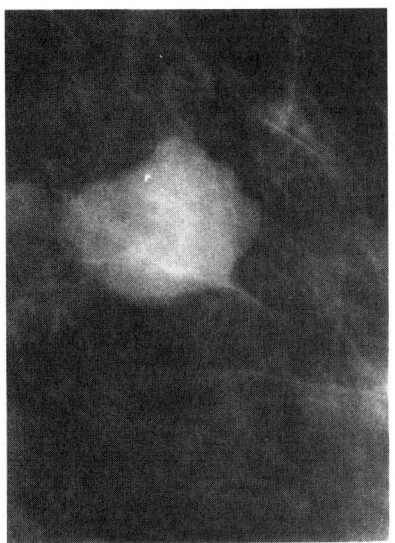

Figure 5.4. Malignant microcalcifications, MLO view, left breast. This film demonstrates a large cluster of pleomorphic microcalcifications distributed within linear branching arrays, suggesting their intraductal location.

Figure 5.5. Malignant microcalcifications, MLO view, left breast (same lesion as Figure 5.3). This spot compression magnification mammogram better depicts the morphology, number, and distribution of these malignant calcifications. This appearance is classic for high-grade intraductal carcinoma (DCIS) and represents calcified necrotic tumor debris within the ducts.

are all similar in size and all round or oval. Studies have demonstrated that this subset of calcifications is "probably benign" and carries a less than 1% chance of malignancy. Many radiologists recommend periodic mammographic surveillance for these calcifications, with short-term interval follow-up mammograms instead of biopsy. If the calcifications remain stable, they can continue to be followed, but change prompts biopsy. This approach reduces the number of benign biopsies but requires careful follow-up. For the remainder of indeterminate calcifications (i.e., those that are amorphous in shape or so tiny the shapes cannot be discerned), malignancy remains a significant possibility and therefore biopsy is indicated.

Architectural Distortion

Architectural distortion is a mammographic finding that refers to an area within the breast where the normal structural architecture is disrupted with no definite mass visible. It may appear as fine linear spiculations that radiate from a point or involve focal retraction or distortion of the interface between fibroglandular tissue and subcutaneous or retromammary fat. There are many causes of architectural distortion, including cancer, postsurgical scarring, trauma with fat necrosis, and radial scar. Unless one can correlate the location of the suspect mammographic findings to a site of prior surgery or trauma, an area of architectural distortion is suspicious for malignancy and should prompt tissue diagnosis. In addition, any area of increasing architectural distortion, despite a history of surgery or trauma at that site, should be viewed as a suspicious finding. Biopsy of areas of architectural distortion reveal an underlying malignancy approximately 15% of the time.

ULTRASONOGRAPHY

Ultrasonography is currently employed exclusively as a diagnostic tool used to evaluate a palpable or mammographic abnormality. It is never used to screen breasts in asymptomatic women because of its low sensitivity. Currently its principal role is to determine the solid or cystic nature of a previously identified mass. Ultrasonography is also utilized to guide percutaneous interventions such as aspiration, fine-needle or core biopsy, and sometimes preoperative needle localization of nonpalpable lesions. It is not used to evaluate or biopsy microcalcifications, as their small size usually precludes sonographic depiction. Although there is some evidence that ultrasonography is capable of differentiating benign from malignant solid masses, this capability has not been convincingly demonstrated and the technique therefore is not employed in most breast imaging centers.

RULE OF MULTIPLICITY

The rule of multiplicity states that any process that is bilateral and diffuse is almost certainly benign. Bilateral multicentric (occurring in two quadrants) cancer is highly unlikely. Thus when mammography demonstrates multiple bilateral masses or bilateral scattered calcifications, it is likely that these findings reflect benign processes. Diagnostic evaluation of each component finding usually is not warranted. However, it is important to distinguish any mass or group of calcifications that appears different from the others and to evaluate them with additional imaging to determine if they are suspicious for malignancy and therefore warrant biopsy.

INTERVENTION PROCEDURES

Several types of intervention breast procedures are performed by the radiologist. Ultrasound or mammographic guidance is utilized to localize nonpalpable abnormalities prior to surgery or to provide a minimally invasive method for obtaining a tissue diagnosis (tissue core-needle biopsy or fine-needle aspiration) instead of an open surgical procedure.

Preoperative mammographically guided needle localization is performed immediately prior to surgery to localize a nonpalpable mammographic abnormality for the surgeon, allowing removal of the targeted lesion. There are several ways to perform needle localization, but all involve placing a needle in the breast and positioning its tip in close proximity to the targeted abnormality. A metallic wire usually is then deployed through the needle and its final position documented with subsequent mammograms. The wire is designed to anchor in place and to resist removal until surgery. This procedure is well tolerated by patients, is safe, and almost always results in surgical sampling of the targeted nonpalpable mammographic abnormality.

Tissue core-needle biopsy of a mammographically or sonographically visible lesion provides a minimally invasive, relatively inexpensive, yet accurate method of obtaining a tissue diagnosis. This technique involves placing a core biopsy needle into the lesion utilizing either ultrasound or mammographic guidance. The needle usually is 14 gauge and requires a small 3- to 5-mm skin incision. Multiple core biopsies, which are small cylinders of tissue, are obtained from the targeted lesion and then sent to pathology for review. This technique can be used to sample both masses and calcifications. Core biopsy specimens allow the pathologist to evaluate both the architecture of the lesion (histology) and its cytologic features and are thus generally considered superior to fine-needle aspiration techniques, which reveal only cytology.

Fine-needle aspiration (FNA) may be performed by the radiologist to obtain a cellular sample from a mammographic, or more typically, a sonographic mass that is nonpalpable. FNA is quick and inexpensive but requires an experienced cytopathologist to obtain accurate results. A small (usually 25 gauge) needle is guided into the mass and then rapidly advanced and withdrawn with 1- to 5-mm strokes, causing some cells from the mass to be drawn into the needle by surface tension. Suction may or may not be applied to the needle. The aspirated cells are then fixed onto glass slides and sent to pathology for review. This technique provides only cytologic information and therefore can determine the benign or malignant nature of the sampled mass but not the nature of associated architectural changes.

CONCLUSIONS

Screening mammography is performed on asymptomatic women to detect clinically occult cancer. Once an abnormality is detected, appropriate diagnostic evaluation should be undertaken to determine if the abnormality is suspicious for malignancy and requires biopsy. This diagnostic evaluation may consist of CBE, diagnostic mammography, ultrasonography, or a combination of these techniques, depending on the abnormality being investigated. Most abnormalities referred for diagnostic evaluation are either benign or are so unlikely to be cancer that they can be safely followed clinically and mammographically. If an abnormality is indeterminate or suspicious for malignancy, tissue diagnosis is indicated to assess for malignancy. Tissue diagnosis can be accomplished by FNA, tissue core-needle biopsy, or surgical excision depending on the type, size, and location of the abnormality.

Recommended Reading

Sickles EA. Breast calcifications: mammographic evaluation. Radiology 1986;160:289–293

Sickles EA. Periodic mammographic follow-up of probably benign lesions: results in 3184 consecutive cases. Radiology 1991;179:462–468

Sickles EA, Kopans DB. Mammographic screening for women aged 40 to 49 years: the primary care practitioner's dilemma. Ann Intern Med 1995;122:534–538

6 MAMMOGRAPHY IN A BREAST CENTER

John G. Pearce

When referring patients for mammography, it is essential to understand what the patient may go through for a successful study to be achieved. Modern film-screen mammographic techniques require significant compression of the breast to spread out internal breast structures and allow the best visualization of all the anatomy. These techniques are one of the major reasons that modern mammography is so efficient in detecting early disease. We are all aware that breast tissue extends into the axillary region, and it is important to ensure that this area is correctly imaged and included on the mammogram.

The pectoral muscle, on which the breasts lie, is the landmark for positioning patients for optimal mammograms. Because of body differences and quirks of anatomy or structure, routine techniques must be modified from time to time. For example, a patient's torso may be too long to fit on the film and allow even compression across the entire breast. Tall patients with long trunks may require the mediolateral oblique view of the breast to be split into an upper component (deep axilla including axillary tail of the breast) and a lower component (mound of breast and inferior mammogram fold). Split filming allows proper compression of all breast anatomic components and enhances the analysis.

The most active component of breast anatomy is the glandular tissue, which often extends into the axillary tail and is the most frequent site for problems. The glandular "envelope" is surrounded by fat and held in place by fibrous tissues. This fibrous latticework, known as Cooper's ligaments (Fig. 6.1), extends peripherally and anchors to the overlying skin.

The basic unit of breast anatomy is the lobule (Fig. 6.1) of which there are some 18 or so, each with its own opening at the nipple. The subunit of anatomy that is the most important is the terminal ductal lobular unit (TDLU) (Fig. 6.2), where most breast pathology is found. Our understanding of the mechanism of disease and the pathophysiology of malignancy is discussed elsewhere in this book (Chapter 3). There is no doubt that the "action" of most clinical breast problems evolves around the TDLU. Within the TDLU occur benign and malignant calcifications, invasive and in situ malignancies, cysts, and other benign conditions. It is thus an important part of the breast anatomy. If the TDLUs are

John G. Pearce

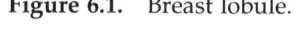

Figure 6.1. Breast lobule.

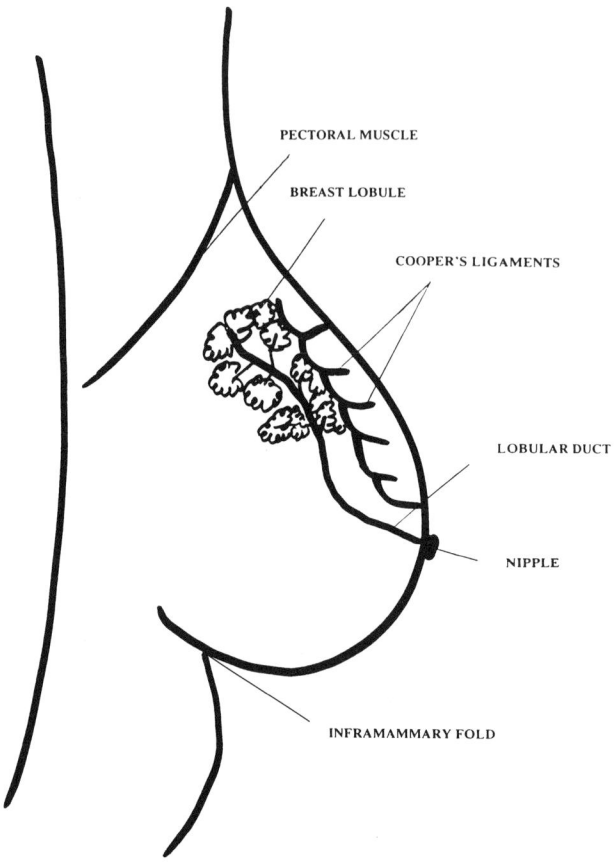

PECTORAL MUSCLE

BREAST LOBULE

COOPER'S LIGAMENTS

LOBULAR DUCT

NIPPLE

INFRAMAMMARY FOLD

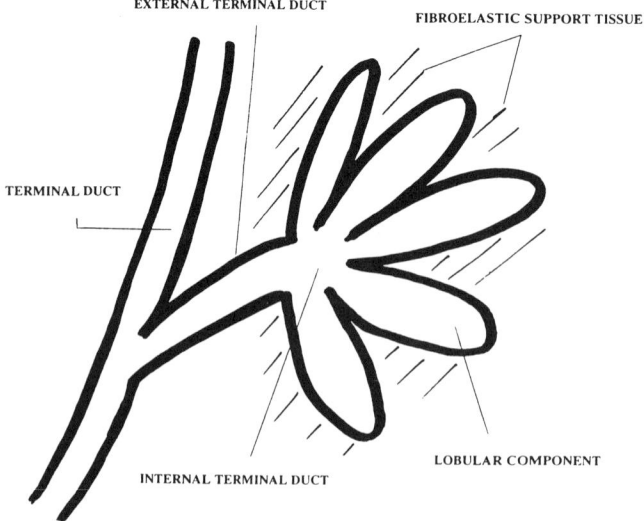

EXTERNAL TERMINAL DUCT

FIBROELASTIC SUPPORT TISSUE

TERMINAL DUCT

INTERNAL TERMINAL DUCT

LOBULAR COMPONENT

Figure 6.2. Terminal ductal lobular unit (TDLU).

all situated in active glandular breast tissue, it makes sense that the goal of basic mammography is to include all such tissue on the film; therefore when such glandular tissue cannot be completely incorporated on the two traditional views, additional views are obtained. Sometimes more views are needed to clarify an area of potential concern. They are usually obtained as part of a diagnostic mammogram (Table 6.1).

Compression of the breast may be uncomfortable, but it should not be painful. Pain is often related to the positioning techniques. It should be remembered that patients in the progesterone phase of their menstrual cycle (1 week before their period) often have significant fluid production within their TDLUs and are somewhat congested. This is not a good time to undergo mammography, particularly when added views with tight focal (small cone) compression are needed. By being aware of this physiology one can often avoid the most sensitive times and thus encourage a positive experience.

Table 6.1. Labeling codes for positioning

Condition	Labeling code	Purpose
Laterality		
Right	R[a]	
Left	L[a]	
Projection/position		
Mediolateral oblique	MLO	Standard view
Craniocaudal	CC	Standard view
90° Lateral		
Mediolateral	ML	Localize, define
Lateromedial	LM	Localize, define
Spot compression		Define
Magnification	M[a]	Define
Exaggerated craniocaudal	XCCL	Localize
Cleavage	CV	Localize
Axillary tail	AT	Localize, define
Tangential	TAN	Localize, define
Rolled		
(Lateral)[b]	RL	Localize, define
(Medial)[b]	RM	Localize, define
Caudocranial	FB (from below)	Define
Lateromedial oblique	LMO	Define
Superolateral to inferomedial oblique	SIO	Define
Implant displaced	ID	Augmented breast

[a] Used as a prefix before the projection. For example, RMMLO = right magnification mediolateral oblique.
[b] Used as a suffix after the projection. For example, LCCRL = left craniocaudal upper breast tissue rolled laterally.

KEY PRACTICE POINTS

Mammography: A "negative" mammogram does *not* rule out cancer.

Abnormal mammogram: A palpable breast mass *must* be definitively diagnosed.

SCREENING MAMMOGRAPHY

In 1996 controversy arose over conflicting evidence promoted by various advisory groups concerning screening guidelines for mammography.[1,2] Reaction from the body of informed mammographers and breast health care physicians has led to much more in-depth analysis of all screening trials. Mammographers were experiencing a significant cancer yield among patients ages 40–49 and were concerned when some advisory groups began discouraging annual mammography in that age bracket. Now that more meta-analyses (statistical analysis of many trials) have been performed and longer-term results from the ongoing Swedish trials are available, it has become clear that a significant impact on women's breast health is achieved by performing frequent screening and annual mammograms in women 40–70 years of age. These large trials now have objective data clarifying approximately 25% increased survival among the patient groups who have had annual screening mammograms since age 40.[2]

At the University of Southern California (USC) we strongly encourage regular mammography for all of our patient groups and do not modify this recommendation on the basis of ethnic influence. Our recommendations continue to be as follows.

Age < 35:   Only for a specific problem (all patients under age 30 are reviewed by a radiologist before continuing to mammography)
Age 35–40:   baseline mammogram
Age 40–70:   annual mammograms
Age 70+:   continue annually if there is dense parenchyma, if much active glandular tissue remains, or if there are risk factors in history; otherwise every 1–2 years

All age brackets are moved 5 years earlier (e.g., from 40 to 35) if there is a family history of breast malignancy. All patients are encouraged to have interval examinations and imaging if a specific new problem arises that is appropriate for the imaging workup.

There is no question that early diagnosis is the key to a better outcome. The changes seen in life expectancy rates and quality of life after breast malignancy have been significantly affected by the use of regular high quality mammography and its ability to find early disease often before it is suspected or remotely palpable on physical examination. Once a diagnosis of cancer is suspected patients benefit from information in printed material covering options for diagnosis and treament such as the pamphlet developed by The California Department of Health Services.[3]

It is essential that primary care physicians understand their role in breast health care. Aligning a medical practice with quality mammography services is essential. Medicolegal activity is busy in this area of medicine, and primary care providers are regularly involved. Thus communication with a radiologist and a foolproof follow-up system to detect abnormal reports and recommendations is essential. The effective teams are those that support and complement each other's roles and interactions with the patients. Radiologists at USC often proceed with added views and other forms of imaging and procedures when needed to expedite an answer for the patient. Ensuring adequate follow-up is the role of primary care physicians and consultants, including radiologists.

For screening we begin with two views per side: the mediolateral oblique (MLO) and the craniocaudal (CC). If these views do not cover all active glandular tissue, we add views as needed (e.g., an exaggerated craniocaudal lateral, or XCCL, view, which accentuates visualization of the axillary tail and lateral glandular tissues in a modified CC projection).

DIAGNOSTIC MAMMOGRAPHY

Diagnostic mammography requires additional views and the use of any other imaging modalities required to achieve a reasonable interpretation (Table 6.1). For analysis of mammographic findings, one often needs to clarify certain features. For example, definition of the borders of masses or better definition of the shapes and calcifications or their distribution may be essential to the correct interpretation.

When well defined by additional views, many mammographically benign masses (Table 6.2) can be interpreted and correlated with the definitive diagnosis with reliability and confidence. Other mammographic lesions such as benign spiculated masses can mimic the mammographic characteristics of cancer (Table 6.3) and require histologic confirmation for definitive diagnosis.

Table 6.2. Mammographically benign breast masses

Calcified cyst
Calcified fibroadenoma
Cyst confirmed by ultrasonography
Foreign body
Galactocele
Intramammary lymph node
Lipoma
Microcyst with milk of calcium
Oil cyst

Table 6.3. Spiculated mass lesions that can mimic
cancer on mammography

Biopsy scar
Fat necrosis
Granular cell myoblastoma
Papillomatosis
Pseudotumor
Radial scar
Sclerosing adenosis

Deciding on the need for added views is the province of the radiologist, and he or she should be given a free hand to complete the examination as necessary. The primary care physician should be secure in the knowledge that the patient is completely imaged so an appropriate diagnosis can be reached. With both screening and diagnostic mammography, any recommendations for recall and added views or supplemental imaging made by the radiologist should be followed by the primary care physician. Lack of follow-up can lead to delay in diagnosis, a common source of medicolegal action.

The American College of Radiology has developed a mammographic interpretation coding system (BI-RADS) in an effort to standardize terminology.[4] Under this system, when a mammogram and augmented imaging suggest the need for tissue confirmation, the BI-RADS codes 4 (suspicious) and 5 (highly suspicious) are used. These and other codes will soon appear on reports, as they are being incorporated into the new final regulations of the Mammography Quality Standards Act (MQSA). These regulations include an on-going practice audit which formalizes the recommendations of prior mammography quality assurance protocols such as suggested by Sickles.[5]

FOLLOW-UP MAMMOGRAMS

Screening

Patients under age 30 with generalized breast pain have almost zero yield on mammography. Specific focal signs and symptoms in this age group should be evaluated with ultrasonography first and limited mammography (MLO view only) if ultrasonography yields pathology. Because of the active hormonal status of such patients, their breast tissues are usually dense, and routine screening mammography is of little use. One should not be lulled into a false sense of security. Malignancies, though rare, do occur in young patients. This author has seen wild, poorly differentiated invasive breast malignancy in a 12-year-old and in several patients between 16 and 25 years of age. Careful clinical evaluation remains essential.

Diagnosis

Diagnostic mammography is clearly left to the expertise of the radiologist. Referring physicians must recognize that this province belongs to the radiologist and let the expert utilize a high-yield, efficacious use of the imaging armamentarium to arrive at the diagnosis.

The use of added views, magnification views, ultrasonography, nuclear medicine, magnetic resonance imaging (MRI), and positron emission tomography (PET) scanning are useful tools in the diagnostic workup of breast problems. One should be clear that no one modality replaces the value of quality mammography. Advances in high-resolution ultrasonography have expanded the role of this technique in the diagnostic process, although ultrasound scans do not surpass quality film-screen mammograms.[6]

Interventional imaging breast studies have proved to be cost-effective. It is the radiologist's job to map the extent of disease and to assume a major role in preliminary tissue diagnosis by use of ultrasound-guided or stereotactic tissue core-needle biopsy (TCNB). Whenever possible, the use of TCNB assists in the correct planning and discussion of all options (as required, for example, by the California Standards of Care Act) with the patient. Conservative management and changing guidelines for the treatment of ductal carcinoma in situ (DCIS) require accurate knowledge of all areas of both breasts before any planned surgery. At USC, following a clinical fine-needle aspiration (FNA) procedure with immediate mammography has not been a significant concern: mammographic analysis has not been hindered.

ABNORMAL MAMMOGRAMS

With Physical Findings

An area of concern located by clinical examination must be imaged completely with full diagnostic mammography and augmented imaging (e.g., ultrasound scans) as needed. A complete study is essential and one *must not* short-circuit the full workup of both breasts. Patient management decisions often depend on this complete study. For example, mammography may reveal an unexpected second lesion that, if malignant, usually mandates mastectomy rather than conservative lumpectomy.

It is essential that specific areas of clinical concern, found either by the referring physician or the patient herself, be communicated to the radiologist. Indicating the site with an overlying radiographic marker (e.g., a beebee) at the time of mammography signals the radiologist that it is an area requiring careful analysis.

The standard of care requires that any area of clinical concern be examined by mammography and, if negative, by ultrasonography. These two examinations together ensure thorough imaging of the area of concern.

Without Physical Findings

Routine follow-up should include quality two-view mammography of each breast. Routine ultrasonography is not appropriate in this situation.

An accurate breast-oriented patient history is extremely helpful to the radiologist, especially in high-risk situations. The history should include the patient's hormone status and information about her current use of exogenous hormones.

Having prior films available at the time of the reading is helpful. Studies verify about a 7% increased yield of findings—not necessarily bad—when there is direct comparison with old films at the time of reading. Every attempt should be made to have old films available, even if at a later date. A comparative addendum could then be issued. However, a policy of never reading without old films can lead to mistakes because unread films may be filed accidentally, resulting in adverse delays in diagnosis; several court cases have reflected this scenario. The cost of producing an addendum report may be an issue, but delay in diagnosis can be much more costly. Everyone involved with women's breast health should encourage that old films be available to the radiologist at the time of follow-up or annual mammography.

ROLE OF ULTRASONOGRAPHY

We have moved beyond "cyst versus solid" as the only use for ultrasound scans of the breast. The role of ultrasonography as a significant adjunctive breast imaging modality is changing[6,7] as newer high-resolution equipment becomes more readily available. High resolution with variable focus and variable aperture transducers is allowing visualization of great detail from the skin to the chest wall. It is now sometimes possible to visualize with ultrasound scans such anatomic structures as TDLUs. This increased detail, even with large breasts, has made intervention and ultrasound-guided core biopsies much easier and quicker. Ultrasonography is now the leading modality, followed by stereotactic devices, utilized for TCNBs.

Ultrasound criteria for malignancy are controversial. They are sensitive, and, although often not as specific as one would prefer,[6-8] they are useful. It is the standard of care to evaluate a palpable area of clinical concern with ultrasonography when a mammogram shows no specific abnormality in the area. In clinical practice an ultrasound evaluation is done first in patients under 30 years of age, often revealing cystic structures and answering the clinical question. If ultrasound reveals a discrete solid mass in a patient under age 30, the mass is further characterized by mammography.

Ultrasonography is helpful in young patients whose dense breast parenchyma makes mammography not particularly sensitive.[1] The intrinsic subject contrast between the mass and the dense fibroglandular tissues within the breast itself often does not allow detailed characterization of a lesion.

In older patients, where varying levels of mammographic density may occur from natural or medically induced hormonal variations and from age and menopause, mammography is an excellent tool for characterizing breast problems.[9] In this group, high-resolution ultrasonography is a valuable adjunct, especially when all modalities have congruent findings.

When mammography fails to correlate with an area of clinical concern, it is considered the standard of imaging care to evaluate the same area with ultrasonography. High-resolution ultrasonography may reveal a focal area that corresponds to the clinical area, and the altered echogenicity may prompt tissue sampling by FNA or TCNB. These mammographically vague areas may conceal a malignancy, frequently lobular carcinoma, and they should be evaluated by ultrasound scans.

Thus high-resolution ultrasonography has taken on a completely new role in the imaging of breast lesions. Ultrasound-guided breast biopsies (especially TCNB) are accurate and of great clinical utility.[10,11] They are a relatively inexpensive way of securing accurate tissue confirmation of an imaged area of concern. They are less expensive than open biopsy, but even so should be used judiciously to avoid negating their overall cost savings.[12,13] The techniques are described in the literature,[10,11,14] and it is essential that facilities develop consistency with respect to indications, techniques, and pathologic specimen handling. Well performed FNA, coupled with expert cytopathologic interpretation, is invaluable.[14] TCNB affords more tissue for easier processing and evaluation of prognostic markers on the tissue samples. The key to the utility of both procedures lies in the consistency and accuracy of the way samples are collected and processed.

CONSULTATIONS AND REFERRALS

The most effective breast health care is practiced by a team of professionals, including the primary care physician, surgeon, radiologist, pathologist, and treatment team members. They complement each other. An effective breast clinic utilizes all available expertise.

Consultation and referrals for mammography require that the radiologist be given not only information on the physical findings but a complete breast-oriented history, including risk factors. Nevertheless, many mammographic and ultrasonographic observations come down to a judgment call. Experience is essential and should never be underutilized.

The availability and rereading of prior films assist in evaluating a breast health situation. The full use of the diagnostic imaging armamentarium is essential to complete the diagnostic evaluation and should be carefully overseen by the radiologist, who is the clinician with the most experience in this area.

It is a major mistake to request or give "curbside" consultations without proper viewing conditions and complete clinical information. Many lawsuits evolve from such practice. Primary care and referring clinicians should avoid doing so and insist on a formal written review of any "outside films" that may be submitted. Too often the quality of such studies is suboptimal. This situation occurs less often these days since the introduction and enforcement of the MQSA of 1992 and involvement of the U.S. Food and Drug Administration, but it still can be a factor. Incorrectly identified or poor-quality films should not be interpreted; they should be repeated. Physicians should remember that if you pass judgment on a poor-quality or incomplete study, you are held accountable and to the same standard as if it were a quality study. As this area is one of considerable medicolegal activity, it is unwise to plan clinical management based on technically inadequate studies.

MENSTRUAL AND HORMONE THERAPY EFFECTS: MAMMOGRAPHIC CHANGES IN DENSITY

Mammographic densities reflect the presence of various tissues, the most common of which is active glandular tissue. Breast glandular activity involves the production and reabsorption of fluid in the active glandular component of the TDLU. When reabsorption does not keep up with production, cysts may form. The fluid produced within the breast glandular tissues increases radiographic densities. The cyclic fluid production activity is influenced by hormones. The progesterone phase of the cycle (approximately 1 week before the menstrual period) is a highly active time when breast tissues are more involved in fluid production. There is increased mammographic density, and glandular tissue is congested, making breast compression more uncomfortable. Hence one should schedule mammography, and especially added views, for the first 2 weeks of the menstrual cycle.

Hormone manipulation via the use of exogenous hormones can significantly alter mammographic studies. At different points in any patient's menstrual cycle, a mammogram can show significant differences in the densities of the glandular tissues. Increased density may make visualization of subtle mammographic features more difficult. Technique correction may be required.

Methods of attempting to quantify changes in mammographic densities have long been of interest to mammographers.[15,16] Efforts to correlate mammographic density with variable risk factors are controversial.[9,16] Theoretically, hormone manipulation of mammographic density could alter patient risk.[17,18] This area is being revisited by several investigators.[15,17–19]

References

1. Feig SA. Strategies for improving sensitivity of screening mammography for women aged 40–49 years [editorial]. JAMA 1996;276:73–74

2. Editorial. Mammography screening for ages 40–49. Cancer Lett 1997;23

3. California Department of Health Services. Women's Guide to Breast Cancer Diagnosis and Treatment. Breast Cancer Early Detection Program, State of California Early Detection Program, State of California, Medical Board of California, Sacramento, CA, 1995

4. American College of Radiology. Breast Imaging Reporting and Data System (BI-RADS™). (2nd ed). Reston, VA, American College of Radiology, 1995

5. Sickles EA. Quality assurance: how to audit your own mammography practice. Radiol Clin North Am 1992;30:265–275

6. Rubin E. Ultrasound of the breast: basic concepts. Contemp Diagn Radiol 1994;17:1–6

7. Fornage BD. Ultrasound of the Breast. Ultrasound Q 1993;11:1–39

8. Stavros AJ, Thickman D, Rapp C, et al. Solid breast nodules: use of sonography to distinguish between benign and malignant lesions. Radiology 1995;196:123–134

9. Feig SA. Hormonal reduction of mammographic densities: potential effects on breast cancer risk and performance of diagnostic and screening mammography. J Nat Cancer Inst 1994;86:408–409

10. Bremer RJ, Fajardo L, Fisher PR, et al. Percutaneous core biopsy of the breast: effect of operator experience and number of samples on diagnostic accuracy. AJR 1996;166:341–346

11. Parker SH, Burbank F, Jackman RJ, et al. Percutaneous large core breast biopsy: a multi-institutional study. Radiology 1994;193:339–364

12. Gisvold JJ, Goeliner JR, Grant CS, et al. Breast biopsy: a comparative study of stereotaxically guided core and excisional techniques. AJR 1994;162:815–820

13. Liberman L, Fahs MD, Dershaw DD, et al. Impact of stereotaxic core breast biopsy on cost of diagnosis. Radiology 1995;195:633–637

14. Jackson VP, Bassett LW. Stereotatic FNA biopsy for nonpalpable breast lesions. AJR 1990;154:1196–1197

15. Ursin G, Astrahan MA, Salane M, et al. The detection of changes in mammographic densities. Submitted for publication

16. Wolfe JN. Breast patterns as an index of risk for developing breast cancer. AJR 1976;126:1130–1139

17. Pike MC, Spicer DV, Dahmoush L, et al. Estrogens, progestogens, normal breast cell proliferation and breast cancer risk. Epidemiol Rev 1993;15:17–35

18. Spicer DV, Ursin G, Parisky Y, et al. Changes in mammographic densities induced by a hormonal contraceptive designed to reduce breast cancer risk. J Natl Cancer Inst 1994;86:431–436

19. Saftlas AF, Hoover RN, Brinton LA, et al. Mammographic densities and risk of breast cancer. Cancer 1991;67:2833–2838

7 PRACTICAL DIAGNOSTIC BREAST ULTRASONOGRAPHY

Yuri Parisky

Breast ultrasonography has been utilized for several decades to augment findings by physicians on mammography and clinical examinations. Early breast ultrasonography was limited in its utility. The technology was rudimentary and the results not particularly beneficial. Patients were placed supine in a waterbath, and sector imaging was performed with fairly insensitive imaging equipment. Tremendous advances have occurred since the early 1990s in technology and our ability to understand and appreciate the utility of ultrasound as a diagnostic tool.

As a general screening procedure, ultrasonography is not particularly useful, with inadequate yields for specificity and sensitivity in the detection of early breast cancer. However, it has evolved into an important complementary diagnostic examination that is indicated in specific clinical situations. It is useful for (1) evaluating an abnormal mammographic finding, and (2) evaluating an abnormal clinical finding. Diagnostic breast ultrasonography may be used to determine whether a mammographically apparent mass is a cyst or solid and to identify characteristics of a palpable finding that is not mammographically apparent. It is paramount to remember that should ultrasonography fail to yield appropriate diagnostic answers in the case of a mammographic or clinical abnormality, the radiologist or clinician is required to continue the diagnostic workup. A negative ultrasound scan (showing no abnormality) should not supersede the perception of a mammographic or clinical breast abnormality.

TECHNICAL FACTORS

The ultrasonography operator, whether physician or technologist, should have a thorough understanding of basic ultrasound technique, the equipment employed, and normal and abnormal ultrasonographic breast anatomy. At least a rudimentary knowledge of mammography is important, as mammographic abnormalities may be the indication for diagnostic breast ultrasound scanning. Pertinent mammographic images and/or clinical history should be available to the technologist prior to scanning the patient.

KEY PRACTICE POINTS

Ultrasonography: An adjunct to mammography, it can confirm the presence of a mass that is vague on mammography. It is used to localize lesions. It is *not* an appropriate test for screening. It can distinguish a cyst from a solid mass. It is useful for guiding the draining cysts and abscesses.

Breast ultrasound equipment has evolved significantly over the past two decades. Ultrasound transducers have been developed by numerous manufacturers specifically to facilitate imaging of the breast. Ultrasonographic breast imaging should be performed in real time with a linear array transducer with high-frequency capabilities. At present, commercially available transducers with 7- to 12-megahertz (MHz) frequency capability are available. These types of transducers have numerous advantages over earlier annular array transducers and mid-frequency transducers. The linear array transducers have significant capabilities that mechanical sector transducers did not. Among the many benefits included are multiple focal zones that can be adjusted to the depth of interest. Linear array transducers facilitate interventional breast procedures. They have wider near-field imaging resolution.

Ultrasonographic equipment ranges in price and technical features. It is preferable to utilize a sophisticated ultrasound device, for which the appropriate breast ultrasound transducer can be purchased as an attachment. The select breast ultrasound transducers cost about $10,000. When utilized with a sophisticated ultrasound machine, they provide greater control of imaging parameters. Some have Doppler color flow vascular imaging which, although still in the early research phase, may prove to be of benefit for defining certain lesions.

SCANNING TECHNIQUE

The patient should be scanned in real time in the supine position with her ipsilateral wrist behind her head to elevate the breast and offer access to the axilla. Scanning should be performed in a quiet environment which protects the patient's privacy.

At the University of Southern California/Norris Breast Center (USC/NBC), we prefer first to image the entire breast, with additional images then demonstrating any identified pathology. In the area of clinical or mammographic concern, additional images should be obtained to document the presence or absence of underlying pathology. If ultrasonography discovers a lesion, its exact location should be documented and images demonstrating its dimensions in both radial and antiradial planes recorded. The exact geographic location of the lesion can be documented using clockface notations with appropriate measurements from the nipple or by utilizing concentric circles radiating from the nipple (the inner circle being assigned "A" and the farthest outer circle being assigned "C"). The depth of the lesion can also be described in thirds, labeled from 1 (superficial) to 3 (deep). A combination of the clockface notation and the concentric depth measurement is preferred, as it allows accurate localization of the lesion and is easily reproducible on subsequent examinations.

If clinical examination, mammography, or ultrasonography suspects a malignant lesion, evaluation of the axillary contents is strongly recommended. In addition to capturing representative and appropriate images on either film or print, the ultrasonographer should document findings on a breast diagram.

Commercially available ultrasonic gels should be utilized to provide appropriate acoustic coupling. If a lesion is close to the surface of the skin, a standoff pad may be utilized. These devices are either fluid-filled or are of a solid material that allows optimal transmission of acoustic energy. Liberal amounts of ultrasonic gel should be used to obtain appropriate coupling of the interface between the skin and the transducer. The images displayed on the screen and recorded on film or paper show cystic structures as black anechoic masses and fibrous structures as echogenic white areas. Any and all recorded images and notations become part of the patient's permanent medical record and should be appropriately preserved.

Normal Anatomy

High-frequency ultrasonography of the breast allows visualization of all of the breast parenchyma except in some women with extremely large breasts. Figure 7.1 illustrates the normal breast ultrasound pattern. Normal ducts can be seen at the outer edge of the areolar complex and extending several centimeters proximally. The ducts appear as tubular hypoechoic structures. The terminal duct lobular units of the breast appear as relatively homogeneous hypoechoic structures separated from one another by thin echogenic extralobular fibrous connective tissue. Extralobular fat has almost the same hypoechoic appearance and may be difficult to differentiate from normal intralobular glandular tissue. If the mammogram is dense owing to increased accumulation of fibrous tissue, this condition may appear as increased echogenicity on the ultrasound scan; however, the hypoechoic glandular and fat components can be differentiated. For this reason ultrasonography is well suited for the evaluation of mammographically dense fibrous breasts. Normal glandular structures and most pathologic lesions are more conspicuous against the echogenic background. Intramammary lymph nodes and axillary lymph nodes can usually be identified as discrete structures with an oval or kidney bean appearance, with echogenic fat in the hilum or even replacing most of the lymph node.

CLINICAL INDICATIONS FOR DIAGNOSTIC BREAST ULTRASONOGRAPHY

Clinically Palpable Abnormality

For women age 30 and younger, it may be more desirable to evaluate a palpable abnormality with ultrasonography than with mammography. This practice is prudent for several reasons. Young women tend to have dense breasts, which limits the effectiveness of mammography. Furthermore, there may be some resistance to using radiation in this age group. Ultrasonography is particularly suitable for young women, as most palpable lesions found at this age are either cysts or fibroadenomas. These lesions have readily identifiable ultrasonographic characteristics, which in most cases alleviate the concerns of the clinician. The area of palpable abnormality should be identified (for instance, with a topical marker) on the woman's breast prior to the ultrasonographic examination so this area can undergo extensive evaluation to detect any underlying pathology. Following identification of the lesion responsible for the concern, a less detailed evaluation of the entire breast may be performed. Evaluation of the remainder of the breast is not a screening process to detect the unlikely occult malignancy but may be useful for identifying other lesions, such as cysts or fibroadenomas, commonly found in women. This scan then serves as a further reference if in fact any of those additional lesions becomes clinically apparent (palpable) at a later time. Although appropriate evaluation should be performed both clinically and ultrasonographically of every subsequent palpable abnormality, the initial ultrasound scans may serve as a baseline.

Patients age 35 and over who have a palpable abnormality should first undergo diagnostic mammography. The location of the lesion should be marked prior to ultrasound examination. Scrutiny should be performed in the area of the palpable abnormality and a survey done of the remainder of the breast. It is preferable to have the ultrasound and mammographic findings reviewed by a physician who has expertise in both areas of imaging.

A negative diagnostic ultrasound scan showing no abnormality, especially in the setting of dense breasts, should never overrule the clinical findings. If the abnormality is not perceived on the ultrasound scan, the physician should proceed with fine-needle aspiration (FNA) or other diagnostic procedures.

Mammographic Abnormalities

Breast ultrasonography is most commonly used to complement the mammographic imaging evaluation. Ultrasonography can characterize a dominant mass as cyst, fibroadenoma, or malignancy and can identify many of the less common abnormalities that may present as masses. When a diagnostic ultrasound scan is indicated by the mammographic findings, it is imperative that the area in question be marked on the breast and the mammogram films provided so the ultrasonographer may correlate the imaging examination. An imaging protocol similar to that for evaluating palpable abnormalities should be employed, with careful scrutiny given to the mammographically suspicious area. If a lesion seen mammographically is difficult to detect on ultrasonography, the patient may have a repeat mammogram with a lesion localization grid placed over the mammographic abnormality. Once the exact area is identified, diagnostic breast ultrasonography can be performed. If a pathologic lesion is identified, it should be appropriately characterized. If ultrasonography does not identify the lesion, the mammographic findings for a nonpalpable mass should determine the next step. Common mammographic findings that indicate the need for ultrasonography include single or multiple masses, areas of increased density, architectural distortion, suspected infection or inflammatory process, and postprocedure or postsurgical complications. Ultrasound evaluation of ductal disease is not commonly utilized. Although mammary duct ectasia (periductal mastitis) and other benign ductal disease can be demonstrated and documented by ultrasound scans, the diagnosis of ductal carcinoma in situ remains outside the scope of general clinical breast ultrasonography. Likewise, ultrasonographic evaluation of ductal calcifications, although they may be demonstrated with certain high-frequency transducers, is not within the purview of general ultrasonography.

Breast Abnormalities

Mammographically Apparent Mass Density or Clinically Palpable Mass

During the infancy of breast ultrasonography, masses confirmed mammographically by two views (e.g., craniocaudal and mediolateral oblique) or that were clinically palpable were evaluated by ultrasound scans to determine whether they were cystic or solid. This was the limit of the ultrasound evaluation. Considerable progress has been made in diagnostic breast ultrasonography, and mass lesions can now be routinely identified and categorized as benign or malignant (Table 7.1). Specific criteria have been developed to assess the likely

Table 7.1. Ultrasound imaging of breast masses
Benign masses
Abscess
Cyst
Fibroadenoma
Fibrosis
Hamartoma
Hematoma
Lymph node
Malignant masses
Intracystic carcinoma
Lymphoma
Metastasis
Phyllodes tumor
Primary adenocarcinoma
Sarcoma

Table 7.2. Breast ultrasonography: benign findings

Finding	Specificity (%) (if absent)	Sensitivity (%) (if absent)	Negative predictive value (%)
Thin echogenic capsule	76	95	99
Ellipsoid shape	51	98	99
<Four lobulations	19	99	99
Hyperechoic	7	100	100

Table 7.3. Breast ultrasonography: malignant findings

Finding	Sensitivity (%)	Positive predictive value (%)
Angular margins	83	68
Hypoechoic	69	60
Shadowing	49	65
Taller > wider	42	81
Spiculated	36	92
Branch pattern	30	64

benignity (Table 7.2) or malignancy (Table 7.3) of a particular lesion detected by ultrasound scans.

Cysts

Cysts are common mass lesions found at clinical examination or on mammography. Ultrasonography is the definitive imaging tool for diagnosing the presence of cysts. Its accuracy approaches 100%, although strict criteria must be applied. The lesion should be well defined, have smooth walls and sharp anterior and posterior borders, exhibit posterior acoustic enhancement, and have no internal echoes (Fig. 7.2). Cysts may be compressible by the ultrasound transducer. If these criteria are met, the diagnosis of a simple cyst can be rendered. Some cysts contain internal echoes, which may be a function of artifact or a result of internal proteinaceous material, cellular debris, cholesterol crystals, or a sequel to infection or hemorrhage. These cysts may be deemed complex, and further evaluation may be necessary. With color flow Doppler evaluation, if there is absolute absence of flow within the lesion, and if aside from internal echoes the remainder of the strict criteria for simple cysts are met, the lesion likely represents a complex cyst. Cyst puncture, aspiration, and on occasion pneumocystography can confirm the presence of a simple or complex cyst. It is not uncommon for ultrasound scans to encounter a complex cyst when an incomplete aspiration (FNA) has resulted in partial collapse and bleeding into a cyst.

Intracystic mural nodules are rare (Fig. 7.3). They represent either papillomas or intracystic carcinoma. Papillomas are more common, although the ability to differentiate a benign from a malignant process is beyond the capabilities of ultrasonography. These lesions should be excised.

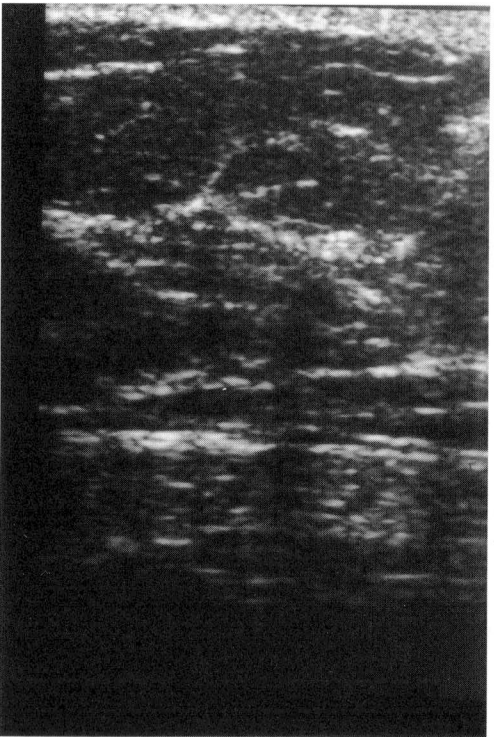

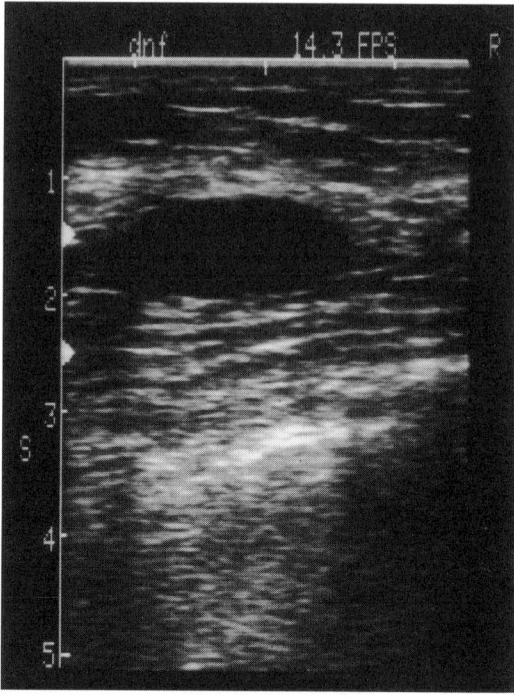

Figure 7.1. Ultrasound scan of normal breast tissue. There is no disruption of the normal sonographic pattern.

Figure 7.2. Ultrasound scan of a typical cyst. The anechoic mass has a linear axis and well defined smooth anterior and posterior borders. There is posterior acoustic enhancement.

Solid Breast Masses

Characteristics of both benign and malignant solid breast masses have been determined (Table 7.1). These criteria unfortunately are not absolute, and there is significant overlapping of some of the features. Nevertheless, ultrasound is a useful tool for confirming the presence of a malignancy and rendering the proper diagnosis of a fibroadenoma. Diagnosing a solid lesion as benign requires both mammographic and ultrasonographic correlation.

Fibroadenoma

A fibroadenoma, which is the most common solid mass found in women aged 20–40, typically has definite ultrasonographic features. These lesions are usually oval, with a smooth or macrolobulated border. They are either isoechoic or hypoechoic internally (Fig. 7.4). Many have posterior sonographic enhancement or are neutral in this regard. On occasion, unfortunately, they may have posterior shadowing, which is a feature not uncommonly seen with a malignancy. Mammographically these lesions may contain calcifications; and if the calcifications are confirmed as areas of echogenic foci with shadowing within the suspected fibroadenoma, a definitive diagnosis may be rendered. It is rare to have a carcinoma coexisting

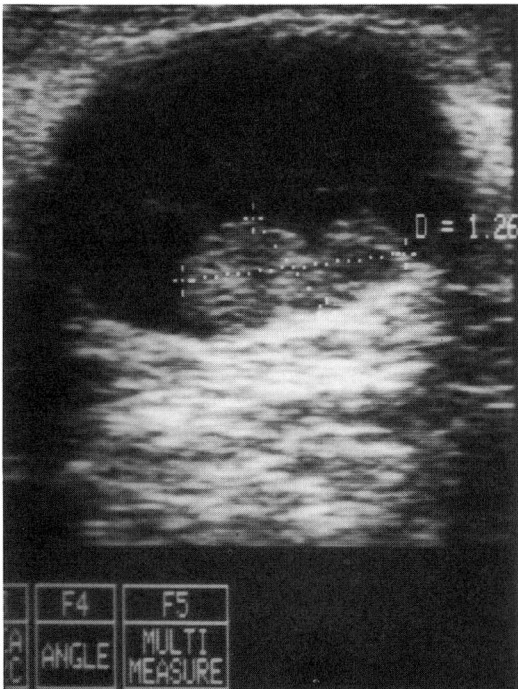

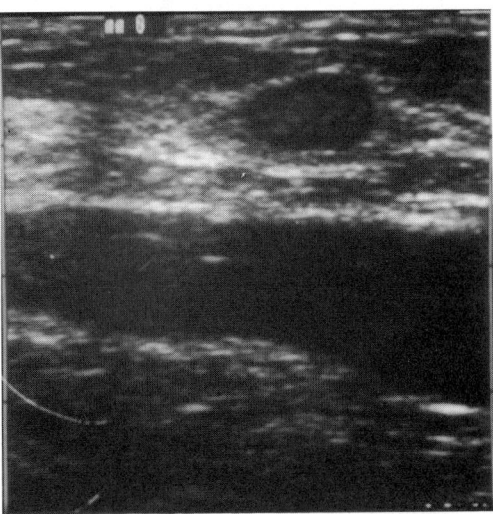

Figure 7.4. Ultrasound scan of a fibroadenoma above a saline-implant prosthesis. The mass above the implant is oval (with a linear axis), is hypoechoic, and has smooth borders.

Figure 7.3. Ultrasound scan of a cyst containing an intracystic nodular cancer at the base.

in a fibroadenoma. Color flow Doppler sonography evaluation of suspected fibroadenomas is still being researched, and the initial reported findings are mixed. Premenopausal women with fibroadenomas may show increased blood flow to the lesion, which is a finding that may also be present in a malignancy. Further evaluation is indicated.

Carcinoma

The criteria for identifying malignant breast lesions are similar for ultrasonography and mammography. The cancers are irregular with angular margins and microspiculations, and they appear to disrupt the normal ultrasonographic anatomy of the breast (Fig. 7.5). The lesions are typically hypoechoic to anechoic and often have posterior shadowing. Any atypical lesion should be considered a malignancy until proved otherwise. Unfortunately, some breast cancers can exhibit benign features on ultrasound scans. This is commonly seen with a medullary carcinoma, which may mimic a fibroadenoma on ultrasonography.

Fibrosis

Fibrosis resulting from an inflammatory process, postoperative changes, or intrinsic benign breast pathology may present as a mammographic density with irregular borders in two projections. Ultrasonographically, fibrosis has no

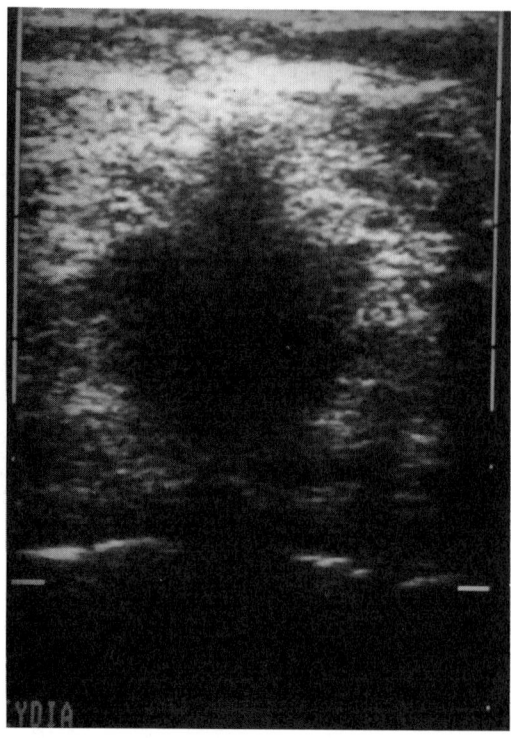

Figure 7.5. Ultrasound scan of an invasive ductal carcinoma. The significantly hypoechoic mass has a vertical axis and a pine tree shape with irregular angular margins and posterior shadowing.

particularly suspicious characteristics and usually presents as an area of focally increased echogenicity without shadowing.

Abscess

Abscesses are usually suspected clinically. Ultrasonographic confirmation may show findings similar to that of a complex cyst. There are often significant internal echoes and through transmission. The border of the abscess is ill-defined and irregular, unlike that of a cyst. The ultrasonographic findings coupled with the clinical suspicion should render the diagnosis. Follow-up ultrasonography should be performed to confirm the resolution of the abscess. Ultrasonography can be utilized to guide an interventional procedure (e.g., 18-gauge or larger needle aspiration) to drain the abscess.

INTERVENTIONAL ULTRASONOGRAPHIC BREAST PROCEDURES

Cyst Aspiration

Inadequate drainage of a palpable cyst can usually be completed with ultrasound guidance. Nonpalpable cysts can also undergo FNA and drainage with ultrasonographic guidance. Once the cyst is identified and the patient appropriately prepared, including betadine cleansing of the skin, the transducer is placed longitudinally along the long axis of the cyst and a 20-gauge needle is introduced at an angle parallel to the long axis of the transducer. With this technique the needle can be observed ultrasonographically as it enters the cyst. After the needle enters the cyst, the cyst can be aspirated dry with manipulations seen in real time by ultrasonography. Pneumocystography may be of questionable value for treating cysts, although there are some centers that advocate its use. Air introduced into the cyst causes the cyst wall to appear as a curvilinear intense echogenic line on the ultrasound scan.

Tissue Core-Needle Biopsy

The optimum use of interventional ultrasonography in breast procedures is with tissue core-needle biopsy (TCNB), which can access lesions identified as malignant or suspicious and fibroadenomas requiring histopathologic confirmation. It is performed with real-time ultrasonography. At USC/NBC, we use a 14-gauge core biopsy needle with an automatic biopsy gun. We prefer a nondisposable spring-loaded automatic biopsy gun, as the device has stronger springs and allows greater penetration of breast tissue upon firing. The technique is similar to FNA, although the skin and subdermal tissues are anesthetized with 1–2% lidocaine with 1:200,000 epinephrine. The epinephrine is employed to provide hemostasis. The 14-gauge needle is inserted into the breast until it touches the lesion (Fig. 7.6). While being observed in real time on the ultrasound scan, the needle is fired by the gun and can be seen penetrating the lesion. Gentle pressure may be applied on the transducer to fix or trap the lesion between the transducer and the needle. Typically, four to six passes are performed to ensure adequate specimen capture. Numerous studies have confirmed the utility, sensitivity, and specificity of this procedure, which can be used for: (1) confirmation of a suspected malignancy, which then allows definitive surgery and axillary lymph

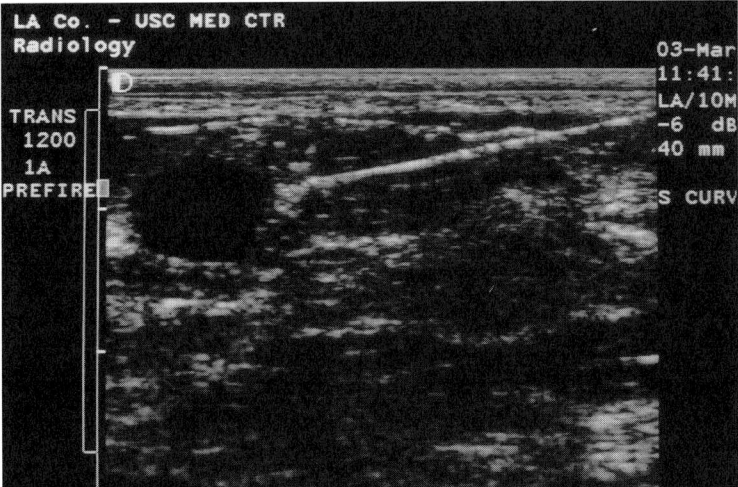

Figure 7.6. Ultrasound scan of a tissue core-needle within the breast in position to sample a hypoechoic mass, which proved to be a fibroadenoma.

node dissection during a single operative procedure; (2) histopathologic evaluation of an indeterminate lesion; (3) histopathologic confirmation of a suspected fibroadenoma.

CONCLUSIONS

Ultrasonography is a useful adjunct to mammography, especially in cases of mammographically dense breasts. As clinically indicated, ultrasonography can also be used to characterize palpable breast lesions, but it is not an appropriate breast cancer screening technique. Furthermore, it has proved useful as guidance for tissue core-needle biopsies of breast lesions, particularly mass lesions. As with all technical procedures, appropriate training and experience should precede the unsupervised clinical use of breast ultrasonography.

8   FINE-NEEDLE ASPIRATION AT THE BREAST DIAGNOSTIC CENTER

William H. Hindle

The first work on needle aspirations to be reported in the United States was by Hayes E. Martin in 1930 at Memorial Hospital in New York.[1] Attempting to secure tissue fragments for histologic diagnosis, he used local anesthesia, a scalpel entry wound, and an 18-gauge needle.

It was not until the late 1950s and early 1960s that fine-needle aspiration (FNA) of a palpable solid breast mass began to be extensively applied in cytology centers in Europe (e.g., at the Karolinska Institute in Stockholm). By the mid-1970s and thereafter, published series of FNAs for cytology of a solid breast mass were being reported from selected medical centers in the United States.

Review of the extensive FNA literature from around the world reveals that a "false-positive" diagnosis is rare. Such an example would be a hypercellular atypical fibroadenoma. Given an adequate cell sample, the frequency of "false-negatives" is said to be less than 10%, and such a report would be followed up because in clinical practice a suspicious mass must always be definitively diagnosed. A histologic diagnosis would have to be obtained from a specimen obtained by tissue core-needle biopsy (TCNB) or open surgical biopsy (OSBx) in cases of FNA uncertainty.

INDICATIONS

The indication for breast FNA is a persistent, palpable, dominant breast mass (Table 8.1). Occasionally, FNA is performed on a localized area if strong concern is exhibited by the patient or her referring physician. However, the diagnostic cytology yield from such an area is minuscule and not generally cost-effective. When (1) the aspirator is certain that the cellular sample is from the exact area of concern, (2) the cytologic evaluation reveals abundant benign ductal epithelial cells, and (3) there is concordance with mammography, the option of close follow-up can be offered. Otherwise, a further diagnostic procedure, consultation, or reevaluation is indicated.

CONTRAINDICATIONS

There are no contraindications to FNA of a dominant breast mass, although theoretically a florid skin infection over the mass is a relative contraindication (Table 8.1). However, such an infection has never been seen in our Breast Diagnostic Center (BDC). Age, even at the ends of the spectrum, is not a contraindication to FNA; nor are pregnancy and lactation.

COMPLICATIONS

Potential, though infrequent, complications are listed in Table 8.2. Ecchymosis (bruising with discoloration) of the skin is an unusual complication of FNA with the technique utilized at the BDC. Nonliquid hematomas have occurred, but they subside spontaneously. Pneumothorax has been reported in the literature but has not occurred in the BDC, where it is our practice to immobilize a mass to be aspirated over a rib.

Dislodged tumor cells (e.g., ductal carcinoma cell clusters) have been described in the histologic evaluations of surgical specimens obtained after FNA. The viability of dislodged tumor cells is questionable. Furthermore, several published series reveal no difference in the local recurrence rate or overall survival whether the malignancy was diagnosed by FNA or OSBx.

Whenever the skin is punctured, it is theoretically possible for infection to occur at the needle site. However, we are not aware of it ever occurring in the BDC experience.

Table 8.1. Indications and contraindications for breast fine-needle aspiration

Indication
    Undiagnosed palpable dominant mass
Contraindications
    Absolute: none
    Relative: florid skin infection overlying the mass

Table 8.2. Complications of breast fine-needle aspiration

Occasional, but rarely a clinical problem at the BDC
    Bleeding from the skin puncture
    Ecchymosis at the site of the needle puncture
    Hematoma within the breast tissue
    Acellular specimens
Reported in the literature but have not occurred at the BDC
    Infection at the puncture site
    Pneumothorax
    Seeding of tumor cells along the needle tract

An FNA reported as "acellular" or "inadequate for cytologic diagnosis" could be considered a complication. In fact, it is as though no FNA had been performed, as no clinical conclusion can be drawn. The BDC practice is to repeat the FNA.

ADVANTAGES

Breast FNA of a palpable dominant mass is an efficient, accurate, cost-effective office procedure. No special equipment is required, although training and experience in FNA technique and slide preparation are essential. With detailed instruction and supervision, the techniques of FNA and slide preparation can be readily learned in a timely fashion (if an adequate volume of cases is available). Properly performed FNA can give prompt, reliable results. Neither anesthesia nor sedation is necessary. Patient acceptance and appreciation of having a quick result (cytologic impression) are almost universal. FNA can be repeated without residual evidence of trauma (e.g., scar formation).

Fine-needle aspiration of a palpable breast mass immediately differentiates a cyst from a solid mass. Therapy is immediate with drainage of the cyst.

A definitive cytologic diagnosis of a neoplasm, when supported by concordance of the clinical impression and mammography, can lead to immediate reassurance if benign or the initiation of timely treatment if malignant.

INFORMED CONSENT

By BDC protocol and policy, informed consent is obtained before breast FNA is performed. Information is given, and the discussion is held in the patient's native language (which in the BDC is usually Spanish). The indications, complications, and potential advantages are reviewed. Breast FNA is compared to a venipuncture, and obtaining and interpreting the cellular sample are likened to a Papanicolaou smear, procedures with which most women are familiar.

At the BDC the process of obtaining informed consent not only properly prepares the patient but serves as an educational experience for the resident physicians obtaining the consent. The discussion is held in private, but the presence of a family member or "significant other" is encouraged.

FNA EQUIPMENT

The typical medical office already contains all the essential equipment for breast FNA (Table 8.3). At the BDC the basic equipment and material used for breast FNA are (1) a prepackaged sterile alcohol wipe for the skin; (2) a 22-gauge 1-inch needle with a transparent plastic hub; (3) a 10-cc prepackaged disposable sterile syringe; (4) a prepackaged sterile 4 × 4 inch gauze; and (5) a clean emesis-type plastic basin for carrying the materials in and out of the patient's examination room and to the cytotechnician, a procedure for the protection of all concerned. The syringe is available should the mass be a cyst that requires drainage. A

Table 8.3. Fine-needle aspiration equipment

Antiseptic skin wipe (or equivalent)
Needle with a transparent hub: 22-gauge, 1-inch
Gauze sterile 4 × 4 inches
Band-Aid-type wound covering
Prepackaged disposable sterile syringe, 10 cc
Slides with a frosted end for patient identification
Smear fixative (95% ethanol) or equivalent spray

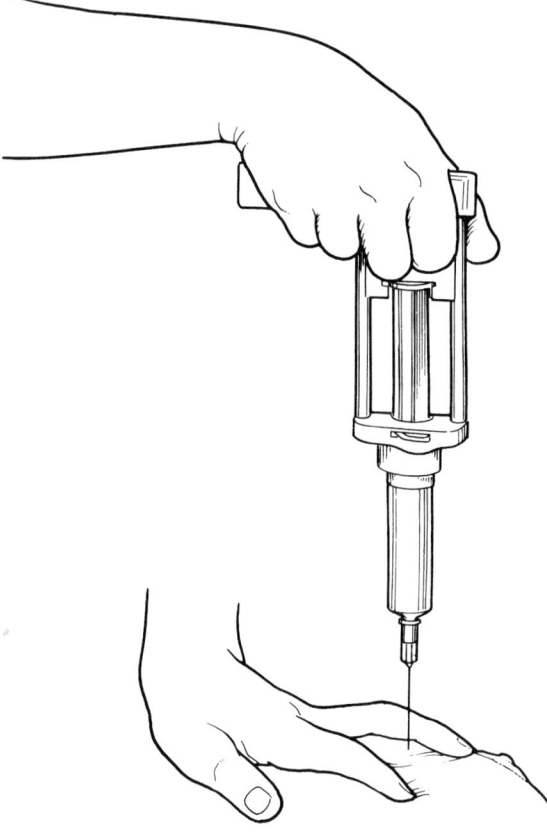

Figure 8.1. Fine-needle aspiration using the Cameco syringe holder and a 20-cc disposable syringe. This technique was popularized by the Karolinska Aspiration Clinic, Stockholm, Sweden.

Band-Aid to cover the FNA site is optional. A pistol-type syringe holder that fits into the aspirator's palm is available for those who prefer the negative pressure technique for FNA.

A variety of FNA devices (Figs. 8.1–8.5) are available commercially (often prepackaged), such as the original Karolinska-type syringe holder, a hand-held plastic reusable pistol-type syringe holder (used in the BDC), a three-finger control syringe, a plain syringe, and a needle alone, which is used with the BDC preferred FNA technique. Each aspirator develops a personal preference, which should be for the equipment that yields an abundant cell sample for that aspirator.

Figure 8.2. Fine-needle aspiration with an Inrad syringe holder and a 10-cc disposable syringe.

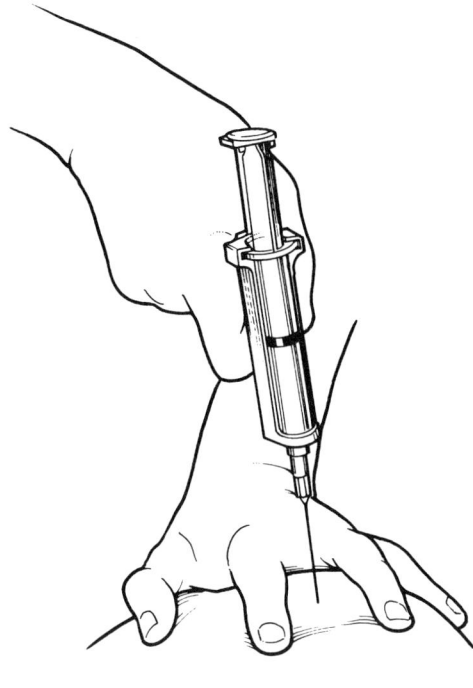

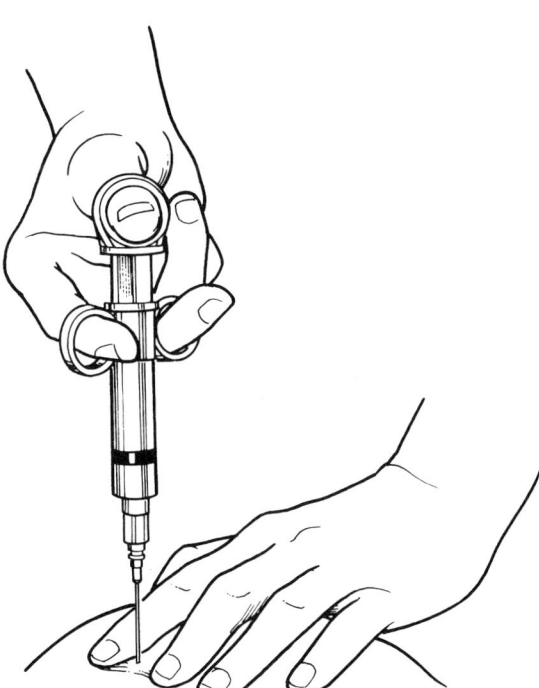

Figure 8.3. Fine-needle aspiration with a disposable 10-cc three-finger-control syringe.

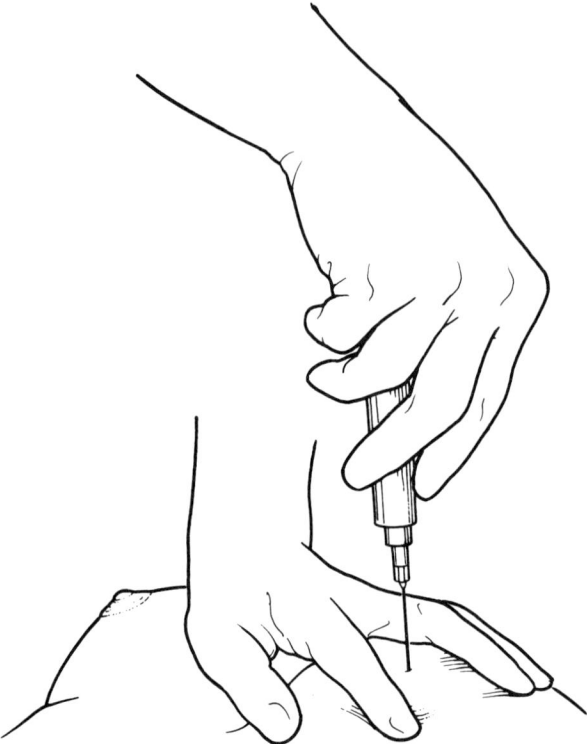

Figure 8.4. Fine-needle aspiration with a disposable 10-cc syringe.

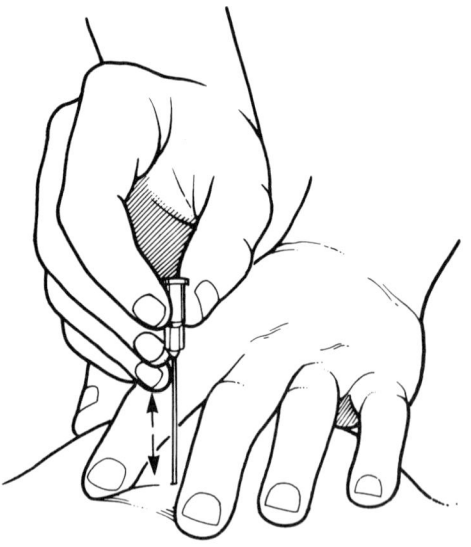

Figure 8.5. Fine-needle aspiration using a needle alone and no suction for negative pressure.

FNA Technique

At the BDC the needle-alone FNA technique[2] (without negative pressure in a syringe) is preferred because (1) it is readily learned, (2) it affords intimate control of the needle, and (3) information can be gained from feeling the resistance of the mass to the needle.

With all the FNA techniques, the most difficult and exacting portion of the procedure is immobilization of the mass. A mass of 4 cm diameter or larger can be held in any fashion that is comfortable for the aspirator. Some masses are so large (or fixed) that the mass need not be held in position. Many of the palpable lesions seen in the BDC are 1–2 cm in diameter and require careful positioning and immobilization.

Needle-Alone Technique

The following is the step-by-step FNA procedure used in the BDC (Table 8.4).

1. The mass is palpated to be certain it is a distinct dominant breast mass (Fig. 8.6).

2. A mobile mass is moved by the fingers of the nonaspirating hand (i.e., the left hand of a right-handed aspirator) to a position over a rib (Fig. 8.7).

3. The mass is positioned between the index and middle finger, and the fingers are pressed downward (Fig. 8.8), which brings the mass closer to the skin.

4. The skin is then stretched tautly over the mass, immobilizing it on top of the rib (Figs. 8.9, 8.10). When the mass is immobilized over the rib, many aspirators, particularly when learning the procedure, palpate the mass with the dominant (aspirating) hand to be certain the mass is in position under the tented skin and to assess its depth relative to the skin. From this point on until the FNA procedure is completed, the nonaspirating hand remains firmly in position, immobilizing the mass.

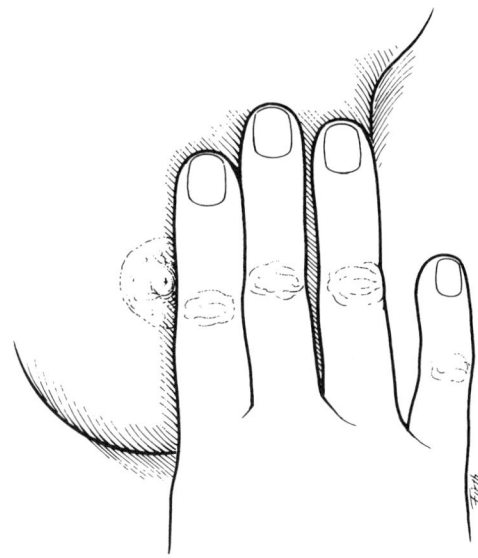

Figure 8.6. Palpation to locate the dominant breast mass.

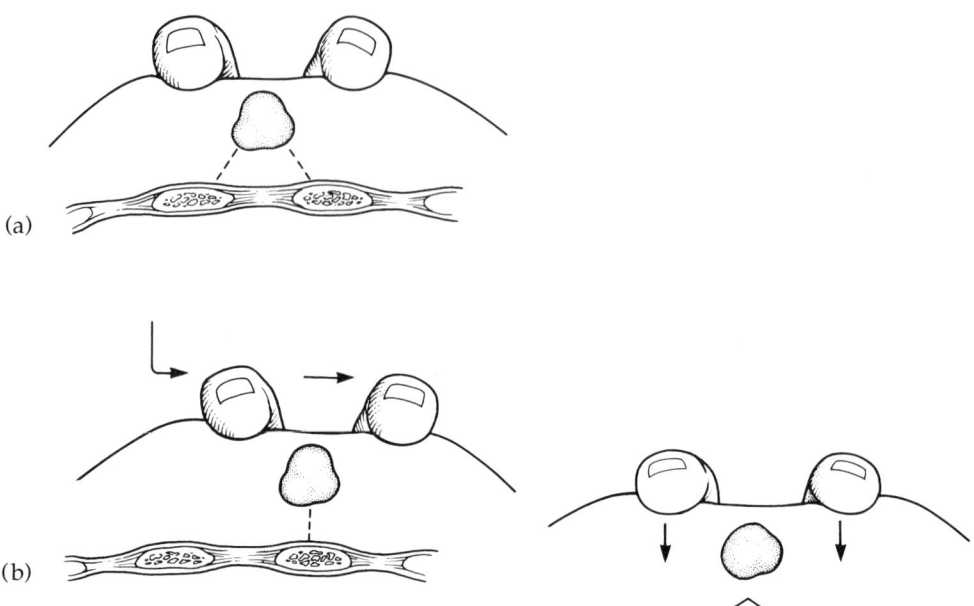

(a)

(b)

Figure 8.7. (a) Mass is localized between the pads of the index and middle finger. (b) It is then moved laterally to a position over a rib.

Figure 8.8. Pressing down with the fingers brings the mass closer to the skin.

5. The skin over the mass is cleansed with the alcohol skin wipe.

6. With the needle hub held between the thumb and index finger, the aspirator gently but firmly thrusts the needle through the skin and downward (by wrist, not arm, action) while noting changes in tissue resistance. When a neoplasm is encountered there is a distinct change in the resistance to the needle, and useful clinical information is gained by characterizing that resistance and the sensation perceived as the needle enters the mass.

7. The hub of the needle is watched to see if any fluid has accumulated. With a cyst the fluid is usually obvious and abundant. In that case, a syringe is attached to the needle hub, and gentle suction is used to drain the fluid until the cyst is completely "dry" (Figs. 8.11, 8.12). If at any time gross blood appears in the needle hub, the FNA should be discontinued, the bloody fluid smeared and fixed, and the FNA repeated at another skin site. Because most adenocarcinomas are vascular, blood often appears in the needle hub, and even with repeated attempts all samples of a carcinoma may be grossly bloody. Therefore smears are made in an attempt to identify cancer cells in the bloody fluid.

8. If no fluid appears in the needle hub, the needle tip is moved up and down within the mass in sharp jackhammer-like thrusts up to 30 times. Because breast neoplasms are homogeneous by FNA cytology, representative cellular samples can be obtained with multiple needle thrusts at the same angle. Changing the direction of the thrusts serves no purpose and increases the potential for bleeding.

9. When the thrusting is completed, the needle is removed from the skin, placed in the plastic emesis-type basin, and immediately taken to the cyto-technician for slide preparation and fixing (or air-drying in some cases).

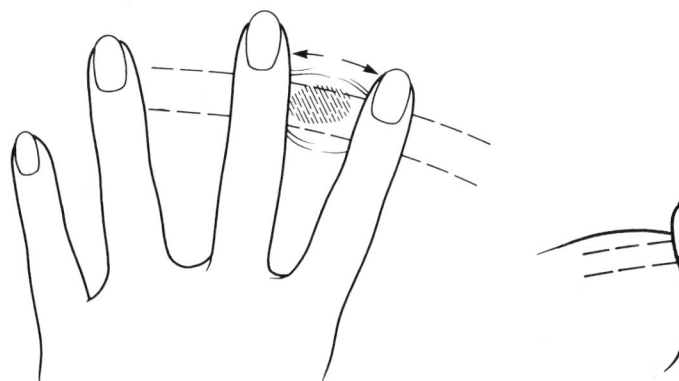 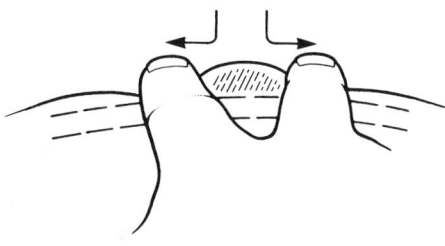

Figure 8.9. Trapping the mass over a rib as seen from above.

Figure 8.10. Trapping the mass over a rib, viewed horizontally.

Table 8.4. Steps for fine-needle aspiration (for a right-handed person)

1. Palpate the breast to locate the mass.
2. Trap the mass between the index and middle fingers of the left hand and push to a position over a rib.
3. Press down with the fingers.
4. Stretch the skin over the mass by spreading the index and middle fingers on each side of the mass.
5. Keep the fingers of the left hand stable, immobilizing the mass over the rib for the remainder of the aspiration.
6. Check the position and stabilization of the mass with the fingers of the right hand.
7. Clean the skin over the mass with an antiseptic skin wipe.
8. Hold the needle hub between the thumb and index finger of the right hand.
9. Insert the needle gently but firmly into the skin.
10. Feel the needle tip as it advances through the subcutaneous fat and breast tissue toward the mass.
11. Note the resistance to the advancing needle tip as it enters the mass and moves within the mass.
12. If gross fluid appears in the needle hub, indicating a cyst, attach a syringe and completely drain the cyst.
13. If the mass is solid, move the needle up and down within the mass with sharp jackhammer-like thrusts, exfoliating the cells into the bore of the needle.
14. Repeat the sharp downward thrusts as many as 30 times unless gross blood appears in the needle hub.
15. If gross blood appears, discontinue the aspiration and repeat the procedure at a different angle.
16. Remember to keep the needle tip within the mass while completing the 30 thrusts.
17. Remove the needle and place a 4 × 4 inch gauze pad folded into quarters over the needle puncture.
18. Quickly attach a syringe to the needle and eject the cellular specimen from the bore onto a slide and then immediately fix the slide.
19. Have the patient (or an assistant) continue firm pressure on the gauze over the puncture site for at least 2 minutes.
20. If desired, cover the puncture site with a Band-Aid type dressing.

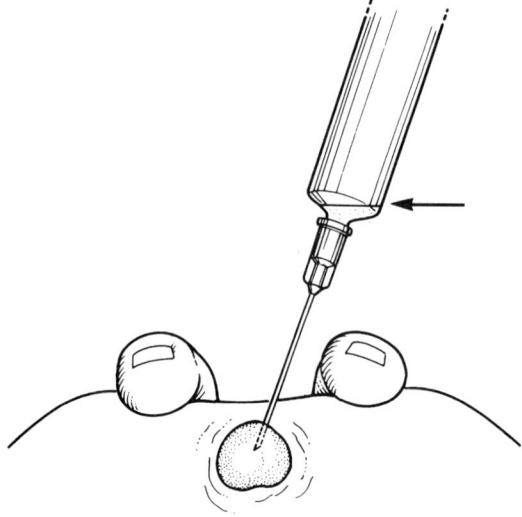

Figure 8.11. Diagnosis of a cyst by fine-needle aspiration is immediate when fluid appears in the hub of the needle or the barrel of the syringe.

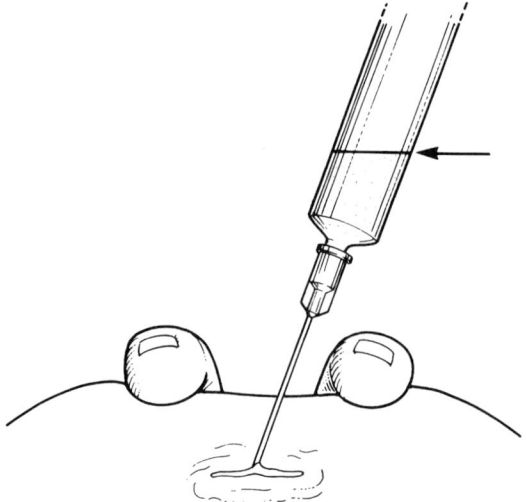

Figure 8.12. Therapeutic drainage of all fluid from a cyst by negative pressure in the syringe produced by drawing back (up) on the barrel of the syringe.

10. Immediately a 4 × 4 inch sterile gauze folded into quarters is placed over the FNA site. The patient is instructed to apply firm pressure on the gauze pad with the three middle fingers of the hand opposite the FNA (e.g., right hand to left breast) for a period of at least 2 minutes.

11. A Band-Aid-type dressing may be placed on the FNA site if desired.

It is important to take ample time when beginning an FNA to immobilize the mass precisely over a rib (Fig. 8.13), which gives a firm surface to press against and avoids the possibility of pneumothorax. The aspirator should mentally visualize the needle tip so that throughout each up-and-down movement the needle tip remains within the mass. The cell sample is exfoliated into the bore (barrel) of the

Figure 8.13.   Pushing and compressing a mobile mass over an underlying rib.

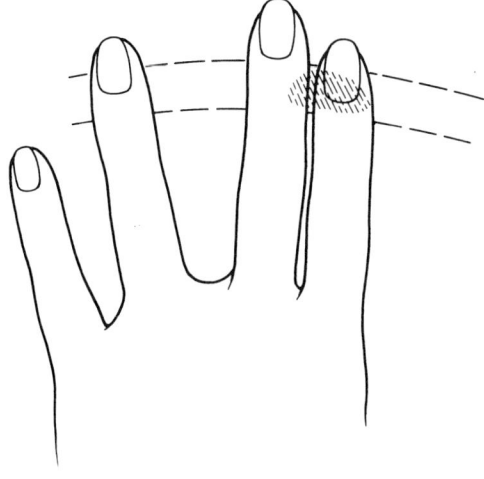

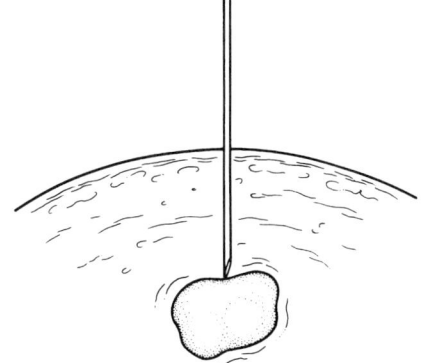

Figure 8.14.   Initial probing of a solid mass by the needle, with tactile sensation of the needle tip hitting the mass.

needle during the downward thrust. Usually the entire cellular specimen is collected within the bore of the needle, and no material or fluid appears in the needle hub. An inadequate cellular sample can result from inattention to the exact needle tip placement (sampling error) or from a lack of multiple sharp thrusts.

Assessment of tactile resistance to the advancing needle can yield clinically useful information (Fig. 8.14). There is little or no resistance in normal breast tissue. With fibrocystic changes, the aspirator may perceive intermittent irregular resistance from fibrous bands. The resistance encountered in a fibroadenoma is described as rubbery, similar to the eraser on a pencil. The aspirator may sense a pop when a cyst is entered. An adenocarcinoma usually produces a gritty resistance, likened to raw potato. With a neoplasm, the aspirator usually perceives a distinct change in resistance as the needle penetrates and enters the mass.

Negative-Pressure Technique

The traditional and most commonly used technique for breast FNA is performed with a needle, syringe, and syringe holder. The classic Karolinska technique, which uses a relatively large syringe holder and forceful arm strokes, is effective but requires considerable practice to learn and perform properly. Frequent use of the technique is usually necessary to achieve consistently abundant cellular samples. Because multiple punctures (passes) are commonly used, many aspirators using this technique inject local anesthesia into the skin prior to the procedure.

This method utilizes negative pressure in the syringe and potentially results in an abundant cellular specimen. However, when blood is present it rapidly accumulates in the needle hub and syringe, and the FNA must be redone. The initial steps and immobilization of the mass are the same as for the needle-alone technique. The specific steps of the negative pressure technique are diagrammed and sequentially numbered in Figure 8.15.

1. The needle is thrust through the skin.
2. The needle moves toward the mass.
3. Resistance is assessed when the needle enters the mass.
4. Then, and only then, negative pressure is created in the syringe by withdrawing the inner barrel to about the 3- to 5-cc mark. Up-and-down thrusts are made while the needle tip remains within the mass. If no fluid is obtained, up to 20 trusts are made (compared to the 30 trusts used for the needle-alone technique).

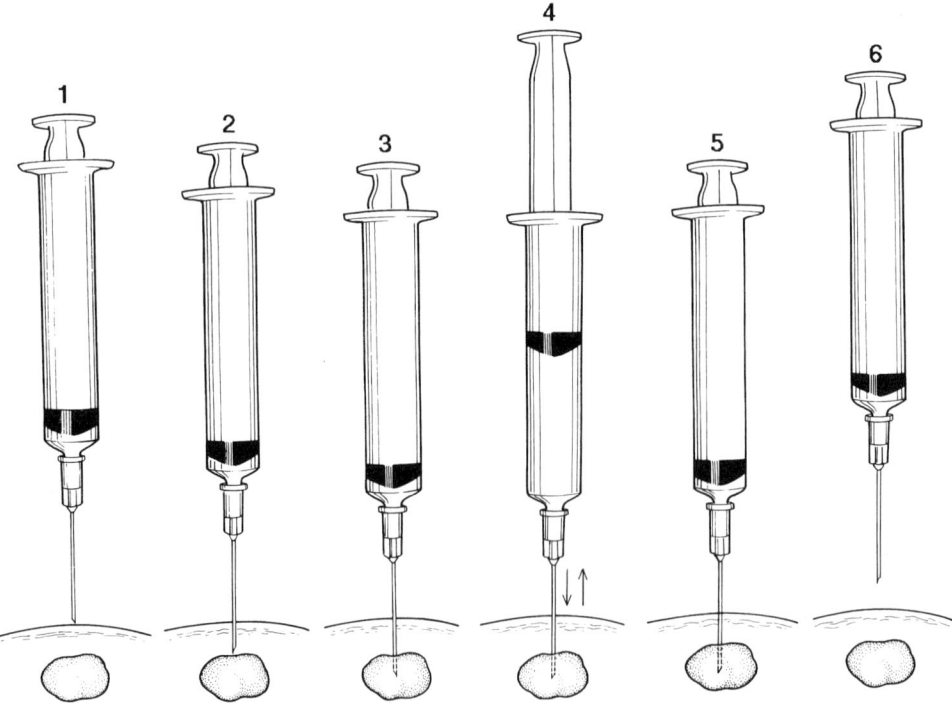

Figure 8.15. Sequential steps (1–6) of the traditional fine-needle aspiration technique utilizing suction by negative pressure created by drawing back on the barrel of the needle when (and only when) the needle tip is in the mass to be aspirated.

5. The negative pressure in the syringe is released (the inner barrel of the syringe automatically returns to the neutral position). It is critical to release all the negative pressure before the needle tip is removed from the breast. Otherwise, air sucks the tissue juice up into the syringe where it rapidly dries and cannot be recovered for cytologic evaluation.

6. Finally, the needle is withdrawn from the breast.

FNA Slide Preparation

In the BDC a cytotechnician, trained and supervised by the Department of Pathology, is present to prepare and stain the slides. This practice ensures uniformity and quality control while giving staff and resident physicians the opportunity to view the slides and have almost immediate feedback on site. If the cell sample on the slide is inadequate, a repeat FNA is performed. By BCD protocol no more than three FNAs are performed on a patient at a single visit, although three FNAs are rarely necessary. Because new physicians are continuously being instructed in the FNA technique, about 20% of the initial FNAs are repeated. It is not cost-effective to send a paucicellular or acellular slide to a cytopathologist for evaluation.

The clinician in an office setting should be capable of preparing and fixing the slides but should contact the consultant cytopathologist before initially performing an FNA to discuss preferences of slide preparation and staining.

As soon as possible after an FNA is performed, a syringe filled with 7 cc of air is attached to the needle. The needle is touched to a prelabeled slide (with the patient's name and identification) at a 45-degree angle with the bevel of the needle down toward the slide (Fig. 8.16a). The air is forcefully ejected down through the needle, expelling a drop of tissue juice on the slide. The material on the slide is then spread with another slide using either the pull-apart technique (Fig. 8.16b) or the spread technique, similar to preparing hematology slides. When the slides are to be fixed, both sides are immediately dropped in the fixative (Fig. 8.16c). A paper clip on one slide keeps them apart in the fixative. (Alternatively, the slide can be sprayed with fixative.) The slides should remain in the fixative for 2 minutes and then inspected for the presence of cellular material. A rapid stain such as toluidine blue [or Diff-Quik (Harleco, Gibbstown, NJ) for an air-dried slide] is useful for assessing whether adequate cellular material has been obtained. Toluidine blue stain is stable, and after a drop is placed on the slide (and covered with a slide) the amount of cellular sample is assessed under the microscope. The toluidine blue stain is bleached out when placed in the fixative bottle, but the slide can be restained with the cytopathologist's choice of stain. In the BDC we use a rapid Papanicolaou stain. If there is inadequate cellular material on the slide, the FNA is repeated. Once fixed, the slides can be sent to the cytopathologist at leisure. When a slide is to be air-dried, the smearing is the same but no fixative is used. (See Chapter 10 for a detailed and illustrated description of BDC slide preparation and staining.)

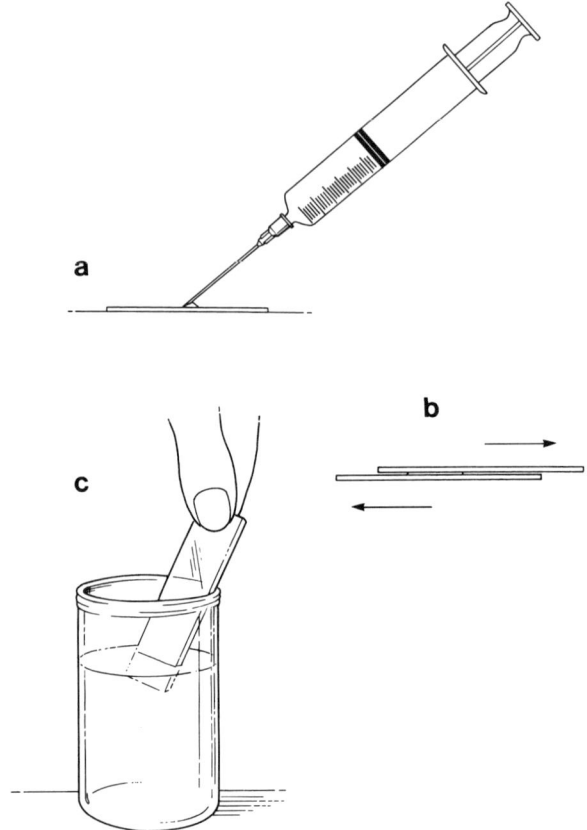

Figure 8.16. Smearing and fixing a fine-needle aspiration slide by (a) ejecting air down the needle so a drop of aspirated fluid appears on the slide, (b) smearing the cellular specimen by placing a second slide on top and pulling the slides gently but firmly apart, and (c) dropping the slide to be fixed into the Papanicolaou smear fixative.

CYTOLOGY REPORT

The formal cytologic interpretation and written report must be made by a cytopathologist who has been trained and is experienced in evaluating breast cellular aspirates. Potentially, the results can be obtained rapidly. When an abundance of well preserved cellular material (e.g., epithelial cells) is present on the slides, the cytologic diagnosis is accurate and reliable. An anxious patient can be told the specific cytologic diagnosis, and expedient treatment can be arranged. If the cytopathologist is on site, the result can be obtained within an hour. In any case, given a normal work week, a phone report should be available within 24 hours.

The written FNA cytology report should follow the lexicon and form suggested in *Acta Cytologica*.[3] Although the specific cytologic diagnosis is of paramount importance, it is essential that a written description of the cellular material (e.g., "small clusters of benign ductal cells are noted") be included so the clinician can use that information when deciding on appropriate clinical management.

Likewise, the cytopathologist should insist on having the pertinent clinical data (e.g., "a 28-year-old nonpregnant woman with a 2 × 2 cm firm mobile left breast mass consistent with a fibroadenoma") before making the final cytologic diagnosis. When the cytologic diagnosis is cancer (or suspicion thereof), the cytopathologist should notify the clinician in a timely manner directly by phone. The use of the terms "positive" and "negative" is discouraged in the written cytology report, as the terms are nonspecific and can be confusing or may be misinterpreted by the clinician and the patient. The final cytologic diagnosis should be specific and succinct (e.g., "adenocarcinoma," "fibroadenoma," or "consistent with fibrocystic change"). When indicated, the suggestion that tissue histology by TCNB or OSBx be obtained for confirmation is welcomed by clinicians.

When an adequate cell sample is obtained, the FNA cytologic diagnosis is accurate and has been shown to be clinically reliable as a basis for patient management in more than 90% of histologically verified palpable breast neoplasms. In many comprehensive breast centers, a concordant diagnosis of the diagnostic triad (clinical breast examination, FNA, mammography) approaches 99% accuracy for both benign and malignant breast neoplasms as confirmed by tissue histopathologic diagnosis. Many breast FNA cytology centers report >95% sensitivity and >90% specificity for carcinoma diagnosis.

TIMING OF FINE-NEEDLE ASPIRATION

The phase of the woman's menstrual cycle at the time of FNA has not been demonstrated to alter the cytologic interpretation of FNA. However, some women have considerable breast tenderness at certain times during their menstrual cycles, and if possible such times should be avoided for the patient's comfort.

Traditionally it was recommended that mammography be done before FNA or 2 weeks (or more) after. This guideline was based on work by Klein and Sickles[4] and Sickles et al.[5] The potential difficulty of interpretating mammographic findings may be a function of different FNA techniques as well as the time interval (i.e., number of hours) between the FNA and mammography. At the BDC mammograms are usually obtained on the same day and usually within hours of an FNA with no critical difficulty in mammographic interpretation or patient management.[6] In any case, it is essential that the mammographer have the clinical information (date, exact location, and result, if available) when an FNA has been performed within a month prior to mammography.

INADEQUATE OR NONDIAGNOSTIC FNAS

A breast FNA report of "acellular" or "inadequate for cytologic diagnosis" is *not* a "negative" report and does *not* rule out malignancy. No clinical conclusions about the mass can be drawn from such a report. It is as though the FNA had not been performed.

According to BDC protocol, if an initial FNA performed by a resident physician is inadequate or acellular, that resident physician repeats the procedure. If this second FNA is also inadequate or acellular, a third FNA is done by a staff physician or the cytopathologist. If the third FNA is inadequate or acellular, tissue samples for histologic diagnosis are obtained by TCNB or OSBx. The TCNB is performed by staff or the cytopathologist usually at the same patient visit, and three samples are taken. An 18-gauge, disposable, prepackaged, spring-loaded, cutting needle/syringe (TEMNO Biopsy Needle; Bauer Medical, Clearwater, FL) is used for the TCNB. If the histology is not diagnostic, the patient is scheduled for an OSBx. Similar successive steps for definitive diagnosis can be carried out by primary health care providers, although they may prefer to refer the patient to a breast specialist trained and experienced in these subsequent diagnostic procedures.

Occasionally in the BDC with an FNA final report of "inadequate for cytologic diagnosis," clinical management can nevertheless proceed when the results of the remainder of the diagnostic triad correspond with the written description of the cellular material submitted. For example, when there is a clinical impression of lipoma, mammography consistent with a lipoma, and the descriptive portion of the cytology report indicates that only adipose tissue was present on the slide, a management decision can be made.

References

1. Martin HE, Ellis EB. Biopsy by needle puncture and aspiration. Ann Surg 1930;92:169–181

2. Zajdela A, Zillhardt P, Voillemot N. Cytological diagnosis by fine needle sampling without aspiration. Cancer 1987;59:1201–1205

3. Logrono R, Kurtycz DF, Inhorn SI. Criteria for reporting fine needle aspiration on palpable and nonpalpable masses of the breast [editorial]. Acta Cytol 1997;41:623–627

4. Klein DL, Sickles EA. Effects of needle aspiration of the mammographic appearance of the breast: a guide to the proper timing of the mammography examination. Radiology 1982;145:44

5. Sickles EA, Klein DL, Goodson WH III, et al. Mammography after fine needle aspiration of palpable breast masses. Am J Surg 1983;145:395–397

6. Hindle WH, Chen EC. Accuracy of mammographic appearances after breast fine-needle aspiration. Am J Obstet Gynecol 1997;176:1286–1292

9 ASPIRATION CYTOLOGY OF BREAST CANCER: DEVELOPMENT AND ACCEPTANCE AS A DIAGNOSTIC PROCEDURE

William H. Kern

The use of aspiration biopsy smears to diagnose palpable masses, particularly breast tumors, was first developed in this country during the mid-1920s by Martin and Ellis at Memorial Hospital in New York and was described by them and by Stewart during the early 1930s. These authors reported in 1934 on their positive diagnoses of 280 breast cancers. They listed indications and advantages that we still accept, including the simplicity of the procedure, the lack of significant surgical complications, the minimal risk of tumor dissemination, the rapidity of the diagnosis, and the ability to reassure an anxious patient based on a negative diagnosis or to plan and proceed with definitive treatment if the diagnosis is positive. They also offered advice that is still pertinent today: "In our laboratory no diagnoses are rendered from aspirated material without reasonably full clinical data since an accurate knowledge of the exact source of the material is of major importance."

Despite the good results reported from Memorial Hospital, the procedure was not widely accepted for several decades. The reasons are that initially only 18-gauge needles were used to produce what essentially were "squeezed tissue preparations" rather than thin films. This practice was at least moderately uncomfortable for patients. At the same time, intraoperative frozen section techniques had been developed by surgical pathologists in the United States and were available at most major hospitals. Pathologists preferred this technique to a diagnosis based on the more limited sample of an aspiration smear.

The second impetus for the acceptance of aspiration cytology came from Europe. It was based on the experience of hematologists with fine-needle aspirations (FNAs) and was furthered by a relative lack, at most European hospitals, of readily available surgical pathologic services with rapid diagnoses. The FNAs produced thin films that could be air-dried and stained with Giemsa or wet-fixed and stained with the Papanicolaou technique. Franzen and Zajicek were prominent among the clinicians and pathologists who developed this procedure, and they established the first FNA clinic at the Karolinska Hospital in Stockholm in 1960. It was devoted primarily to tumor diagnosis and was staffed by full-time cytopathologists. FNA cytology quickly became popular in Europe and soon afterward was introduced more widely in the United States as well.

By 1979 I was able to compile 17 reports from the literature on the results of aspirations from 4687 breast cancers, with a rate of only 8.4% false-negative results and, based on aspirations of 7135 benign breast lesions, 1.1% false-positive results. At that time, to the best of my knowledge, the surgeons at my own institution (The Hospital of the Good Samaritan) were the only ones in Los Angeles who routinely performed mastectomy for breast cancer based on an FNA diagnosis without frozen section confirmation. This approach, of course, did and still does require strict cytologic criteria for a definitive diagnosis. Classifications such as "atypical" or "suspicious—biopsy recommended" must be used when indicated. During this period aspirations of 559 breast cancers and 349 benign lesions were performed: 306 (55%) of the cancers were classified as cytologically malignant and 114 (20%) as suspicious. The relatively high number of "insufficient material" or negative reports was at that time mainly due to the inexperience and sometimes inadequate technique of some of the physicians performing the aspirations, emphasizing the need for close cooperation between clinicians and pathologists. There were no false-positive diagnoses.

A great deal of experience has now been accumulated. At many other institutions in Los Angeles and throughout the United States, FNA of the breast is widely used and accepted as an important diagnostic procedure.

10 FINE-NEEDLE ASPIRATION CYTOLOGY OF THE BREAST

Barbara Florentine

Juan C. Felix

Fine-needle aspiration (FNA) has evolved as a standard procedure for the initial evaluation of a palpable breast mass. Ideally, the patient presents to a comprehensive breast diagnostic clinic where a multidisciplinary team, composed of a primary care provider, a cytopathologist, an imaging technician and radiologist, and an "on-call" surgeon evaluates her breast symptoms.

ROLE OF THE CYTOPATHOLOGIST

The cytopathologist may either perform the FNA procedure or assist the aspirator in obtaining a diagnostic cellular specimen. The major advantage of having the cytopathologist present is so each cellular sample may be assessed under the microscope until he or she is confident that a satisfactory specimen has been obtained. In addition, valuable information can be gained about the size, shape, and consistency of the mass from the way it "feels to the needle." The clinical impression is also helpful to the cytopathologist when performing the cytologic analysis. Cytopathologists who are isolated from the clinical scene may interpret FNA smears obtained by other physicians with extreme caution either because of receiving a less than optimal specimen or having inadequate clinical information.

Not all institutions and clinics have the luxury of a multidisciplinary breast team or a trained cytopathologist available under one roof. In these situations the primary care clinician should take responsibility for procuring the specimen and then sending it to be interpreted by a cytopathologist. This system is less than ideal but can work if (1) a complete and accurate history and physical description of the mass accompanies each sample; (2) well prepared slides of specimens taken from representative areas of the mass are submitted; and (3) open communication is established between the aspirator and cytopathologist. If these three practices are adhered to, the cytopathologist can render a definitive cytologic diagnosis in most cases.

It is of paramount importance to establish and maintain a collegial relationship with the cytopathologist who interprets your FNA biopsies. Before starting an

---

KEY PRACTICE POINTS

Breast fine-needle aspiration cytology: FNA cannot definitively differentiate ductal carcinoma in situ from invasive ductal carcinoma. FNA is not reliable for diagnosing benign or malignant sclerosing lesions or invasive lobular carcinoma. FNA does *not* definitively diagnose atypical ductal hyperplasia, atypical lobular hyperplasia, ductal carcinoma in situ, hamartoma (fibroadenolipoma), lipoma, lobular carcinoma in situ, papillary neoplasms, or sclerosing adenosis.

FNA service, it is highly recommended that you introduce yourself to the cytopathologist and establish open communication. The cytopathologist should feel comfortable notifying you if he or she has any difficulty with the sample preparation or has any questions concerning the patient. Alternatively, if your institution supports an FNA service, you can send the patient directly to the clinic where the lesion can be aspirated by the cytopathologist.

DIAGNOSTIC TRIAD

When the cytopathologist viewing a breast FNA slide under the microscope makes a diagnosis, he or she not only considers the cytologic findings but relies on the clinical and radiologic evidence submitted to support the diagnosis. This constellation of clinical, radiologic, and FNA results is popularly known as the diagnostic triad, or triple test. It has been shown to approach a diagnostic sensitivity and specificity of 100% when all three parameters of the triad are in concordance. Primary care providers are sometimes unaware that the cytopathologist needs information concerning the clinical and imaging studies. The cells on the FNA slide often do not give a conclusive diagnosis but present the cytopathologist with cytologic clues, which can support the clinical impression. Presenting relevant clinical information to the cytopathologist ensures an optimal cytologic diagnosis.

SLIDE PREPARATION AND FIXATION

It is critical to the value of FNA cytology to have well prepared slides made from representative samples of the breast mass. Poorly prepared slides and slides with scant cellularity can give inaccurate cytologic diagnoses. A cytopathologist presented with such slides tends to write an ambiguous report (e.g., "atypical cells present—could be a fibroadenoma, carcinoma, or even normal breast; recommend excision biopsy for definitive diagnosis"). These "nondiagnoses" are not helpful; and when FNA is used in this manner it loses its clinical purpose and becomes a superfluous layer in the diagnostic algorithm. Furthermore, the aspirating clinician who reads the diagnosis of "atypical cells" is obligated to evaluate the lesion further, even though he or she may be convinced that the lesion is clinically benign. Thus the patient is forced to have an additional procedure, most often a tissue core-needle biopsy (TCNB) or an open surgical biopsy (OSBx) to prove the lesion is benign. The frustrated primary care provider may be tempted to abandon the FNA technique in the future because he or she incorrectly concludes that the procedure is clinically useless.

Once a cellular specimen has been obtained, the next task is to prepare the smears properly. This step is crucial because no matter how well the FNA is performed the results can be useless if the slides cannot be interpreted owing to artifact caused by crushing or drying.

To prepare the specimen, the aspirator first attaches a 10-cc syringe partially filled with air to the needle containing the specimen (Fig. 10.1). Next, with the bevel of the needle tip on the slide close to the frosted end, the material is blown out in one drop onto the slide (Fig. 10.2). It is important to place the needle tip

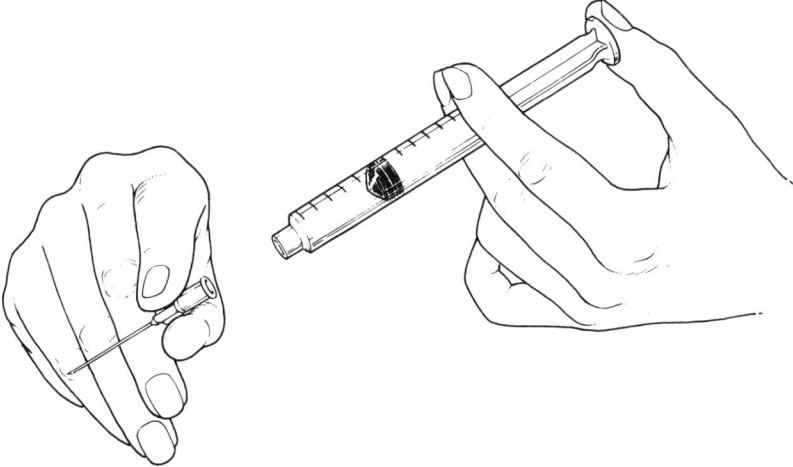

Figure 10.1.   Syringe is partially filled with air and then attached to the needle containing the FNA cellular specimen.

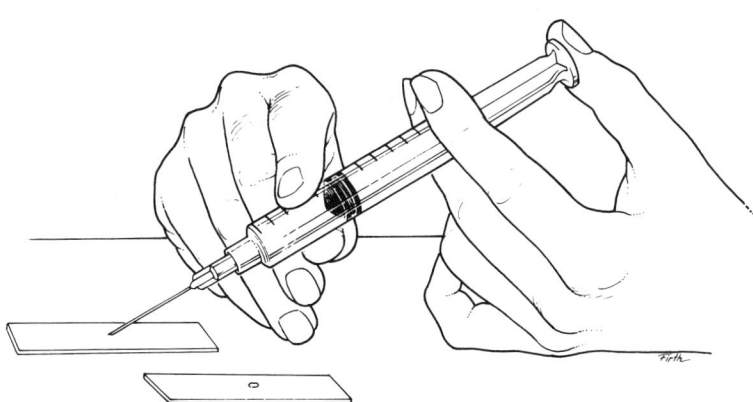

Figure 10.2.   With the needle held bevel-down at about a 45-degree angle to the slide, air in the syringe is forcefully ejected, depositing a drop of fluid containing the cellular material on the slide.

directly on the slide to prevent splattering and air-drying of the specimen. After the material is expressed, a quick look can determine if an additional FNA "pass" (puncture) is necessary to ensure adequate cellular sampling of the mass. For example, if the drop appears oily (suggesting that fat is present) with no evidence of cellular material, it may indicate that the mass has been missed, a sampling error.

To prepare the smear, a second slide is placed over the first (Fig. 10.3), and the drop of specimen (which may be no larger than a pinhead) is allowed to spread evenly between the two slides as they are gently pulled apart with an easy sliding motion (Fig. 10.4). Alternate methods of slide smearing/preparation are depicted in Figure 10.5 showing the pull method of spreading the cellular material (Fig. 10.5A) and the open air-dried slide (Fig. 10.5B).

The next step depends on which type of stain is used on the slides. Most cytopathologists like to have one or two slides stained with Romanowsky-type (Wright-Giemsa) stains, and one or two with the Papanicolaou stain because each stain highlights different cellular and nuclear characteristics. In our Breast Diagnostic Center (BDC) an ultrafast Papanicolaou stain is used primarily.[1]

Preparation for Romanowsky-type stained slides is straightforward. After smearing, these slides are placed on a clean flat area, allowed to air-dry completely, and then placed in a slide folder suitable for secure shipment to the cytopathology laboratory. Preparation of the smear for the Papanicolaou stain is more complicated. This stain requires that the slides be "fixed" (preserved)

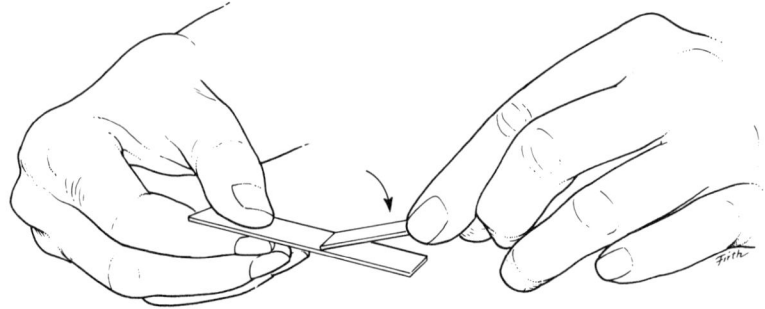

Figure 10.3.   A second slide is placed over the drop of cellular fluid.

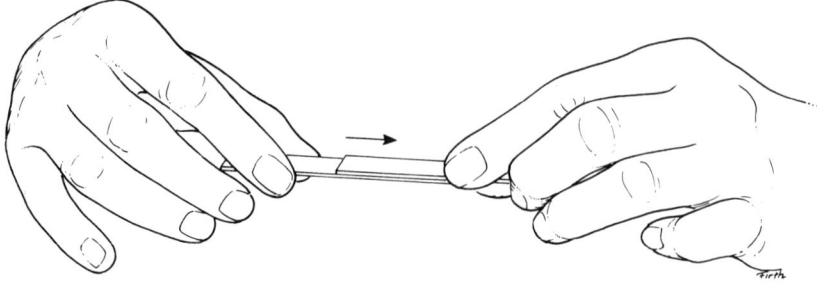

Figure 10.4.   The two slides are gently pulled apart, smearing the drop between them.

immediately after being smeared; otherwise the cells begin to dry out, causing artifactual cellular distortion. There are two ways to "fix" the slide for the Papanicolaou stain: (1) the immersion method and (2) the spray fixative method. The immersion method involves placing the slides directly into a jar of 95% alcohol, or "Pap fixative" (Fig. 10.6) and shipping the entire container to the cytopathology laboratory. If this method is to be used, the top of the jar should be removed before beginning the FNA procedure so the specimen may be smeared and immediately dropped into the fixative container to prevent air-drying and resultant cytologic artifact. Paper clips can be attached to the top of each slide to prevent the slides from sticking to each other in the jar (Fig. 10.7).

The spray fixative method uses the same principles that are used to fix a cervical Papanicolaou smear. If this method is used, the spray is applied to each slide

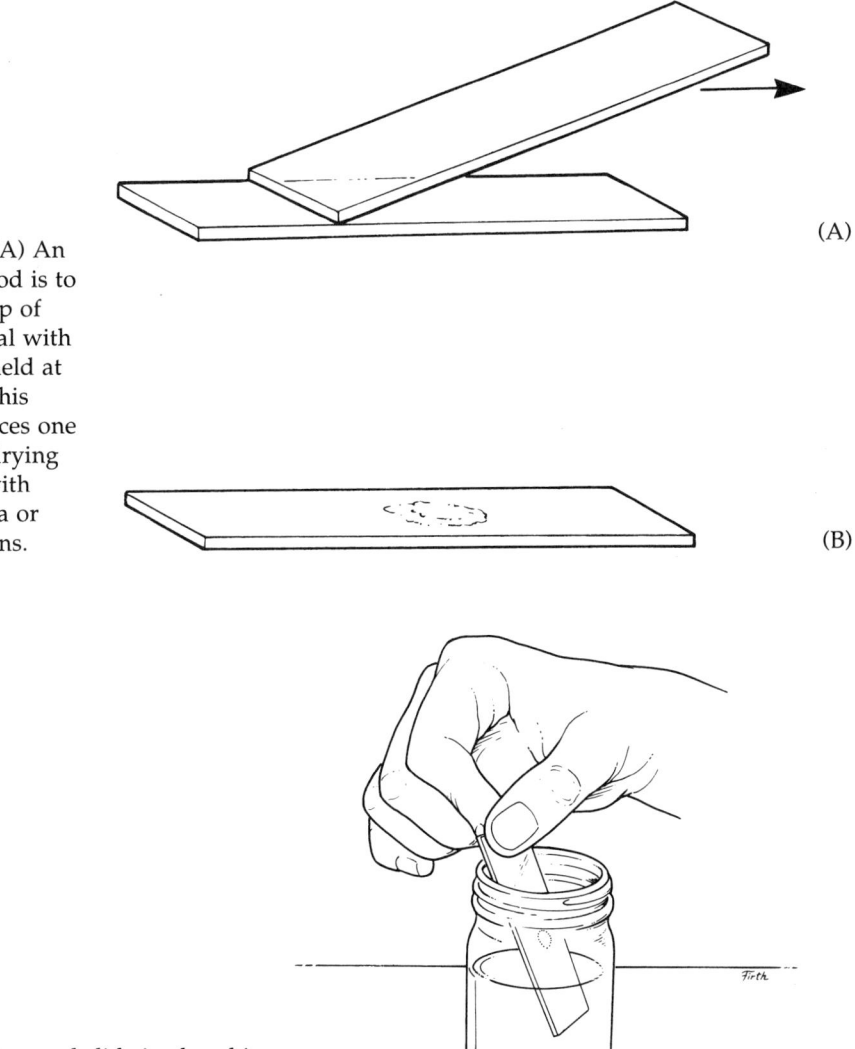

(A)

Figure 10.5. (A) An alternate method is to spread the drop of cellular material with another slide held at an angle. (B) This practice produces one smear for air-drying and staining with Wright–Giemsa or equivalent stains.

(B)

Figure 10.6. Smeared slide is placed in a bottle of 95% alcohol (Papanicolaou fixative).

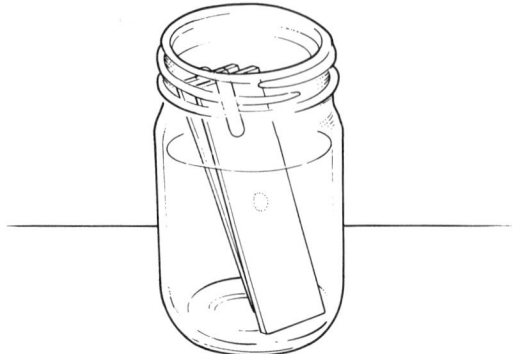

Figure 10.7. Paper clips attached to the upper end of each slide keep the slide surfaces separated in the fixative.

immediately after it has been smeared (use of an assistant expedites the process). Spray fixatives produce more cellular smears than the immersion technique, but the cells are not as well preserved.

After the slides are smeared, the sample adequacy can be assessed by holding the slides up to a light to see if small "tissue fragments" are visible on the slide. If so, the specimen is probably adequate for cytologic evaluation. If the immersion technique is used, observe the slides through the glass jar but do not remove them. Examining the slides outside of the fixative is discouraged, as drying artifact can occur rapidly and may be irreversible.

Rapid assessment of an FNA smear to check for adequacy of the cell sample can be performed on air-dried smears stained with Diff-Quik, a stable commercially available stain (Baxter Scientific, Irvine, CA). An alternative approach is the use of toluidine blue–eosin stain, which takes less than 2 minutes.[2]

If, despite following the above suggestions, the primary care provider finds it difficult to make high quality smears, an alternative method is to rinse the needle directly into a fluid-based collection system (e.g., 50% alcohol or Saccamono's carbowax fixative) and then send the liquid containing the cellular specimen to the cytopathology laboratory for processing. The laboratory centrifuges the liquid specimen and makes a slide from the cell button that accumulates in the bottom of the centrifuge tube. The liquid-based cytology collection solutions, such as those used by ThinPrep (Cytyc Corporation, Boxborough, MA) or Cytorich (AutoCyte, Elon College, NC) procedures, provide excellent collection media and produce equally high quality slides with few or no artifacts. The advantage of these systems is that they do not require skill in slide-making. Unfortunately, they do not allow immediate assessment of cell sample adequacy at the time of the FNA.

Cytology of the Breast

The physiologic functional unit of the breast is the terminal duct lobular unit (TDLU), which architecturally resembles a hollow bunch of grapes, where the ducts are the stems and the lobules are the grapes. In the nonpregnant state the lobules are rudimentary and not developed to maturity. During lactation the lobules evolve into true acini, which secrete milk. The ducts act as a conduit to the nipple where the milk is discharged. The TDLUs are embedded in the adipose and stromal (fibrous) connective tissue of the breast.

Cytology of Normal Breast Cells

There are four main cell types in the breast: epithelial, myoepithelial, adipose, and stromal (fibrous). The ducts and lobules are lined by one or sometimes more layers of epithelial cells. The lobular cells have secretory and absorptive roles. The myoepithelial cells are contractile and surround the ducts and lobules; they are responsible for squeezing the milk out of the lobules and into the major collecting ducts. Stromal cells (fibroblasts) and adipose (fat) cells make up most of the breast volume and provide support for the TDLUs.

Epithelial, Foam, and Apocrine Cells

Benign ductal epithelial cells seen in breast aspirates are usually cohesive, small, and relatively uniform. The nucleus is round to oval and is about twice the size of a red blood cell. The cytoplasm is usually scanty. In benign lesions, ductal cells may be seen in sheets, with branching tree-like or antler shapes, or in papillary configurations. The sheets represent ducts that have been sheared apart during preparation of the smear, and the antler shapes represent intact three-dimensional branching ducts that have been aspirated.

Foam cells (histiocytes) are derived from either duct cells or macrophages. They are found singly in both benign and malignant aspirates. The foam cell is so named because of its abundant foamy cytoplasm.

Apocrine cells represent metaplasia of the lobular epithelium into a sweat gland ("apocrine") type and are found in benign conditions such as fibrocystic changes, fibroadenoma, and cysts. They can be found singly or in sheets. They have abundant finely granular, pink cytoplasm (with hematoxylin and eosin or Papanicolaou stains) and contain centrally or eccentrically placed nuclei with prominent nucleoli.

Myoepithelial cells are represented in breast FNA smears by football-shaped ("bipolar") nuclei that are stripped of cytoplasm. These "naked" or "bare" nuclei (without attached cytoplasm) are usually scattered around singly throughout the smear. The presence of numerous bipolar cell nuclei on a smear is a good indication that the lesion is benign. Hence these nuclei are sometimes called "sentinel" nuclei.

Stromal and Adipose Cells

Stromal cells (fibroblasts) contain elongated nuclei and secrete a myxoid to collagenous extracellular material seen most often in fibroadenomas or as a desmoplastic reaction in carcinomas. Adipose cells appear as clusters of large round to polygonal cells with clear cytoplasm. Usually small blood vessels can be seen within the fatty fragments.

The characteristic microscopic appearance of FNA cytology from normal breast tissue is depicted in Figures 10.8 and 10.9 and Color Plates 3 and 4. The cellular elements commonly seen in fine-needle aspiration smears of normal breast tissue are listed in Table 10.1.

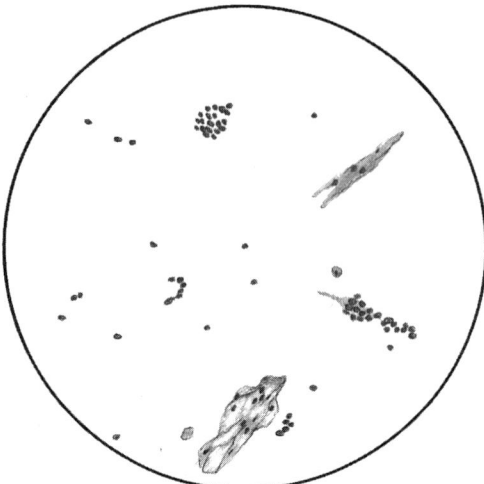

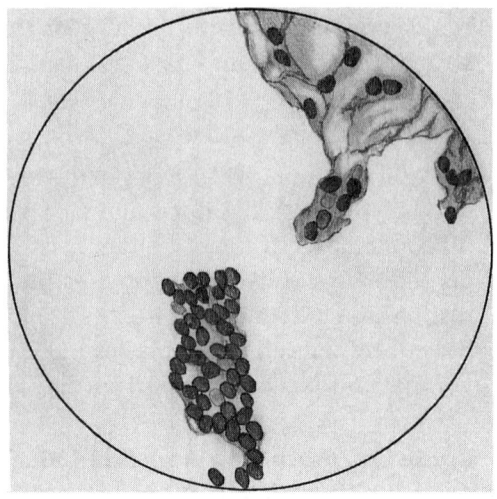

Figure 10.8. Low-power magnification of an FNA smear obtained from normal breast tissue depicting small cohesive clusters of normal breast components.

Figure 10.9. High-power magnification of an FNA smear from normal breast tissue depicting a small cohesive aggregate of benign ductal epithelial cells and a cluster of adipose cells with their typical clear cytoplasm.

Table 10.1. Cellular elements characteristic of an FNA smear from normal breast tissue

Widely scattered cellular elements

Small clumps of benign ductal epithelial cells

Stroma (connective tissue fragments)

Adipose tissue (fat)

Inflammation

An FNA slide of tissue taken from a patient with an acute breast infection or abscess shows neutrophils, macrophages, scattered epithelial cells, and debris. Bacteria may be present. The subareolar fistula or abscess, a specific subtype of infection, contains squamous material in addition to the inflammatory cells. These subareolar lesions tend to recur and require excision for definitive therapy.

Granulomatous inflammation of the breast is most often idiopathic. An etiologic agent is only rarely identified (e.g., *Mycobacterium* or fungus). The hallmark of granulomatous mastitis is finding granulomas or multinucleated cells.

Fat Necrosis

Fat necrosis can be seen after trauma or, rarely, accompanying a carcinoma. It represents the reaction of the body to traumatized fat. Cytologically, large foamy macrophages, calcifications, and dead (necrotic) fat cells are seen.

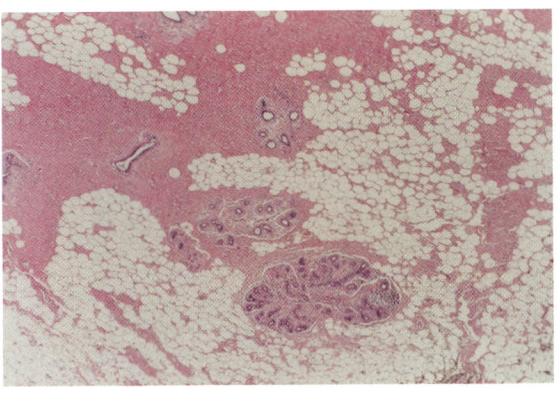

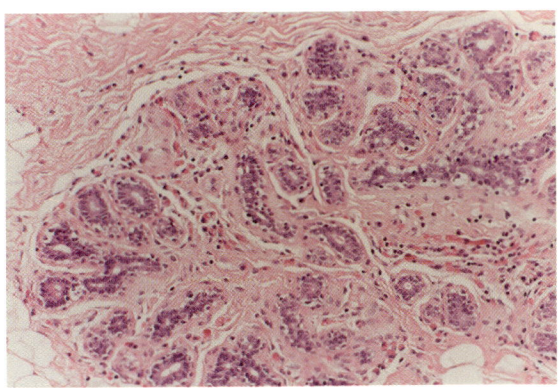

Plate 1. Normal breast histology, low power (original magnification ×40). Normal breast components are present including terminal ductal lobular units imbedded in fibrous and adipose tissue. Fat cells compose the majority of the breast tissue volume.

Plate 2. Normal breast histology, high power (original magnification ×200). A single layer of ductal cells sparsely encircled by elongated myoepithelial cells forms the acini within surrounding fibrous tissue. A well-demarcated terminal duct lobular unit is seen on the left.

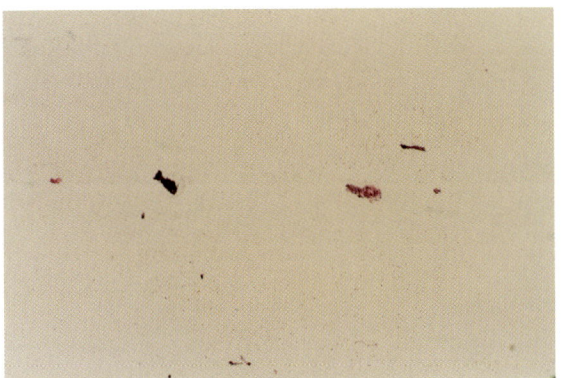

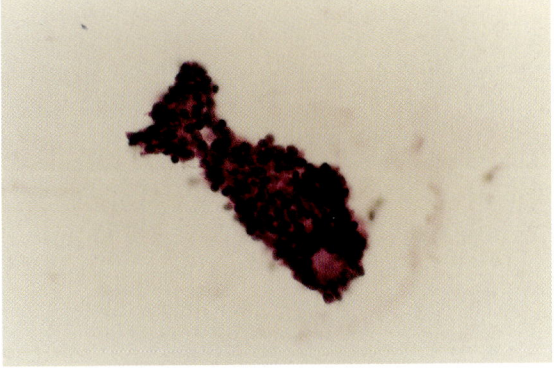

Plate 3. Normal breast cytology, low power (original magnification ×40). The smear is characteristically hypocellular with small cohesive clusters of adipose tissue (center-right) and of ductal cells (center-left).

Plate 4. Normal breast cytology, high power (original magnification ×200). The benign ductal cells are compact, uniform, and cohesive in a tight cluster.

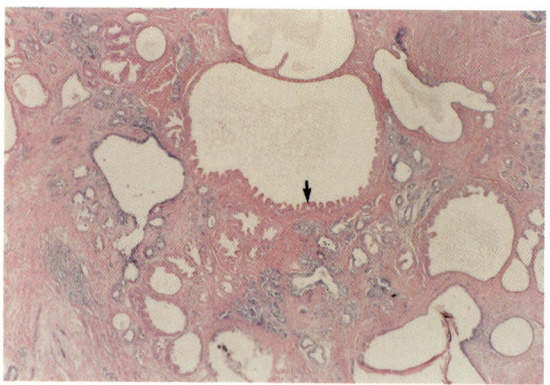

Plate 5. Fibrocystic changes, histology, low power (original magnification ×40). Microcysts and mild degrees of epithelial ductal hyperplasia are seen with increased fibrosis in the surrounding stroma. Many of the microcysts are lined by the typical apocrine metaplasia of ductal cells (solid arrow).

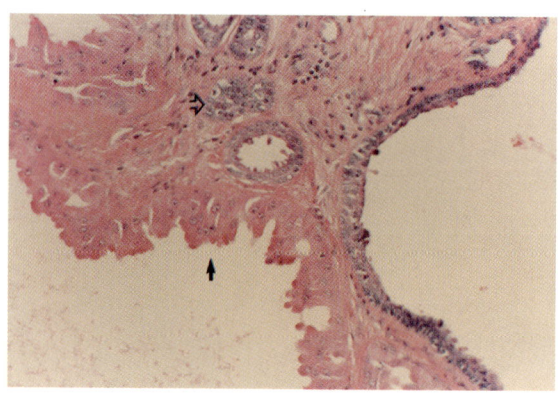

Plate 6. Fibrocystic changes, histology, high power (original magnification ×200). Apocrine metaplasia (solid arrow) of ductal cells is prominent with characteristic abundant eosinophilic cytoplasm (on the left). A central duct (hollow arrow) shows mild epithelial hyperplasia. A dilated duct or microcyst lined with the usual ductal epithelium is seen on the right. The surrounding stroma is fibrotic.

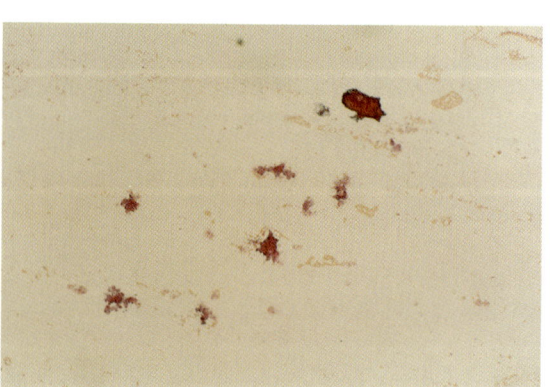

Plate 7. Fibrocystic changes, cytology, low power (original magnification ×40). Scattered clusters of dense fibrous tissue and of apocrine (ductal) cells are seen. Large histiocytes (foam cells) are present in a clear background.

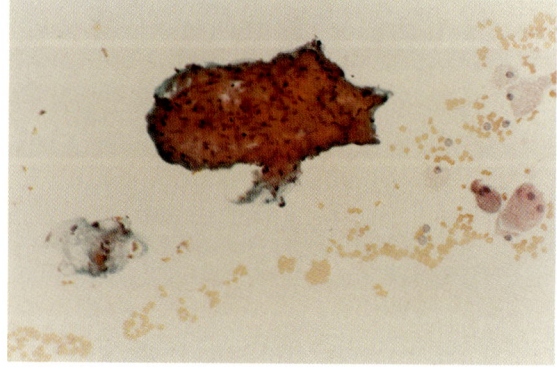

Plate 8. Fibrocystic changes, cytology, high power (original magnification ×400). Dense fibrous tissue often predominates in a smear. Foamy histiocytes (at the right) are frequently seen. Benign ductal cells should be identified elsewhere in the smear to confirm the benign nature of the lesion. In this picture, there are numerous small brownish-colored red blood cells in the background.

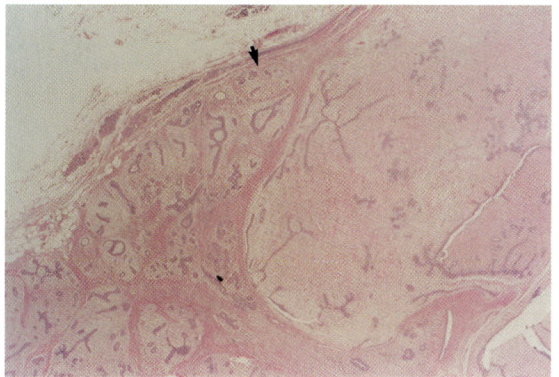

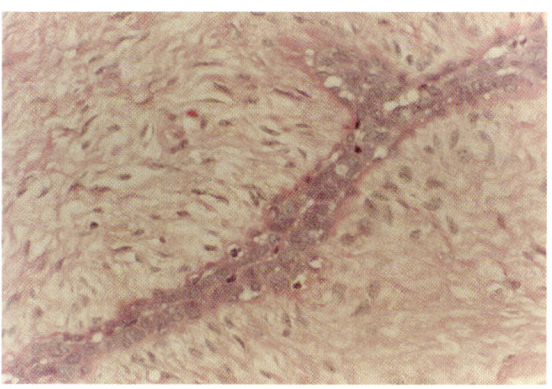

Plate 9. Fibroadenoma, histology, low power (original magnification ×40). There is a well-demarcated border (solid arrow) separating the solid fibroadenoma from the normal breast tissue. The fibroadenoma has the characteristic elongated branching glandular pattern of ductal cells surrounded by pale, hypocellular stroma.

Plate 10. Fibroadenoma, histology, high power (original magnification ×400). The elongated slit-like glands contain a single layer of uniform ductal epithelial cells with occasional outer small* elongated myoepithelial cells. The surrounding stroma is formed of finely arranged collagen bundles with interspersed small* fibrocytes. [*compared to ductal cells]

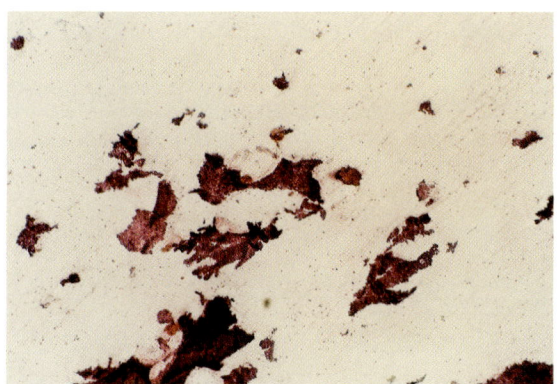

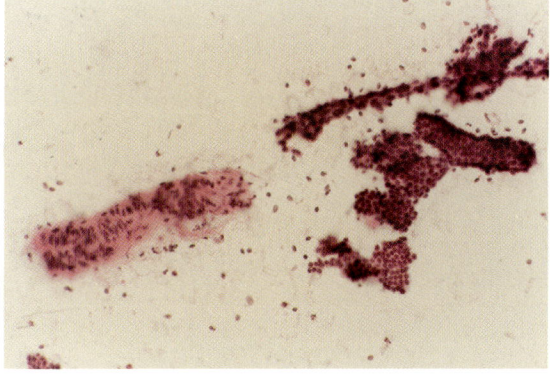

Plate 11. Fibroadenoma, cytology, low power (original magnification ×40). There are numerous monolayer clusters of extremely cohesive ductal epithelial cells with antler-like formations. The background is filled with scattered, single, small, naked (without cytoplasm), elongated (bipolar) nuclei.

Plate 12. Fibroadenoma, cytology high power (original magnification ×200). The epithelial monolayer clusters are composed of uniform, small, evenly spaced ductal cells that are delineated sharply at the cluster edge. A fragment of characteristically cellular stroma and numerous scattered myoepithelial cell naked nuclei (bipolar/elongated shape without attached cytoplasm) are present.

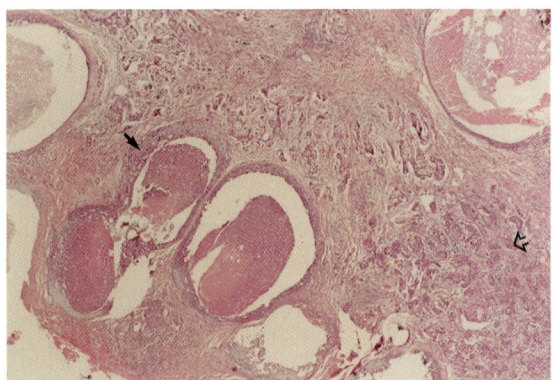

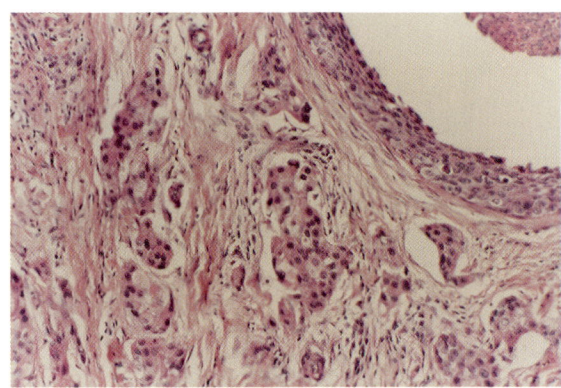

Plate 13. Invasive ductal carcinoma, histology, low power (original magnification ×40). This tumor is composed of infiltrating ductal carcinoma and areas of in situ ductal carcinoma (solid arrow) with typical necrotic centers within the intact duct. Dilated ducts lined by proliferating epithelial cells, which are delimited by the basement membrane, characterize the in situ component. The invasive component (hollow arrow) presents as small aggregates of malignant cells and single malignant cells infiltrating through the stroma.

Plate 14. Invasive ductal carcinoma, histology, high power (original magnification ×200). Invasive clusters of enlarged, irregularly shaped, hyperchromatic ductal epithelial cells are infiltrating the benign stroma. A portion of a duct containing in situ ductal carcinoma is present in the upper right corner of the picture.

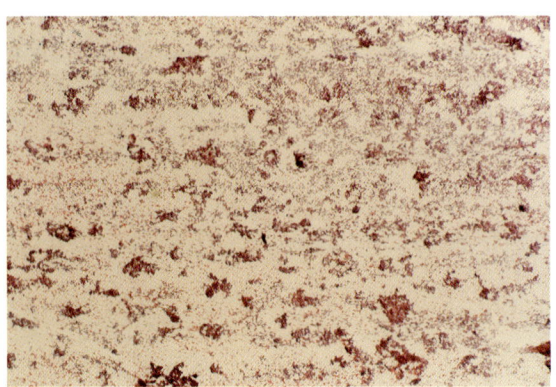

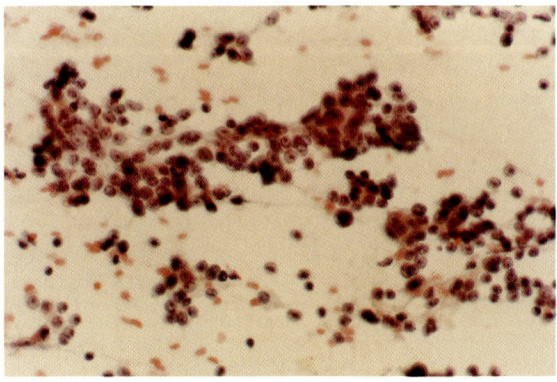

Plate 15. Invasive ductal carcinoma, cytology, low power (original magnification ×40). The entire smear is covered with abundant, poorly cohesive, malignant ductal cells with a "dirty" background of blood and necrotic debris.

Plate 16. Invasive ductal carcinoma, cytology, high power (original magnification ×200). Numerous poorly cohesive (dyshesive) clusters of malignant ductal cells as well as abundant, characteristic single, malignant cells are present. The malignant ductal cell nuclei are enlarged and irregularly sized with prominent macronucleoli.

Hyperplastic Lesions

Hyperplastic lesions are masses that are presumed to develop because of hormonal influences (e.g., lactational adenoma and lactation-associated epithelial hyperplasia). The most common hyperplastic lesions are pregnancy-associated breast lesions and fibrocystic changes. If the hormonal stimulus is removed, many of the lesions regress.

Pregnancy-Associated Breast Lesions

A lactating adenoma presents as a discrete breast mass in a pregnant or lactating woman. Lactation-associated epithelial hyperplasia is often less discrete and poorly demarcated. Both conditions are presumed to represent a localized hypersensitivity response to the pregnancy hormones, rather than a benign neoplasia as its name suggests. Typically the FNA smear shows abundant cellular material and contains intact and disrupted lobules which, because they are actively secreting milk, are fully developed or "hyperplastic." Many single dyshesive epithelial cells are seen. The nucleoli are prominent, especially in the lobules where protein (in this case milk) synthesis occurs. Numerous single epithelial cell nuclei devoid of cytoplasm are scattered on the slide as the fragile cytoplasm filled with milk bursts when it is smeared, giving rise to a "dirty" background on the slide. The features of abundant cellularity, dyshesion of cells, prominent nucleoli, and a dirty background are shared with cancer. Therefore it is important to convey the history of pregnancy or lactation to the cytopathologist.

Fibrocystic Change

In the past, fibrocystic change (FCC) of the breast was referred to as "fibrocystic disease." It is now appreciated that FCC is not a disease at all but a constellation of physiologically induced changes that are present in varying degrees in almost all premenopausal women.

Tissue with FCCs is aspirated when some of the elements coalesce to form a dominant mass discovered by palpation that becomes worrisome to the clinician or patient. FCCs are composed of three elements in varying proportions: cysts, fibrosis, and epithelial proliferation. Each element is described separately below, although all three are often found in the same aspirate. The cellular elements commonly seen in FNA smears of FCCs are listed in Table 10.2. Examples of FNA of FCCs are pictured in Color Plates 7 and 8.

Table 10.2. Cellular elements characteristic of an FNA smear from fibrocystic changes

Widely scattered cellular elements
Small clumps of benign ductal epithelial cells
Apocrine metaplasia of benign ductal cells
Histiocytes (foam cells)
Stroma (connective tissue)
Proteinaceous debris (cyst fluid)

Cysts

Cysts associated with the spectrum of FCC are called simple cysts (to differentiate them from complex cysts, which may be neoplastic). Simple cysts vary in size from microscopic to several centimeters and may be single or multiple. A cyst can enlarge to a size that is readily palpable and most commonly presents as a smooth, mobile, sometimes tender mass. When aspirated, the cyst usually yields clear serous to murky yellow-green fluid. Because such fluids are rarely (<1:1000) neoplastic, most clinicians question the value of examining cyst fluid cytologically. In fact, cyst fluid cytology has been shown not to be a cost-effective method for detecting neoplasms and rarely alters clinical management. When cytologic examination of cyst fluid is performed, the picture is often acellular or reveals foam cells and sometimes apocrine cells.

Following complete aspiration of a cyst, the area should be palpated to determine if a residual mass is present. Any such mass should be reaspirated and the cellular specimen sent for cytologic examination because this finding points toward a neoplastic (complex) cyst or may represent a neoplasm that was underneath the aspirated cyst. Bloody (nontraumatic) fluid is usually from a complex cyst and therefore should be sent to the cytopathology laboratory for analysis and potential cellular diagnosis.

Fibrosis

The fibrous component of FCC is underrepresented or not present in most FNA specimens. This type of dense tissue does not aspirate easily. Therefore an aspirate obtained from an area of FCC composed mainly of fibrous tissue yields a paucicellular aspirate. Such specimens are difficult to assess and may be assigned a diagnosis of "unsatisfactory" by the cytopathologist unless he or she is confident the lesion was adequately sampled.

Epithelial Hyperplasia

Epithelial hyperplasia refers to a piling up of more than two cell layers in the lumen of the breast ducts. It occurs less often in lobules. Epithelial hyperplasia is subclassified according to its architectural and cytologic severity as mild, moderate, or severe (florid). With severe hyperplasia the duct lumen is filled with a proliferating polyclonal epithelial cell population. Atypical hyperplasia refers to hyperplasia that shares some cytologic features with carcinoma. Epithelial hyperplasia, particularly the atypical type, places a woman at increased risk for the development of carcinoma. However, most women with proliferative fibrocystic changes never develop breast cancer.

A smear of ductal hyperplasia shows sheets and antler configurations composed of cohesive, mildly to moderately crowded epithelial cells. The sentinel myoepithelial cells are seen scattered in the background. Sometimes the differential diagnosis between ductal hyperplasia and fibroadenoma cannot be made by cytology with certainty. In that situation, the diagnosis relies on the clinical impression from the clinical breast examination (CBE). However, if the FNA suggests atypical ductal hyperplasia, a specific definitive diagnosis should be confirmed by tissue histology obtained by TCNB or OSBx.

Tumors of the Breast

Fibroadenoma

A palpable fibroadenoma presents as a discrete, mobile, three-dimensional mass consisting of both epithelial and stromal proliferation. The FNA aspirate is cellular and typically shows the triad of ductal epithelial cells, myoepithelial nuclei, and stromal fragments. Although the cytologic triad is not present in all aspirates of fibroadenomas, when all three elements are present it ensures the definitive cytologic diagnosis of fibroadenoma.

The ductal epithelial cells are numerous and are found in extremely cohesive monolayer sheets and antler configurations. Abundant bipolar nuclei (representing myoepithelial cells) are often prominent and scattered throughout. Stromal fragments are usually present and consist of fibromyxoid stroma with embedded spindle cells. Stromal fragments may be particularly difficult to detect in FNA specimens of older women, as the stroma becomes more fibrotic with aging and extremely difficult to aspirate.

The characteristic microscopic appearance of the FNA cytology from a fibroadenoma is depicted in Figures 10.10 and 10.11 and Color Plates 11 and 12. The cellular elements commonly seen in FNA smears of a fibroadenoma are listed in Table 10.3.

Papillomas

Papillomas usually arise from the large ducts underneath the areola. The patient characteristically presents with a serosanguineous or bloody nipple discharge emanating from a single duct opening on the nipple. Although a smear of bloody

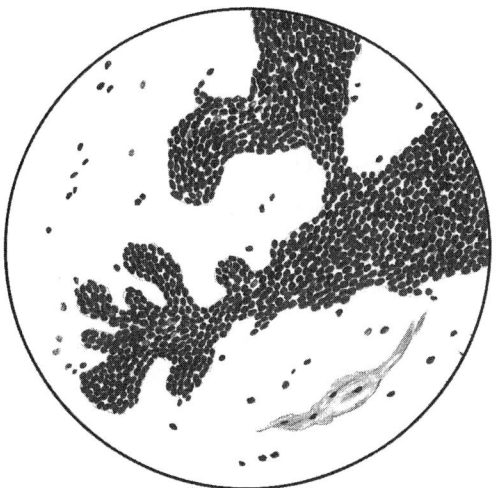

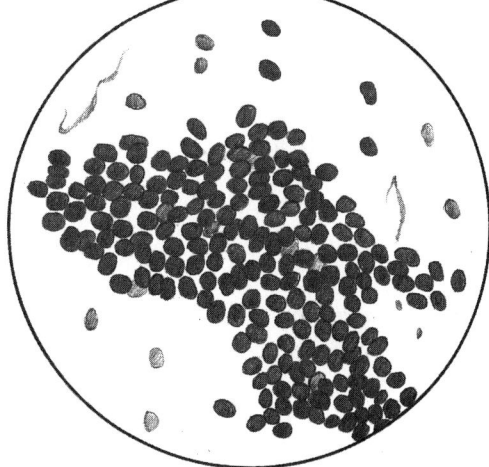

Figure 10.10. Low-power magnification of an FNA smear from a fibroadenoma depicting the typical antler-like sheets of cohesive ductal epithelial cells surrounded by "naked" nuclei.

Figure 10.11. High-power magnification of an FNA smear from a fibroadenoma depicting the uniformity in size and shape of the ductal cell nuclei.

Table 10.3. Cellular elements characteristic of an FNA smear from a fibroadenoma

Abundant cellular elements

Abundant sheets (monolayers) of cohesive benign ductal
    cells

Abundant bare (naked) bipolar nuclei

Stroma (connective tissue)

No adipose tissue (fat)

nipple discharge can be sent to the cytopathologist for examination, it seldom produces a definitive cytologic diagnosis. Further diagnostic procedures are usually required. Finally, nipple smears of nonbloody discharge have been shown not to be cost-effective and rarely influence clinical management.

An FNA of a palpable papilloma is usually bloody. The lesion grows within the duct lumen and may block the duct, causing formation of a complex cyst. The aspirator should aspirate as much fluid as possible and then aspirate any residual solid areas.

Cytologically, a papilloma shows spherical aggregates of epithelial cells (cell balls) and papillary clusters. Hemosiderin-laden macrophages are often present and indicate prior bleeding.

Ductal papillomatosis refers to small, multiple papillomas that arise within peripheral ducts. These lesions are rarely palpable.

It may be difficult to differentiate between a papilloma and the less common papillary carcinoma by FNA cytology. Thus it is recommended that these lesions be diagnosed as "papillary lesions" and that they be excised (OSBx) for a definitive histologic diagnosis.

Cancer

The most common malignancy of the breast is adenocarcinoma. Carcinomas, by definition, are malignant tumors arising from epithelial cells. Most carcinomas of the breast arise in the TDLUs and are called either ductal or lobular type, depending on the morphology of the cancer cells. About 80% of adenocarcinomas are infiltrating ductal carcinomas. Although most of the ductal carcinomas are of the "usual" type ("not otherwise specified," or NOS), there are several subtypes of ductal carcinoma, including medullary, colloid, apocrine, tubular, and metaplastic. The various subtypes of carcinoma generally have a better prognosis than those of the usual (ductal) cell type. However, subtyping cancers on FNA smears can be difficult. It is generally advisable to base the definitive classification on histology.

Lobular carcinomas comprise fewer than 10% of all breast carcinomas. However, it is important to diagnose this specific type because lobular carcinoma is more likely to be bilateral and multicentric.

Most invasive (infiltrating) carcinomas begin in the TDLU and then cross the basement membrane to invade the surrounding stroma and adipose tissue. The term "ductal carcinoma in situ" (DCIS) is used to designate those malignant ductal neoplasms that are confined to the ducts and TDLUs. In situ carcinomas removed at this stage have an excellent prognosis. Most DCIS are nonpalpable lesions and are discovered by mammography (often by the presence of irregular, dense, clustered microcalcifications). In the United States 14-gauge stereotactic mammographically guided TCNB, rather than FNA, is usually performed to diagnose nonpalpable lesions. Nonetheless, some breast cancer centers in the United States with high volumes of cases are using FNA cytology to diagnose nonpalpable masses, with excellent results.

The two cytologic hallmarks of malignant epithelial tumors are the loose attachment of the cancer cells to each other (dyshesion) and the variability in the size and shape of the nuclei (pleomorphism). With rare exceptions, FNA smears of a cancer have abundant cells that can be seen in loosely coherent clusters or that are individually scattered throughout the smear. The cells generally show variability in size and shape within a smear. The cytology of moderately to poorly differentiated carcinomas reveals an FNA cellular aspirate consisting of large, pleomorphic cells exhibiting dyshesion. The nucleus/cytoplasm ratio is increased, and the nuclei appear dark (hyperchromatic). Bipolar "naked" nuclei are not present. Necrosis and mitotic figures are often identified.

The characteristic microscopic appearance of the FNA cytology from invasive ductal adenocarcinoma is depicted in Figures 10.12 and 10.13 and in Color Plates 15 and 16. The cellular elements commonly seen in FNA smears of breast adenocarcinoma are listed in Table 10.4.

Well differentiated carcinomas are sometimes more difficult to diagnose by cytology alone because of their bland features and resemblance to normal ductal

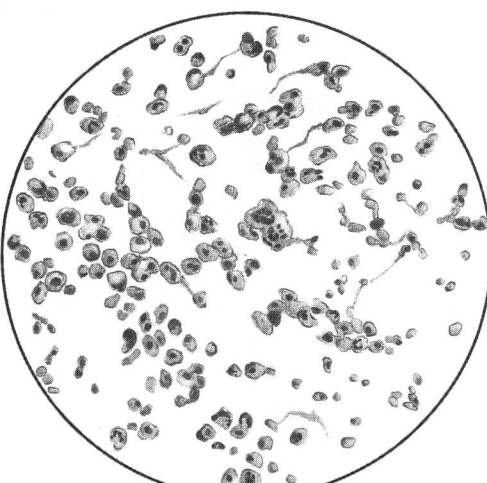

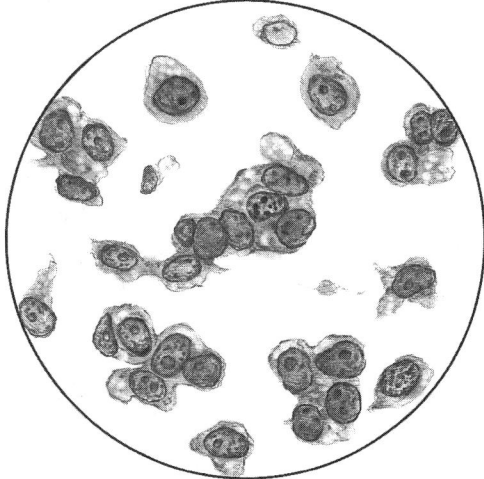

Figure 10.12. Low-power magnification of an FNA smear from an invasive adenocarcinoma depicting the typical dyshesive pattern of carcinoma.

Figure 10.13. High-power magnification of an FNA smear from an invasive adeno-carcinoma depicting the typical irregularity of nuclear size and shape, increased nuclear size, and increased nucleus/cytoplasm ratio seen with carcinoma.

Table 10.4. Cellular elements characteristic of an FNA smear from invasive adenocarcinoma

Abundant cellular elements
"Dirty" background containing abundant and various debris
Abundant dyshesive cells with pleomorphic nuclei
Variable hyperchromasia of the pleomorphic nuclei
Prominent nucleoli in the pleomorphic malignant nuclei
Abundant single cells with malignant nuclear features
Blood (RBCs and WBCs)
Occasional stroma
Adipose tissue may be present from the tissue surrounding the cancer

cells. In these instances the cytopathologist notes only mild nuclear irregularities or subtle degrees of hyperchromasia that are disturbing yet not fully diagnostic of carcinoma. In these instances a diagnosis of "atypical ductal cells" is rendered, and further diagnostic studies are generally recommended.

Lobular carcinomas are often more challenging to diagnose by FNA, as the cells are small and more regular than those of ductal carcinoma. Furthermore, the smears may be paucicellular due to the associated fibrosis, which is often present in these cancers. Again, a high index of suspicion for these lesions should be entertained upon a cytologic diagnosis of ductal cell atypia.

Nonepithelial Tumors

Nonepithelial malignant tumors of the breast include malignant phyllodes tumors, sarcomas, and malignant lymphomas. The cytology of a phyllodes tumor requires keen attention and a detailed clinical history. The low-grade phyllodes tumors may be indistinguishable from fibroadenomas by FNA cytology. Clinical features (e.g., the size or rapid growth of the lesion) can raise the suspicion of the diagnosis of a phyllodes tumor. Like fibroadenomas, phyllodes tumors are biphasic and contain sheets of benign ductal cells and stromal fragments. Generally, the increase in the cellularity of the stromal component and the occasional atypia of the fibroblasts suggest the cytologic diagnosis.

Sarcoma and malignant lymphomas are usually obvious to both clinician and cytopathologist. Their FNA smears frequently exhibit abundant, extremely high-grade malignant cells.

Conclusions

The successful application of breast FNA relies heavily on close communication between the clinician (primary care provider) and the cytopathologist. FNA cytology, the clinical impression, and the imaging report comprise the diagnostic triad, which, when the results are concordant, yields a reliable, accurate diagnosis that can be used with confidence as the basis for clinical management.

References

1. Yang GCH, Alvarez II. Ultrafast Papanicolaou stain: an alternative preparation for fine needle aspiration cytology. Acta Cytol 1995;39:55–60
2. Ducatman BS, Hogan CL, Wang HH. A triage system for processing fine needle aspiration cytology specimens. Acta Cytol 1989;33:797–799

11 PATHOLOGY OF THE FEMALE BREAST

Juan C. Felix

INFLAMMATORY LESIONS OF THE BREAST

Inflammatory conditions of the breast can be divided into two general categories: acute mastitis and chronic mastitis. Acute mastitis is seen predominantly during lactation. During this time the nipple may develop cracks and fissures, which may become colonized or infected by bacteria, predominantly of the *Staphylococcus* species. The ensuing infection affects predominantly the ducts, although inflammation of the surrounding soft tissues and skin may occur. The lesions are characterized by an acute inflammatory infiltrate involving, or centered on, the ductal system. Failure to treat this acute process, or inadequate treatment, may result in the formation of an abscess. This latter entity is characterized by large accumulations of inflammatory cells and amorphous necrotic debris with destruction of the underlying tissue. Correct diagnosis of breast abscesses is important, as they may not respond to antibiotic therapy alone and may require incision and drainage.

Chronic mastitis is generally thought to be the result of ductal obstruction with subsequent accumulation of secretions resulting in tissue irritation and destruction. Less commonly, chronic mastitis can arise as the sequela of severe or unresolved acute mastitis. Chronic mastitis is characterized by accumulations of chronic inflammatory cells, predominantly lymphocytes and plasma cells around irregularly dilated ducts and lobules, with a fibrotic stromal response. A distinct subset of chronic mastitis, known as mammary duct ectasia, is characterized chiefly by dilatation of ducts, inspissation of breast secretions, and marked periductal and interstitial chronic granulomatous inflammation. This disorder tends to occur in the perimenopausal age group and is thought to result from the obstruction of ducts due to inspissation of secretions. This lesion is clinically important because it may be mistaken for a carcinoma clinically, grossly, or by mammography.

Another chronic inflammatory lesion that may be clinically confused with carcinoma is fat necrosis. As the term implies, fat necrosis is characterized by focal necrosis of the fat cells, or adipocytes, and a pronounced infiltration of macrophages. Fibrosis of the fatty tissue ensues, producing induration of the affected fatty tissue, which can mimic the "feel" of a carcinoma. The process is highly associated with a history of trauma to the breast.

FIBROCYSTIC CHANGES OF THE BREAST

The term fibrocystic change (FCC) of the breast is applied to a constellation of morphologic changes in the female breast, ranging from those that are entirely innocuous to those that are associated with a significant increase in the risk of carcinoma. As its name implies, the pathologic features of fibrocystic change include fibrosis and cyst formation.

Color Plates 5 and 6 show the characteristic histology of FCC. These plates can be compared with the normal breast histology shown in Color Plates 1 and 2. Fibrosis is characterized by an increase in dense stromal fibrous tissue. When fibrosis predominates, the term fibrous mastopathy is used.

Cysts are common and are thought to result from a distal duct obstruction. They vary greatly in size from microscopic dilatation to several centimeters in diameter. These cysts are lined by ductal epithelial cells, which often undergo apocrine metaplasia. The latter change is characterized by enlargement of the epithelial cells, with distinctive abundant pink cytoplasm and decapitation (pinching-off of the intraluminal portion of the epithelial cell) type secretion. Neither a cyst nor apocrine metaplasia is related to a risk of breast cancer.

The third, most significant component of fibrocystic change is epithelial hyperplasia, which is associated with a significantly increased risk of breast cancer. The risk of developing carcinoma is directly proportional to the amount and severity of the epithelial hyperplasia: the more severe and atypical the hyperplasia, the greater the risk of cancer. Ductal epithelial hyperplasia sometimes coexists with fibrocystic changes but on occasion comprises the predominant pattern.

Epithelial hyperplasia is common in its mildest form. It is characterized by a mild proliferation of epithelial lining cells resulting in slight multilayering of both lobules and ducts. The epithelial cells in mild hyperplasia show little or no increase in nuclear enlargement or atypism. This mild epithelial proliferation probably carries minimal or no increased risk of the development of breast carcinoma.

In its moderate or severe forms, epithelial hyperplasia is characterized by dilatation of the ducts and significant multilayering of the epithelial lining cells, which often cause epithelial tufting and complex epithelial patterns without supporting stroma within a duct. The latter change is referred to as cribriforming. The degree of epithelial proliferation is generally paralleled by an increase in the cytologic atypia of the epithelial cells, a change characterized by an increase in the size and irregularity of the nuclei within these cells. In its most florid state, the epithelial hyperplasia, tufting, and cribriforming seen with atypical hyperplasia closely resembles the changes seen with ductal carcinoma in situ. Atypical ductal epithelial hyperplasia is associated with a four- to fivefold increased risk of developing breast carcinoma, a risk that nearly doubles if the patient has a family history of breast cancer.

'A subset of epithelial hyperplasia known as sclerosing lesions is important to recognize. These lesions are characterized histologically by extensive intralobular fibrosis and proliferation of small ductules, acini, or both. The two best recognized lesions in this subset are sclerosing adenosis and the radial scar. With both of these conditions small, often irregular ducts and acini are enmeshed in dense fibrotic stroma. The fibrous reaction often distorts the small ducts, producing a histologic pattern that closely mimics the pattern of invasive ductal carcinoma and in particular the pattern of tubular carcinoma. The salient feature distinguishing benign sclerosing lesions from invasive carcinomas is preservation of a more normal architectural pattern in the benign lesions; carcinomas tend to alter the surrounding breast tissue irregularly. Neither sclerosing adenosis nor radial scar is associated with a significant increase in the development of carcinoma, underscoring the importance of recognizing and distinguishing these lesions from their malignant counterparts.

BENIGN TUMORS OF THE BREAST

Lactating Adenoma

Lactating adenomas are found almost exclusively during pregnancy or lactation. They are well circumscribed, discrete, nodular lesions that in the gross state readily express a white milky fluid. Microscopically, lactating adenomas consist of a florid accumulation of hypersecretory acini and terminal ductules arranged in an arborizing pattern. The architectural features are virtually identical to those of the benign tubular adenoma of the breast. This latter resemblance has encouraged some authors to suggest that (1) the lactating adenoma represents lactational changes of a tubular adenoma rather than a distinct tumor, or (2) it is merely a hyperplastic response of normal breast tissue to pregnancy.

Fibroadenoma

Fibroadenomas are the most common tumor of the breast. Although they occur at all ages, they are most frequently diagnosed during the early reproductive years. Grossly, fibroadenomas are sharply demarcated, nodular, rubbery tumors. They vary in size from less than 1 cm up to giant forms measuring 10–15 cm in diameter. On average, fibroadenomas are detected and surgically removed when they are 2–4 cm in diameter. On section, they appear firm, rubbery, and grayish white, and they are easily separated from the surrounding breast tissue.

Histologically, fibroadenomas are composed of a variably cellular fibroblastic stroma that surrounds duct-like structures. These ducts vary greatly in size and architectural features: they may be round, oval, or slit-like. In the usual fibroadenoma the stromal cells are small and evenly spaced, and they show no cytologic atypia and little or no mitotic activity. Likewise, the glandular elements are most often lined by a single layer of epithelial cells with an underlying myoepithelial layer. Examples of the histology of a typical fibroadenoma are shown in Color Plates 9 and 10.

Occasionally, ductal epithelial hyperplasia or lobular hyperplasia arises within a fibroadenoma and may be associated with a slight increase in risk for the development of breast cancer. Exceptionally, carcinomas arise within a fibroadenoma. Of the carcinomas arising in fibroadenomas, more than 50% represent lobular carcinoma in situ. Invasive carcinomas within fibroadenoma are rare, and the world literature has described only a few metastatic cases.

Controversy as to whether fibroadenomas are true tumors rather than hyperplastic lesions has recently been stirred. Several studies have uncovered the presence of telomerase activity in a significant percentage of fibroadenomas, a finding that seems to support the belief they are tumors. However, in one study fibroadenomas were found to be polyclonal, a finding that may be explained by the large number of glandular elements, which are thought not to be neoplastic, thereby casting some doubt on the tumor theory.

Tubular Adenoma

Grossly, the tubular adenoma is indistinguishable from a fibroadenoma. Most authors believe that the tubular adenoma represents a variant of the fibroadenoma in which the glandular component greatly predominates over the stromal elements. Microscopically, the tubular adenoma is characterized by an arborizing pattern of ducts and lobules enmeshed in a fibrous stroma. Like the fibroadenoma, the epithelial cells lining the ducts and acini are single and have an underlying myoepithelial layer.

Intraductal Papilloma

As its name implies, the intraductal papilloma is a neoplastic papillary growth within a major breast duct. Most of the lesions are solitary and found within the principal lactiferous ducts, or sinuses. They present clinically as a result of serous or bloody nipple discharge or as a small subareolar nodule, generally a few millimeters in diameter. Histologically, the tumor is composed of multiple papillae, each having a connective tissue core lined by two layers of cells: an epithelial layer and a myoepithelial layer underneath. In rare cases the distinction between a benign intraductal papilloma and an intraductal papillary carcinoma is difficult. In general, cytologic atypia and the absence of myoepithelial cells, together with increased mitotic activity and pseudostratification, are seen in malignant papillary carcinomas but not in benign papillomas. Less commonly, intraductal papillomas are multiple. This distinction is important, as multiple intraductal papillomas are more likely to recur and are associated with an increased risk of carcinoma.

Phyllodes Tumor

Phyllodes tumors, like fibroadenomas, are composed of glandular elements admixed with a cellular fibrous component. They vary from fibroadenomas in that they are generally larger, tend to be lobulated rather than spherical or elliptical, and have a greater tendency to form cysts than the fibroadenomas. Microscopically, the stroma of phyllodes tumors tends to have a more "myxoid," or edematous, appearance and higher cellularity than that of fibroadenomas. The aggressive or malignant potential of the phyllodes tumor arises in this cellular stroma. Increased stromal cellularity, stromal cell nuclear anaplasia, and high mitotic activity in stromal cells are associated with an increase in malignant potential.

Although most phyllodes tumors follow a benign course, rare tumors are locally destructive or even frankly malignant. Malignant transformation is generally accompanied by a rapid increase in size, usually with an invasion of adjacent breast tissue by malignant stroma. Microscopically, frankly malignant phyllodes tumors are characterized by aggressive expansion of the stroma, which overruns or even obliterates the benign glandular elements. Generally, stromal overgrowth is accompanied by marked nuclear anaplasia and an increased mitotic rate. It should be noted that even malignant lesions tend to follow a slow progression, with most lesions recurring only locally. Metastases are rare, occurring in fewer than 15% of malignant cases.

MALIGNANT LESIONS OF THE BREAST

In Situ Carcinoma

In situ carcinomas of the breast are malignant epithelial growths that are limited to the acini, terminal ductules, or ductal system of the breast without any demonstrable invasion into the surrounding breast stroma. Although all breast carcinomas are thought to arise from the terminal ductule, they are generally classified as either ductal or lobular, depending on their morphologic similarity to those normal cellular components. Tumors classified as lobular are composed of small uniform cells resembling the lining cells of the acinar lobules. Tumors classified as ductal have larger, more irregular cells that more closely resemble the epithelial cells lining the ductal system.

Lobular Carcinoma In Situ

Also referred to as lobular neoplasia, lobular carcinoma in situ is characterized by a marked proliferation of small, uniform cells closely resembling normal lobular cells. They fill and distend the normal lobule, obliterating the lumen of at least one lobular acinus or terminal duct. Lobular carcinoma in situ is multifocal in 70% of cases and is seen bilaterally in 30–50% of instances. Unlike its ductal counterparts, lobular carcinoma in situ does not produce a palpable lesion and is not apparent on mammography. It is usually discovered incidentally in breast tissue removed for other reasons. The presence of lobular carcinoma in situ is associated with a 10-fold increase in the risk of developing invasive breast carcinoma. Both breasts are at risk for development of an invasive carcinoma, with the ipsilateral side slightly more at risk than the contralateral breast. When a carcinoma develops in a patient with a previous biopsy of in situ lobular carcinoma, the type of invasive carcinoma can be ductal or lobular.

Ductal Carcinoma In Situ

Also known as intraductal carcinoma, ductal carcinoma in situ (DCIS) is a neoplastic proliferation of duct-like epithelial cells that are confined within the basal membrane of the ductal system. Unlike lobular carcinoma in situ, intraductal carcinoma often grows to become palpable and is often detectable by mammography.

Grossly, the tumor is usually poorly demarcated. On cut section, thin cord-like structures that represent neoplastic ducts can be seen coursing through the pale-tan breast tissue. Histologically, the ducts are dilated and are lined by an increased number of neoplastic epithelial cells that form a variety of architectural patterns. The four major patterns recognized are comedo carcinoma, cribriform carcinoma, micropapillary carcinoma, and solid DCIS. Recognition of these subtypes is important, as comedo carcinoma is associated with a higher incidence of occult invasion and a small but significant risk for lymph node metastases. The comedo carcinoma variant of ductal carcinoma in situ is characterized histologically by a markedly atypical population of malignant cells filling and distending the breast duct, which contains a central area of necrosis. It is this central area of necrosis that imparts its name to this entity, as it resembles a comedo which, when squeezed, expresses its yellow necrotic center. In contrast to lobular carcinoma in situ, intraductal comedo carcinoma is multicentric in only one-third of cases and is bilateral in only 10%. As mentioned earlier, intraductal comedo carcinoma may be rarely associated with the presence of lymph node metastases, even in the absence of demonstrable invasion. Similarly, it is this subset of DCIS that is most correlated with the presence of Paget's disease of the nipple (see below).

Microscopically the other variants of DCIS are defined by the pattern of growth seen within the ducts. Micropapillary carcinoma, as the name suggests, is characterized by minute papillary-like epithelial projections lining the duct. The cribriform variant shows an exuberant epithelial growth with an internal lattice of atypical ductal cells within the ductal lumen.

Invasive Carcinoma

Invasive Lobular Carcinoma

Invasive lobular carcinoma accounts for 5–10% of all invasive breast carcinomas. They are of particular interest in that they are more frequently bilateral, with an incidence of bilaterality of up to 20%. In addition, they often tend to be multicentric within the same breast. Grossly, they are poorly circumscribed and typically have a scirrhous or fibrotic morphology. Histologically, they are typically composed of strands of infiltrating tumor cells, which are frequently one or two cells in width, giving this tumor the typical Indian file morphology. The cells are small and uniform, with relatively little pleomorphism. When these small tumor cells are arranged in concentric rings around normal ducts, the pattern is virtually diagnostic of invasive lobular carcinoma.

Table 11.1. Characteristics of invasive carcinoma

Invasive ductal carcinoma
Forms well developed glands and nests
    Large cells with variability in size and shape
    Nuclei are large, irregular, and prone to pleomorphism
    Chromatin is coarse or vesicular; nucleoli are often present
Invasive lobular carcinoma
    Predominantly seen as strands and cords of single cells
    Small uniform cells with high nucleus/cytoplasm ratios
    Nuclei are small and round to oval
    Chromatin may be deceptively bland although occasionally is coarse

Invasive Ductal Carcinoma

Also known as infiltrating ductal carcinoma, invasive ductal carcinoma has a more varied architectural and cytologic appearance than its lobular counterpart (Table 11.1). Grossly, invasive ductal carcinoma occurs as a fairly well demarcated nodule of stony hard consistency that averages 2 cm in diameter and rarely exceeds 4–5 cm. On palpation, there may be infiltrative attachments to the surrounding structures with fixation to the underlying chest wall or dimpling of the overlying skin. On cut section, the tumor exhibits a characteristic stellate, or crab-like, appearance and interfaces with the surrounding softer, normal breast. On palpation of the cut section, the tumor has a coarse, gritty feel and produces a grating sound when scraped.

Histologically, the usual type of invasive duct carcinoma consists of anaplastic duct cells arranged in solid cell nests, tubes, glands, and occasional cords of neoplastic cells. The histology of a typical invasive carcinoma is shown in Color Plates 13 and 14. Cytologically, the cells are larger than those of invasive lobular carcinoma and exhibit marked nuclear variability in both size and shape.

Several well recognized variants of invasive ductal carcinoma are recognized. These variants are important, in that their prognosis differs from that of the usual type of invasive duct carcinoma.

Medullary Carcinoma   Medullary carcinoma is a variant of invasive ductal carcinoma that exhibits distinct gross and microscopic appearances. Grossly, medullary carcinoma presents as a sharply demarcated, fleshy nodule that may be confused grossly with a benign fibroadenoma or tubular adenoma. Microscopically, medullary carcinoma is formed by solid, syncytia-like sheets of large anaplastic cells with vesicular, pleomorphic nuclei containing prominent nucleoli. Frequently mitoses are seen. Most often there is complete absence of microglandular structures; and characteristically the nests and sheets of tumor are surrounded by a marked lymphoplasmacytic infiltrate that surrounds and may divide the aggregates of neoplastic cells. It is thought that the immune response generating this lymphoplasmacytic infiltrate is responsible for the favorable prognosis when compared to the usual type of infiltrating ductal carcinoma. Even in the presence of axillary lymph node metastases, this tumor has a fairly good prognosis with a 10-year survival of 70–90%.

Mucinous (Colloid) Carcinoma An unusual variant of infiltrative ductal carcinoma, mucinous (colloid) carcinoma is seen most commonly in older women. The tumor is extremely soft and has the consistency and appearance of pale, gray-blue gelatin. Histologically, the tumor is characterized by large amounts of lightly staining amorphous mucin that dissects and penetrates adjacent normal breast tissue. The tumor cells in this neoplasm are usually scant and can be found floating within pools of mucin. Cytologically, the cells tend to be smaller and less pleomorphic than the usual ductal carcinoma and are found singly or in small clusters with only occasional gland formation. The survival rate for those with colloid carcinoma is appreciably higher than that for women with the usual infiltrating ductal carcinoma. Lymph node metastases are rare.

Inflammatory Carcinoma of the Breast Inflammatory carcinoma of the breast is a distinct clinicopathologic subset of infiltrating ductal carcinoma. Grossly, it causes swelling and redness of the skin of the breast, closely mimicking an infectious process. Microscopically, inflammatory carcinoma of the breast is characterized by extensive involvement of the dermal lymphatic spaces by tumor emboli. Often the underlying breast tissue shows diffuse induration, frequently without a definite breast mass. Inflammatory carcinoma is associated with a worse prognosis than the usual type of invasive ductal carcinoma, with few patients surviving 5 years.

Paget's Disease of the Nipple Paget's disease of the nipple is a distinct form of ductal carcinoma that arises in the main excretory ducts of the breast and extends to involve the skin of the nipple and areola. Paget's disease of the breast is almost invariably associated with ductal carcinoma, with or without invasion, that is thought to antedate the changes involving the overlying skin. Grossly, the skin of the nipple and areola is frequently fissured, ulcerated, and oozing. The surrounding breast skin is usually red and edematous. An underlying mass is only rarely present. Histologically, the squamous epithelium of the nipple skin is infiltrated in its basal layer by single cells or nests of malignant glandular cells, referred to as Paget's cells. The cells have large, anaplastic, hyperchromatic nuclei that are usually surrounded by a clear zone, or halo. The clear zone represents intracellular mucin, which can be identified with special stains. Because of its involvement of the skin, Paget's disease is thought to have a less favorable prognosis than plain DCIS. Approximately 30–40% of women with Paget's disease have metastases at the time of surgery.

RARE MALIGNANCIES OF THE BREAST

Malignant tumors affecting the breast may arise from the skin of the breast, sweat glands, sebaceous glands, or connective fibrofatty tissues. Malignancies of the stroma include angiosarcomas, liposarcomas, and fibrosarcomas in increasing order of rarity. Also rarely seen are malignant lymphomas involving the breast. As a general rule, these rare tumors produce large, bulky, fleshy masses that cause a rapid increase in breast size with considerable distortion of the breast contour. The histologic picture in each case varies according to the tissue of origin, although in each case the cells are overtly malignant with large, pleomorphic nuclei and extremely high mitotic rates. The clinical outlook for women with these tumors is poor. Angiosarcomas, in particular, are the most rapidly fatal of breast tumors.

TUMOR GRADING

The histologic grading of invasive ductal carcinoma of the breast is an accurate, inexpensive method of predicting tumor prognosis. Although numerous grading schema exist to grade invasive carcinomas of the breast, the Nottingham modification of the Bloom-Richardson system has been shown to be one of the most effective and reproducible systems available.

This system evaluates three histologic features in each tumor and assigns a numeric value of 1–3 in each instance (Table 11.2). When the point scores for each histologic feature are added, a numeric score is assigned to each tumor. A minimum score of 3 and a maximum score of 9 is assigned to each tumor graded. A

Table 11.2. Combined architectural and cytologic grading system for infiltrating duct carcinoma

Feature	Numeric score[a]
Tubule formation	
>75% of tumor	1
10–75%	2
<10%	3
Nuclear pleomorphism	
Small, regular, uniform cells	1
Moderate increase in size and variability	2
Marked variation	3
Mitotic counts at tumor periphery	
0–9/10 HPF[b]	1
10–19	2
20 or more	3

Sources: Gompel and Silverberg, *Pathology in Gynecology and Obstetrics*, 4th ed. Lippincott-Raven, Philadelphia, 1994. As adapted from Elston and Ellis, *Histopathology* 19:403–410, 1991, with permission.
[a] The three scores are added together. A final tally of 3–5 = grade I (well differentiated); 6–7 = grade II (moderately differentiated); and 8–9 = grade III (poorly differentiated).
[b] HPF = high power fields, defined by use of a Leitz Ortholux microscope with wide-angle eyepieces and 25× objective (field area 0.274 mm²). This value must be recalculated for other microscopes.

score of 3–5 points equates to histologic grade I, a score of 6–7 points equates to histologic grade II, and a score of 8–9 points equates to histologic grade III. Numerous studies have shown an increase in lymph node metastases and a decrease in 5-year survival as the grade of the tumor increases.

Prognostic Indicators

Lymph Node Metastases

The presence of metastases to the axillary lymph nodes is the single most important predictor of outcome of invasive breast carcinoma. Both the size and number of lymph nodes involved by metastatic carcinoma have a negative influence on the 5-year survival of patients with invasive carcinoma.

Size

The size of the primary tumor shows an excellent correlation with the incidence of nodal metastases and the survival rate. This relatively simple, inexpensive parameter is one of the strongest predictors of dissemination and rate of relapse among patients with node-negative breast carcinomas. In fact, tumor size is one of the two best criteria for predicting prognosis in the minimally invasive breast carcinoma, which includes all in situ carcinomas and invasive carcinomas 1 cm or less in diameter.

Microscopic Grade

Histologic grade is an effective, inexpensive predictor of nodal metastases and patient outcome.

Molecular Prognostic Indicators

It is now well recognized that the presence or absence of distinct molecular markers has a significant influence on the outcome, or prognosis, of patients with invasive breast carcinoma.

Hormone Receptor Status

Invasive ductal carcinomas that express significant numbers of estrogen or progesterone receptors (or both) have a significantly better prognosis than tumors that lack these hormone receptors. Hormone receptor expression can be analyzed by biochemical hormone-binding assays or by immunohistochemistry. The latter method is currently preferred, as it can be performed on routinely formalin-fixed, paraffin-embedded tissue; and it has been shown in numerous studies to be equal or superior to the binding assays for predicting patient outcome.

Oncogene Expression

Overexpression of the product of the oncogene HER-2/neu is associated with an increased incidence of axillary lymph node metastases, as well as a decrease in 5-year survival. Similarly, accumulation of P53 protein product (presumably as a result of gene mutation), has been recently associated with reduced patient survival. Conversely, demonstration of BCL2 has been associated with better long-term survival of patients with breast carcinoma.

Patient Age

Women younger than 50 years of age at the time of diagnoses have the best prognosis.

Pregnancy

Diagnosis of invasive breast carcinoma at the time of pregnancy or lactation is associated with an overall poor prognosis. The 5-year survival rate in most series ranges from 15% to 35%. However, when controlled by stage, the difference does not reach statistical significance in most series.

Micrometastases

The presence of histologically occult tumor in both axillary lymph nodes and bone marrow has been shown to influence both recurrence and mortality in patients with histologically negative lymph nodes. These microscopic metastases are detected using immunohistochemistry directed against epithelial markers (tumor cells) in lymph nodes and bone marrow, where there is normally a lack of epithelial cells.

12 Biopsy of Benign Breast Masses by Obstetrician-Gynecologists in the Breast Diagnostic Center

Susana G. Gonzalez

A woman with a breast mass keenly fears the possibility of having an undiagnosed cancer. Although a physician may have a reasonable clinical impression that a mass is benign (or malignant) based on physical examination, mammography, and even fine-needle aspiration (FNA) cytology, sometimes there is lingering doubt on the part of the physician or the patient. Open surgical biopsy (OSBx) provides a tissue specimen for histologic diagnosis that can definitively determine or exclude the existence of a malignancy.

Protocol at the Breast Diagnostic Center (BDC), Women's and Children's Hospital, Los Angeles County and University of Southern California (LAC + USC) limits gynecologic surgeons to doing breast excision biopsies on benign lesions, usually fibroadenomas, or on clinically benign lesions with atypical (but not suspicious) cells seen by FNA cytology. The nonmalignant nature of the mass has been previously determined by the preoperative diagnostic triad consisting of clinical breast examination (see Chapter 4), FNA (see Chapter 8), and mammography (see Chapter 6).

When the preliminary cytologic impression is suspicious for malignancy, the patient is counseled and promptly (within a week) referred to the Breast Surgery Clinic at the LAC + USC Medical Center for further evaluation and probable treatment. This process allows immediate attention to a potentially malignant mass, expedites patient and family counseling, and hastens the definitive diagnosis and therapy of a breast cancer. A benign mass so large that its removal would compromise the cosmesis of the breast is also referred to the Breast Surgery Clinic for excision.

When the cytology is benign, the patient is scheduled for follow-up or elective removal by surgical excision at the BDC. Other indications for surgery include a fibroadenoma that continues to increase in size or otherwise becomes symptomatic. In addition, OSBx may be elected by a woman for a painful benign mass that does not respond to conservative, nonsurgical therapy.

BDC Technique of Excision Breast Biopsy

At the BDC, OSBx is performed by the fourth year (senior) resident physicians under the direct supervision and assistance of faculty staff. The final written cytopathology report is reviewed prior to surgery. All patients over age 30 have undergone mammography, a protocol adopted to eliminate the possibility of an undiagnosed nonpalpable lesion elsewhere in either breast.

For logistic convenience, OSBx is performed in the inpatient operating rooms of Women's and Children's Hospital (W&CH), which houses the BDC. In the community the procedure is usually performed in outpatient surgical facilities or in minor surgery rooms at the surgeon's office. At W&CH a circulating operating room nurse is present to assist with instruments, drapes, surgical specimens, and other surgical support functions. A "standby" anesthesiologist is on site and immediately available in the W&CH operating rooms area.

Anesthesia and Analgesia

The OSBx is performed using intravenous sedation and local anesthesia. The demeanor of the surgeon is important, as a pleasant, calm, supportive surgeon is more successful in augmenting adequate analgesia than one who is hurried and does not pay attention to the patient's psychological needs. Approximately 15 minutes prior to the procedure the patient is given meperidine (e.g., Demerol) 50 mg IV followed by promethazine (e.g., Phenergan) 25 mg IV. This combination usually provides adequate conscious sedation. Local analgesia surrounding the surgical site is obtained by infiltrating the breast tissue with 1% lidocaine (e.g., Xylocaine) solution. At the end of the procedure the surgical bed and skin incision area are infiltrated with about 5 cc of 0.25% bupivacaine (e.g., Marcaine) solution, which usually provides a pain-free recovery for up to 6 hours.

Incisions

A pleasing cosmetic result is highly desirable when performing breast surgery. Cosmetic considerations play an important role in deciding on the placement and length of the OSBx skin incision.

Biopsy incisions in the breast should be curvilinear and central, following Langer's or other cosmetically suitable skin lines. If the benign mass is within a 3-cm distance of the areolar border, a circumareolar incision at the areolar border usually provides the optimum cosmetic result. The incision should be placed medially if cosmetically possible, even when peripheral dissection (tunneling) through the breast tissue is necessary to reach the mass (benign only). The exception to this rule is when the mass is near the edge of the medial aspect of the breast. In this instance we use a radial incision in the area, which allows use of a standard mastectomy incision for any subsequent mastectomy, if necessary, without resultant skin distortion. The incision length should be adequate to allow the mass to be removed intact without undue pulling on the skin, which can lead to unsightly marks and distortion. The optimum length of the incision is usually equal to the longest dimension of the benign mass.

OSBx Procedure

1. After sterile skin preparation and draping of the area, the mass is palpated and the final decision on placement of the incision is confirmed. The incision line is precisely drawn with a skin marker pen.
2. Lidocaine 1% (e.g., Xylocaine) solution is injected along the incision line and around the mass (Fig. 12.1). (The skin marking of the incision is not shown in Figure 12.1.)
3. A curvilinear incision is made, and a thick skin flap is developed, preserving 1 cm of subcutaneous tissue. Needle-tip cautery is used to dissect through the breast tissue toward the palpable mass (Fig. 12.2). If bleeding is encountered during the dissection, electrocautery is used to establish complete hemostasis. The entire operative field is kept dry as the dissection progresses, avoiding the difficulty of finding bleeding sites after the mass is removed.
4. When the mass is deep within the breast tissue, it may be necessary to dissect the mammary tissue overlying the mass. This is accomplished by "tunneling" or resecting the tissue overlying the mass by cautery or sharp dissection (Fig. 12.3).

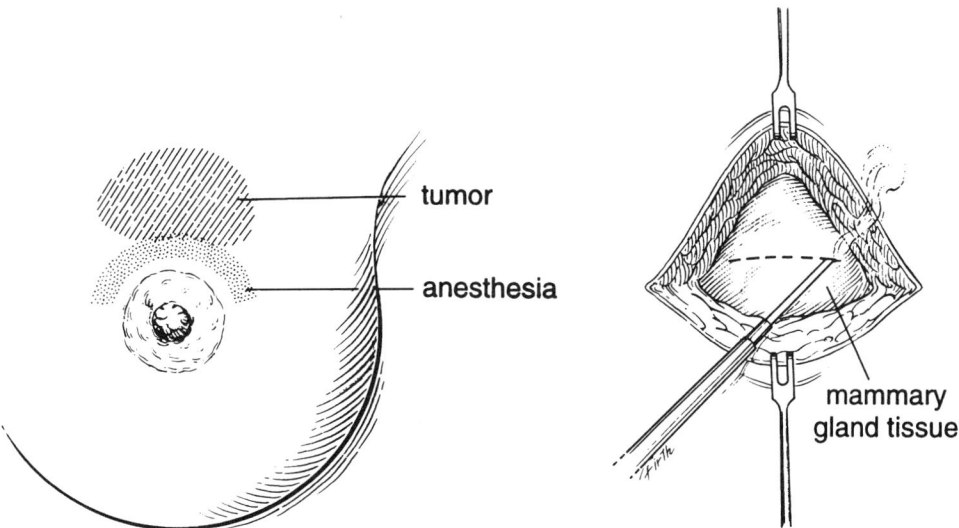

Figure 12.1. (*Left*) Lidocaine 1% (10 cc) is injected along the incision line and around the mass (tumor).
Figure 12.2. (*Right*) Needle-tip electrocautery is used for dissection through the breast tissue toward the palpable mass.

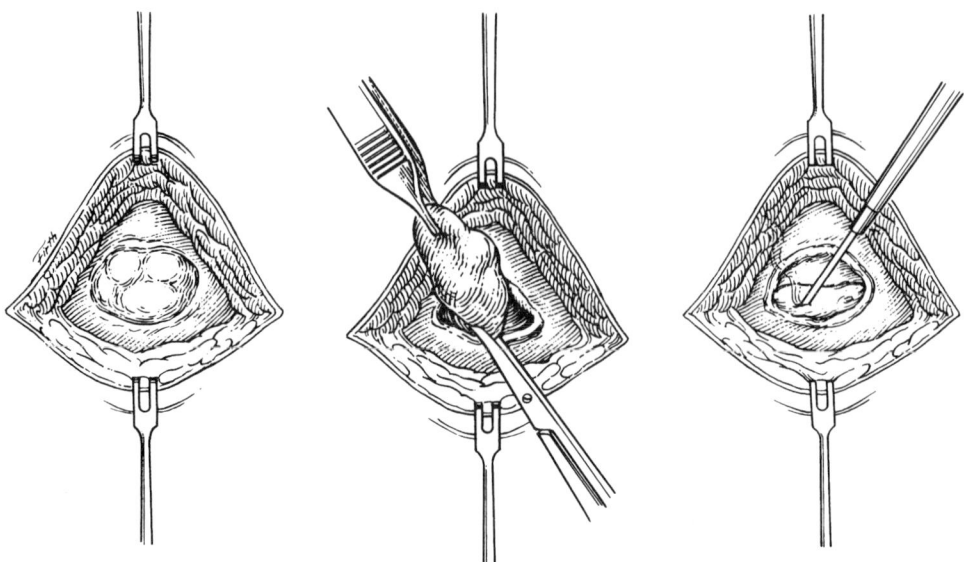

Figure 12.3. (*Left*) When the mass is deep in the breast tissue, "tunneling" through or resecting the intervening breast tissue above the mass may be necessary (if it is certain that the mass is benign).

Figure 12.4. (*Middle*) Once the mass is visible, it is grasped with tissue forceps or a towel clip and put on traction to disclose the borders. The mass is then freed from the attached fat and fibrous bands by sharp dissection.

Figure 12.5. (*Right*) Complete hemostasis is obtained by needle-tip cautery.

5. When the benign mass is visible, a towel clip or tissue forceps can be used to elevate the mass with traction to enhance exposure of the borders (Fig. 12.4). The fat and fibrous connective tissue that hold the mass in place are incised by sharp dissection or needle-tip cautery.

6. After the mass is removed the surgical bed is examined thoroughly for bleeding, and then complete hemostasis with a dry field is accomplished with needle-tip electrocautery (Fig. 12.5).

7. The surgical site is closed using a running subcuticular stitch of 4-0 absorbable synthetic suture, e.g., polyglycolic acid (Dexon) or polyglactin (e.g., Vicryl). (Fig. 12.6) No deep sutures are placed. Bupivacaine (e.g., Marcaine) 0.25% is injected into the skin for postoperative wound analgesia. Steri-strips are placed over the skin incision (Fig. 12.7), and a pressure dressing is applied on top of the incision. The pressure dressing is removed and replaced with a light dressing immediately prior to the patient's leaving the outpatient surgery department.

The surgical specimen of an FNA cytology-diagnosed fibroadenoma is placed in formalin solution and sent to the pathology laboratory for routine examination and reporting. All other surgical specimens are treated in the same manner as lumpectomy specimens (see below).

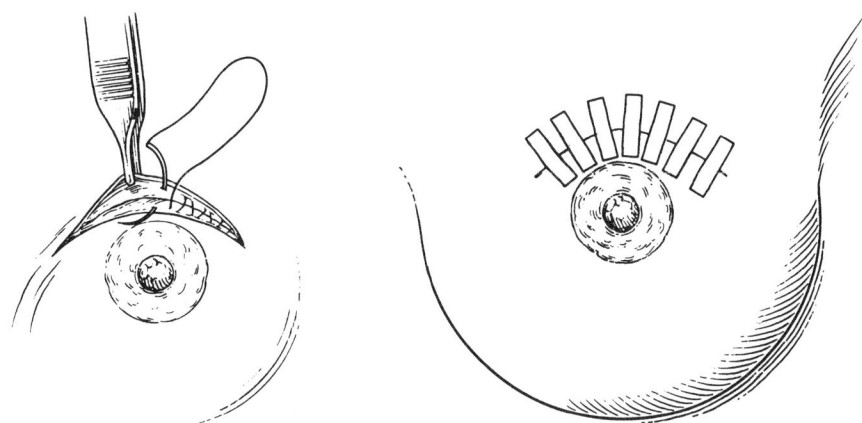

Figure 12.6.   (*Left*) Surgical site is closed with a running subcuticular stitch of 4–0 absorbable synthetic suture.
Figure 12.7.   (*Right*) Steri-strips are placed over the incision, and a pressure dressing is applied.

LUMPECTOMY

If the FNA cytology is reported as "atypia," the previously described excision procedure is *not* followed. Instead, a lumpectomy is performed following the National Surgical Adjuvant Breast and Bowel Project (NSABP) protocol as described by Margolese.[1,2] This lumpectomy procedure is critically different in that the mass is not enucleated as with a fibroadenoma. Instead, the mass is removed en bloc with a 1-cm margin of grossly normal breast tissue surrounding the mass in all directions. This practice allows clear surgical margins should the mass prove to be malignant. The entire fresh en bloc mass is immediately sent to the pathology laboratory for inking and processing. Frozen section examinations are not performed.

COMPLICATIONS

The potential complications of excision biopsies are hemorrhage, hematoma formation, infection, and distortion of the breast size and shape if a large amount of tissue is removed. Hemorrhage and hematoma formation can be avoided if meticulous attention is paid to hemostasis at the time of surgery. Complete hemostasis and the use of a pressure dressing usually prevent ecchymosis.

POSTOPERATIVE CARE

After observation in the postoperative recovery room of at least an hour to allow the effects of the intravenous sedation to pass, the patient is discharged if her vital signs are stable and someone is present to drive her home. Instructions are given to remove the pressure dressing in the evening but to keep the wound site clean and dry. She should call her physician if there is any evidence of active bleeding, fever, or infection. Narcotics for analgesia should not be required. Nonsteroidal analgesic medications such as ibuprofen (e.g., Motrin), acetaminophen (e.g., Tylenol), or aspirin usually provide adequate pain relief. Prophylactic antibiotics are not prescribed. The patient is given an appointment to return to the BDC for routine postoperative followup.

References

1. Fisher B. Reappraisal of breast biopsy prompted by the use of lumpectomy: surgical strategy. JAMA 1985;253:3585–3588
2. Margolese R, Poisson R, Shibata H, et al. The technique of segmental mastectomy (lumpectomy) and axillary dissection: a syllabus from the National Surgical Adjuvant Breast Project workshops. Surgery 1987;102:828–834

13 Excision of a Palpable Breast Mass in Private Primary Care Practice

Audrey J. Arona

Open surgical biopsy (OSBx) of the breast is one of the most common operations in the United States today, and most are performed for what proves to be a benign condition. The patient, however, may endure a tremendous amount of emotional stress due to anxiety, fear, physical discomfort, financial expense, and sometimes breast deformity.

The indications and techniques of breast biopsy have changed considerably from previous years. Because mammography is now widely used, there has been a marked increase in the diagnosis of ductal carcinoma in situ (DCIS). Breast conservation is now more often an option even for patients with invasive breast cancers. Chemotherapy as initial treatment (neoadjuvant therapy) is emerging. Breast biopsy is most often done in outpatient facilities, as local anesthesia is usually used.

All of these factors have contributed dramatically to the alteration of traditional concepts surrounding the diagnosis, management, and treatment of breast cancer. Emphasis is on analyzing the particular pathology present in a given breast cancer and evaluating surgical margins to develop more sophisticated therapeutic strategies. Thus breast excisional biopsy has become a common outpatient surgical procedure.

An excisional biopsy is complete removal of a palpable lesion or of a suspicious lesion perceived by mammography. A single nonfragmented piece of tissue is removed. The technique differs from lumpectomy, which involves excision of an additional 1 cm rim of breast tissue surrounding the mass.

Breast biopsies can be performed by appropriately trained obstetricians/gynecologists (and potentially by other primary care physicians with similar surgical training) for the purpose of removing a benign breast mass or to obtain a definitive diagnosis of a suspicious, possibly malignant lesion. Because most gynecologists treat only benign breast conditions and refer patients with suspicious or malignant breast masses to an oncologic surgeon, this chapter focuses on breast excision biopsy techniques for a palpable benign breast mass. The techniques are similar, with the exception that in cases of possible malignancy closer attention is paid to obtaining adequate surgical margins. Excision of nonpalpable breast lesions perceived upon mammography and localized by preoperative needle-wire placement is discussed in Chapter 22.

At the Breast Diagnostic Center (BDC), where I trained, an OSBx could be done as soon as the mass was diagnosed by fine-needle aspiration (FNA). In private clinical practice, however, it is usually necessary to obtain authorization from a health insurance company before scheduling surgery. This wait can be a trying time for an anxious patient.

INDICATIONS

Breast excisional biopsy may be performed for a number of benign conditions. For example, if FNA of a persistent undiagnosed breast mass is inconclusive, a definitive diagnosis must be obtained by tissue histology. Also, a woman may choose to have a mass removed even if it has been diagnosed as benign by FNA cytology. Many women are bothered by having a palpable breast lump and may prefer to have it removed rather than followed.

In my practice I choose to limit OSBx to fibroadenomas or fibrocystic changes diagnosed by FNA when the patient requests removal of a benign palpable mass. Any mass that shows atypical cells or is suspicious by FNA, and all cancers are referred to an oncologic surgeon.

An excisional biopsy may be elected when a benign breast mass has become so large that the architecture or appearance of the breast is distorted. If a cytologically diagnosed fibroadenoma is larger than 5 cm or has rapidly increased in size, excisional biopsy is recommended to exclude the uncommon phyllodes tumor. If FNA cytology reveals atypical cells and no clearly malignant cells, breast excision biopsy for definitive tissue diagnosis is indicated. Sometimes the cytopathologist interpreting the FNA specimen advises excisional biopsy even though the suspicion for malignancy is low.

WORKUP

The workup for any palpable dominant breast mass is the same: clinical breast examination, FNA, and mammography. FNA should be performed for any mass palpated by the patient or physician even if the mass seems clinically benign to the physician. FNA always precedes OSBx of a palpable breast mass. The FNA procedure is done in my office.

For women 30 years of age and older, a mammogram should be performed for any breast complaint and certainly for a palpable breast mass unless one has been performed within the preceding 6 months and the films are available for review by the physician's consultant mammographer. If possible, mammography is ordered (and performed) before the FNA. If the mammogram is obtained after the FNA no particular delay is specified, but a note on the mammography request form includes the date (and the results, if available) of the recent FNA.

Preoperative Counseling and Consultations

In private practice a breast cancer booklet furnished by the State of California must (by law) be given to the patient before OSBx or FNA. Preoperative consultation (medical or surgical) is not necessary prior to an OSBx unless a patient has a serious medical problem or requires special anesthesia clearance.

Procedure

The OSBx is usually performed in an outpatient surgical center (if allowed by the insurance company). The surgical assistant at OSBx is an operating room technician.

The procedure begins with a careful breast examination to localize and define the mass. Particular attention should be paid to its relation to the margin of the areola and the periphery of the breast, its attachment to or involvement of the skin, the palpated size of the mass, and any other physical findings. Different postures the patient assumes often change the location of the mass. Thus the precise incision site should be determined immediately prior to surgery, which is best done with a skin marking pen while the patient is sitting up so that her particular breast shape and skin lines may be evaluated when determining placement of the incision for the best cosmetic results.

With the patient supine, the incision site is infused with local anesthesia, commonly 1% lidocaine with or without epinephrine. Sharp and blunt dissection then follows, with care taken to cauterize all the bleeding sites encountered. Contrary to some previously held beliefs, electrocautery is beneficial and decreases the risk of subsequent hematoma formation due to unrecognized or retracted bleeding vessels.

Towel clamps are usually placed directly into a benign mass and used for traction throughout the dissection. If the mass is a fibroadenoma, enucleation is readily performed, without removal of surrounding normal breast tissue. Gross inspection is necessary to confirm complete excision of the mass.

Meticulous attention to hemostasis by cautery is essential. A large hematoma can develop into a firm postoperative mass, and although the hematoma eventually resolves the patient often experiences considerable anxiety about it. Sutures are not recommended for hemostasis within the breast unless absolutely necessary, nor is closure of the "deadspace" after the mass is removed. Suture material left in the breast can lead to increased scar formation. Left alone, the space fills with fibrin and reorganizes. This natural healing process provides a more normal contour and consistency of the breast following excision biopsy. A minimal palpable defect in the breast tissue may be present later, but usually it is not visually disturbing or even noticeable.

Drains are not recommended, especially Penrose-type drains. Without drains there is less risk of infection. If a seroma or hematoma forms, it can be drained by needle aspiration with minimal risk of infection.

If gross inspection of the mass after removal indicates any doubt about the histopathologic diagnosis, a pathologist should be consulted immediately. Specimens that have a known cytologic diagnosis are generally fixed in formalin and sent to the pathology laboratory for routine histologic processing.

The skin closure is subcuticular with a small absorbable suture, preferably 4-0 or 5-0, to achieve an optimal cosmetic appearance and little scarring. Braided sutures are not recommended because of tissue drag and possible trapping of bacteria. Steri-strip reinforcement of the skin incision is used for precise apposition and stability. A fluff pressure dressing is applied and left in place for 24 hours to decrease the risk of hematoma formation. Pressure dressings also decrease the patient's postoperative pain and discomfort. Skin clips may be used to close the incision, but if so they should be removed on postoperative day 3 or 4 to avoid clip marks on the skin. Interrupted nylon or silk sutures and, in particular, mattress sutures should not be used. These suturing techniques can cause cross-hatching skin scars. If proper skin closure and proper excision breast biopsy techniques are employed, the resultant scars are thin, flat, and barely visible.

An OSBx takes about 30 minutes total operating room time, and sometimes less.

ANESTHESIA

All breast biopsies can be performed with local anesthesia. Even the most anxious patient can be reassured by the physician's calm appearance, good humor, sympathy, and respect. (Having a nurse present to hold the patient's hand, provide distracting conversation or both can be helpful.) Local anesthesia does not compromise the technique or the adequacy of the specimen removed; moreover, the operative cost is lower, and less time in the recovery room is required.

As stated previously, local infiltration with 1.0% or 0.5% lidocaine with or without epinephrine can be used. Large quantities of low concentrations work best. A field block can be achieved that usually provides adequate anesthesia even for extensive dissection. Narcotics usually are not necessary. Intravenous sedation is optional but is usually not indicated. Longer and more intense postoperative monitoring is necessary if supplemental anesthetic agents are used.

When the surgery is completed, 0.5% bupivacaine (Marcaine) infusion at the skin incision site decreases postoperative pain and lessens any requirement for analgesia.

CHOICE OF INCISION

The main objective of an excision breast biopsy is the removal of all abnormal tissue. Cosmesis, however, is important. The incision should be planned with care and consideration. How and where to make the optimum breast incision is controversial. Generally, circumareolar incisions are best for the most beneficial cosmetic

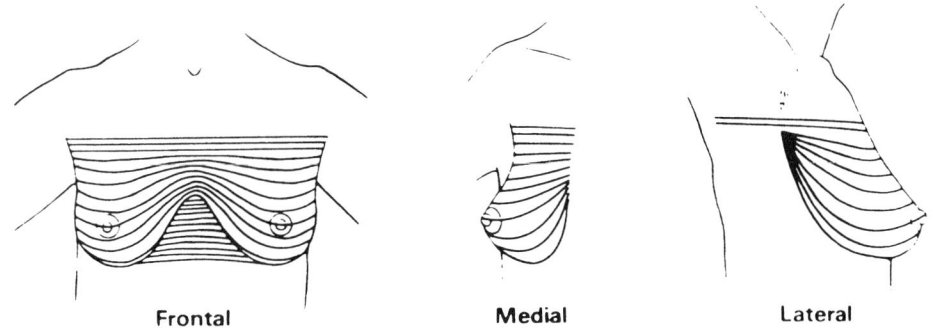

Frontal   Medial   Lateral

Figure 13.1.   Observed breast skin tension lines when the woman is sitting. (From Matory et al.,[1] with permission.)

result. If a benign breast mass is within 3 cm of the areola, a circumareolar incision is the optimum choice. A mass farther than 3 cm from the areola requires tunneling dissection to reach, and extensive tunneling can result in surgical errors and an increased risk of hematoma or breast tissue trauma.

If a circumareolar incision is inappropriate, a transverse or curvilinear incision directly over the mass and parallel to Langer's skin lines of tension usually gives good cosmetic results with little hypertrophy or pigmentary change and minimal scarring. Attention to these skin tension lines takes into account the effects of gravity on the shape of the breast (Fig. 13.1).

If a biopsy is necessary in the lower quadrant of the breast, particularly if some of the skin is to be removed, a radial incision has been found to heal better and is cosmetically acceptable. Otherwise distortion of the breast can occur (Fig. 13.2). The incision length should equal the largest diameter of the mass to be removed.

COMPLICATIONS

Potential surgical complications of excisional biopsy are (1) removal of inadequate or nonrepresentative tissue for diagnosis, (2) wound infection, and (3) wound seroma or hematoma. The risk of complications is minimized if consideration and use of the described techniques are employed. Though the incidence of clinically apparent postoperative breast hematomas is low, subclinical breast hematomas are probably more common. The eventual significance of these occult hematomas is unknown. A hematoma can induce scar tissue formation, which may be painful and can cause difficulty during the interpretation of findings from the physical examination and mammographic follow-up. A hematoma may even be mistaken subsequently for a carcinoma on mammographic follow-up. The presence of blood within the breast tissues can increase the risk of infection. Hence meticulous attention to hemostasis during surgery is necessary.

RECOMMENDED

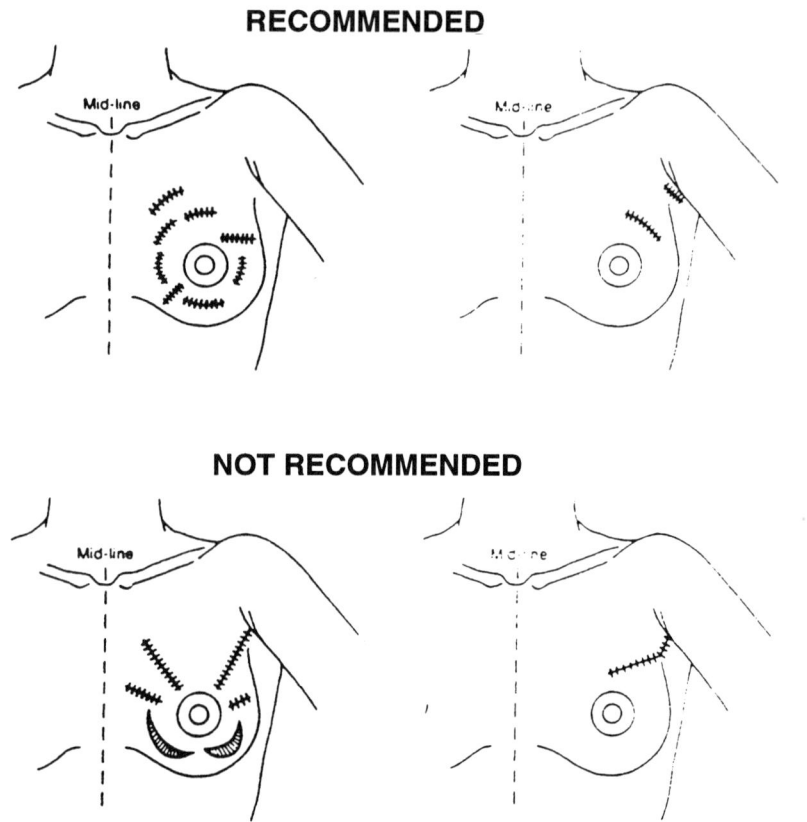

NOT RECOMMENDED

Figure 13.2. NSABP recommendations for breast biopsy incision placement. (From Margolese et al., [2] with permission.)

Postoperative Care and Instructions

The patient remains in the postoperative care area for 1 hour of observation if intravenous sedation is used for the OSBx. Postoperative instructions include (1) no exercises with the upper arm, (2) pressure dressing to be removed within 24 hours, and (3) follow-up appointment in the office at 1 week. Ibuprofen (e.g., Motrin) 400 mg PO q4h PRN is adequate for postoperative analgesia after OSBx. Prophylactic antibiotics are not prescribed or used in the operating room for OSBx.

Other Breast Lesions

The biopsy procedure described above is modified for a suspicious lesion. If feasible, the incision is placed within the boundaries of a possible later mastectomy incision. In suspicious cases a curvilinear incision is made directly over the mass no matter how far from the areola the mass is located. If the mass is superficial and near the skin, an ellipse of the skin is excised over the mass. An incision for a suspicious mass should be 1 cm longer than the largest diameter of the mass.

It is recommended not to cut into a suspicious mass. Complete en bloc excision (not simple enucleation) of the mass, including removal of 1 cm of additional breast tissue surrounding the mass in all directions, is recommended. Once excised, the specimen is marked for orientation by placing sutures on the superior and lateral margins, following the protocol of the National Surgical Adjuvant Breast Project.[2]

The suspicious specimen is sent immediately to the pathology laboratory for inking, sectioning, and fixing. The specimen is not placed in formalin solution in the operating room. Frozen sections and tissue analysis (e.g., estrogen receptor evaluation) are performed at the discretion of the pathologist.

CONCLUSIONS

Approximately 80% of all breast OSBx specimens are found by final histologic evaluation to be benign conditions. Using the techniques described, optimal cosmesis can be achieved with minimal scarring and maximum patient satisfaction. Excision breast biopsy utilizing these techniques should not affect the interpretation of later breast cancer screening procedures. A new finding that develops in the area of a previous breast biopsy should receive the same thorough evaluation as any suspicious breast lesion.

References

1. Matory WE, Wertheimer M, Love S, et al. Partial mastectomy: technical considerations in achieving cosmesis. Breast Dis 1992;5:225–233
2. Margolese R, Poisson R, Shibata H, et al. The technique of segmental mastectomy (lumpectomy) and axillary dissection: a syllabus from the National Surgical Adjuvant Breast Project workshops. Surgery 1987,102:828–834

14 EVALUATION OF A PALPABLE DOMINANT MASS, SOLID OR CYST

William H. Hindle

When a woman complains of a breast lump, it is imperative that the primary care provider (1) confirm the presence of a dominant mass and (2) if one is present, bring about its definitive diagnosis. In addition to the breast-oriented history (see Table 1.6), specific information about the mass should be obtained and recorded. Did the patient find the mass herself, or was it found by her health care provider? How long has the patient been aware of it? Does the mass change at various times in her menstrual cycle (e.g., does it get larger or become more difficult to find prior to menstruation? Is the mass painful? If so, is the pain constant, cyclic, or intermittent?

A palpable dominant breast mass is appropriately evaluated by the primary care provider by applying the diagnostic triad: clinical breast examination (CBE), fine-needle aspiration (FNA), and mammography (Fig. 14.1). When the results of the three procedures are in concordance, the resultant diagnosis can be accepted with confidence and the patient managed accordingly. If any one of the three is suspicious of cancer, a definitive tissue diagnosis, by tissue core-needle biopsy (TCNB) or excisional biopsy (OSBx), is indicated.

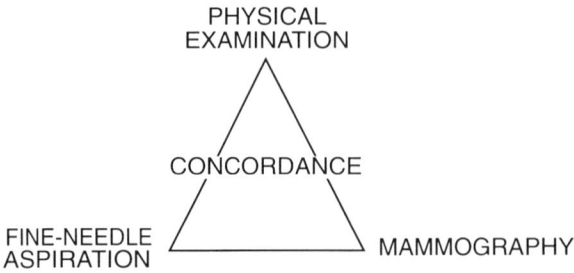

Figure 14.1. Diagnostic triad of a palpable breast mass.

Physical Examination

At the Breast Diagnostic Center (BDC) the protocol is to perform a focused examination of the area of concern and then a complete CBE to evaluate the remainder of the breast and the other breast. Physical characteristics consistent with a benign palpable dominant mass are (1) mobility, (2) smooth borders, (3) distinct borders, (4) soft or rubbery texture, (5) tenderness, and (6) multiplicity (Table 14.1). Multiplicity is the strongest predictor of benignity of a palpable dominant breast mass.

Physical characteristics suggestive of malignancy are (1) fixation, (2) irregular borders, (3) indistinct borders, (4) firm or hard texture, and (5) secondary signs of cancer such as skin changes, dimpling, and nipple retraction (Table 14.2). Fixation to the underlying chest wall or to the skin is a strong predictor of malignancy. Although the primary care provider should be thinking in terms of the histopathology that these physical characteristics represent, none is diagnostic. CBE results in a clinical impression, not a definitive diagnosis.

The paramount function of the CBE is to determine the presence of a dominant palpable mass that by history is persistent. If the lesion is not distinct or definite in a woman who is having cyclic menstruation, it is appropriate to reexamine her in a month—but at another time in her menstrual cycle, preferably shortly after the

Table 14.1. Physical findings usually associated with a benign palpable dominant mass

Distinct margins
Mobility
Multiplicity
Smooth margins
Soft or rubbery texture
Tenderness
Unchanged over time

Table 14.2. Physical findings usually associated with a malignant palpable dominant breast mass

Not freely mobile
Firm or hard texture
Fixation
Indistinct margins
Irregular margins
Nipple retraction
Nontender
Progressive changes
Skin dimpling
Skin peau d'orange

> # KEY PRACTICE POINTS
>
> **Diagnosis of a dominant breast mass:** A persistent palpable dominant breast mass must be definitively diagnosed by fine-needle aspiration cytology or tissue histology.
>
> **Evaluation of a palpable dominant breast mass:** When the results are concordant, the diagnostic triad is 99% reliable: clinical breast examination, fine-needle aspiration, mammography.
>
> **If a cyst** yields nonbloody fluid, clears completely, reveals no residual or underlying mass, and does not refill within 3 months, it may be safely followed.

menstrual flow has ceased. If at the repeat CBE the lesion is not palpable, she should be scheduled for a final reevaluation by CBE in 2–3 months. She should be advised to check the area of concern and to return immediately if she palpates a distinct mass or notices any other changes in her breast.

A focused breast ultrasound examination can be useful if the mass is small (<1 cm) or the primary care provider is unsure if the palpated "mass" (e.g., when it is located in a breast with diffuse prominent nodularity) is truly a dominant mass.

Fine-Needle Aspiration

By BDC protocol, FNA is performed on a palpable dominant breast mass at the initial visit. When an adequate cell sample is obtained, a definitive specific cytologic diagnosis can be made in more than 90% of cases. There is no medical reason to defer or delay FNA of a palpable dominant breast mass. Rather, reassurance or initiation of the appropriate therapy can be expedited by a timely cytologic diagnosis. FNA is cost-effective, efficient, and well tolerated by the patient at the initial visit. Of course, if a specific cytologic diagnosis is not obtained, or if clinical or mammographic suspicion of malignancy persists after FNA, a histologic tissue diagnosis should be obtained by TCNB or OSBx.

Mammography

By BDC protocol, diagnostic mammography is performed on all women over age 30 with a dominant breast mass. While the reported risk of developing invasive breast cancer by age 30 is less than 1:2500, mammography is performed at any age if the clinical impression is cancer. The mammogram gives an impression of the histopathology of the mass, but more importantly it evaluates the remainder of the breast and the other breast, particularly for nonpalpable suspicious abnormalities.

Pregnancy and Lactation

A pregnant or lactating woman with a dominant breast mass is evaluated in the same timely manner using the same diagnostic procedures as for a woman who is not pregnant or lactating.

Cysts

A palpable cyst is readily and rapidly diagnosed by FNA (see Fig. 8.11) and, with drainage of the fluid, the procedure is therapeutic as well (see Fig. 8.12). If the mass is small (e.g., <1 cm), ultrasonography is useful as a guide for cyst aspiration and confirmation that all the fluid has been removed. The cyst fluid should be discarded, as a cytologic evaluation is not cost-effective or useful for clinical management. The exception is grossly bloody fluid (in contrast to traumatic bloody fluid), which might be a sign of an intracystic lesion and which could yield diagnostic cellular material by cell block evaluation. The literature suggests that the presence of an intracystic lesion occurs in about 1:1000 cysts.

A cyst diagnosed and drained by FNA is appropriately followed clinically if: (1) the cyst fluid is not frankly bloody, (2) palpation of the area after the aspiration shows that the cyst has completely cleared, (3) there is no residual (or underlying) palpable mass, and (4) the cyst does not refill within 3 months (Table 14.3). The BDC protocol is to reexamine the patient who has had a cyst aspiration in 2 months. If the cyst has re-formed, it is drained again with ultrasound guidance. If it re-forms a second time, consultation is obtained with consideration of a pneumocystogram or OSBx to rule out the presence of a rare intracystic carcinoma.

Cyst symptoms (e.g., localized pain, tenderness, and size fluctuation) tend to be estrogen-related and vary with changes in estrogen levels. Thus at menopause a palpable (untreated) cyst tends to decrease in size, often becoming nonpalpable and nontender. Likewise, some estrogen-deficient women reexperience their cyst symptoms and have nonpalpable cysts become palpable after estrogen replacement therapy is initiated. However, because the probability of breast cancer correlates with advancing age, the older the woman the more likely it is that the mass is cancer.

Table 14.3. Management of an aspirated cyst

Send frankly bloody fluid for cell block cytology.
Completely aspirate all cyst fluid.
Palpate for a residual mass after aspiration.
Reexamine in 2 months to see if the cyst has refilled.

15 MASTALGIA

Audrey J. Arona

Mastalgia is the most commonly cited complaint of patients with breast problems. Studies have shown the prevalence in working women to be approximately 66% (Table 15.1). Nonetheless, mastalgia is still considered by many physicians to be a trivial complaint and one that is psychological in nature. It is important to know that what brings these patients to us is an underlying fear of breast cancer. Fortunately, only a few patients with breast pain require more than reassurance.

Many terms have been used to describe mastalgia, including mastodynia and mazodynia, but basically it means pain in the breast without any specific pathologic connotation. Mastalgia is an uncommon presenting symptom of breast cancer, but obviously that fact does not exclude its diagnosis. Mastalgia due to cancer, however, differs from the more common patterns of breast pain.

EVALUATION

When evaluating a patient with mastalgia, a comprehensive history is important. It is best to use descriptive terms, such as "tenderness," "heaviness," or a "burning sensation," when questioning the patient. Is the pain continuous or intermittent? What is its duration, distribution, radiation, and timing as it relates to the menstrual cycle? For many patients mastalgia is only one of a number of symptoms associated with the premenstrual syndrome. Because some patients have had a hysterectomy the timing of the pain may be difficult to establish. Are any analgesics being taken that aggravate or relieve the symptoms? Questions relating to any disturbances in occupational, social, or sexual activity should be noted (e.g., sleep loss, marital discord, or disruptions in family life). Has the patient recently been put on any medications such as oral contraceptives or hormonal therapy that may have provoked the onset of mastalgia? Remember to ask about any family history of breast cancer, as it may have heightened the need for reassurance.

The patient presenting with mastalgia should have a complete and thorough clinical breast examination. Any palpable mass requires full investigation using the diagnostic triad—clinical breast examination (CBE), mammography, fine-needle aspiration (FNA) cytology—or a biopsy. Mammography should be offered to patients who are over age 35, as nonpalpable cancers are sometimes picked up by mammography. After a negative mammogram, the patient should be seen again following her next menstrual period; and if her CBE is again normal, reassurance can be given.

CLASSIFICATION

Cyclic Mastalgia

The most common (>80%) pattern is cyclic, so called because of its relation to the menstrual cycle. The mean age for this pattern is 34 years. Patients usually complain that their breasts feel heavy and tender to touch. They occasionally complain of breast swelling. This pattern is almost always premenstrual, and there is usually a component of nodularity present at the CBE that is maximal in the upper outer quadrants (Fig. 15.1). The extent of nodularity rarely correlates with the severity of the pain. Many patients experience 2–3 days of premenstrual breast tenderness or heaviness, which is regarded as normal. Fine nodularity that begins shortly before menses and decreases after menstruation is also normal. The difficulty lies in deciding where normal ends and disease begins. The "pronounced" cyclic pattern means that the symptoms last longer than 1 week. This cyclic pattern is commonly bilateral, and the pain may radiate to the axilla and down the medial aspects of the upper arm (referred pain via the intercostobrachial nerve). These symptoms are

Table 15.1. Prevalence of mastalgia

Population source	Percent[a]
Southampton Breast Clinic	50
Cardiff Breast Clinic	45
General practice	47–52
Working women	66
Screening clinic	70

Source: Hughes et al.,[1] with permission.
[a] Proportions of patients with mastalgia from the given populations as determined by history.

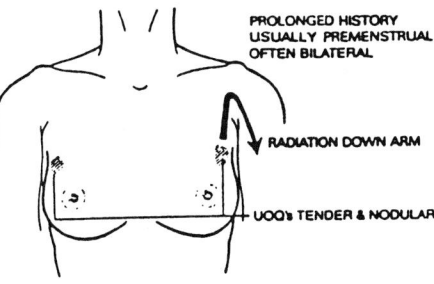

Figure 15.1. Clinical features of cyclical mastalgia. It is premenopausal: mean age 34 years. Descriptive terms are "heaviness" and "tenderness to touch." It is relieved by menstruation and menopause. (From Hughes et al.,[1] with permission.)

usually relieved by menstruation and typically disappear entirely with pregnancy or at menopause.

Mammography is important for identifying nonpalpable lesions but is often not much help for evaluating this pattern of mastalgia. Usually nonspecific changes in density thought to be related to fibroadenosis are seen. No specific appearance correlates with the site of the pain. As previously stated, breast density and nodularity do not correlate well with the severity of pain present. For similar reasons ultrasonography, which helps assess nodularity, has not been found useful for evaluating mastalgia. Magnetic resonance imaging (MRI) reflects tissue metabolism, and it is possible that this procedure may prove useful in the future. MRI is not now a recommended procedure for evaluating mastalgia.

More than 40% of menstruating patients present complaining of a cyclic pattern of mastalgia at some point, and 75% of them require no therapy other than reassurance. Twenty percent request occasional therapy, and only 5% require specific pharmacologic therapy due to severe disruption of their personal lives caused by the breast pain.

Noncyclic Mastalgia

The second most common (12%) presentation of mastalgia is the noncyclic pattern, distinguished primarily by its lack of relation to the menstrual cycle. The mean age at diagnosis for this pattern is 43 years, but it affects both premenopausal and postmenopausal women. Pain charts are helpful (Fig. 15.2) for classifying this type of mastalgia.

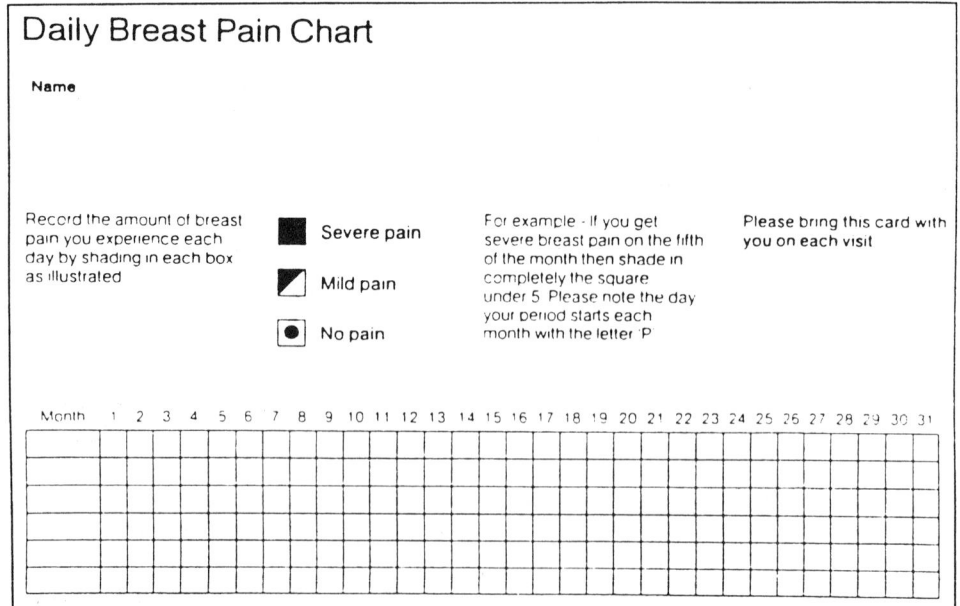

Figure 15.2. Daily breast pain chart (Cardiff).

The pain associated with this pattern is usually more localized, subareolar, and maximal in the inner quadrants (Fig. 15.3). Pain is less frequently bilateral. The patient may describe a burning sensation, transient sharpness, or stabbing pinprick sensation that lasts minutes to days with each episode. The intensity of this pain is usually less than that of the cyclic pain. Nodularity is less prominent with this pattern, and the CBE usually normal at the site of the pain. Unlike cyclic mastalgia, it is not uncommon for this pattern to persist long beyond menopause.

There has been some clinical interest in the mammographic evaluation of patients with noncyclic mastalgia. Mammograms showing coarse calcifications and ductal dilatation thought consistent with duct ectasia or periductal mastitis have been reported, but there has been no histologic evidence for it.

DIFFERENTIAL DIAGNOSIS

Tietze Syndrome

About 7% of mastalgia patients with Tietze syndrome complain of breast pain, but the pain in fact does not originate in the breast. Rather, costochondral pain in the region of the breast overlies tender costal cartilage (Fig. 15.4). It tends to be a chronic condition, occurs more commonly in the medial quadrants of the breast, and on examination one or more costal cartilages are found to be tender and somewhat enlarged. The pain is usually reproducible with pressure over the affected cartilage. Treatment commonly consists of lidocaine or prednisone injections at the site of the tender costal cartilage. Radiologic examination reveals no abnormality.

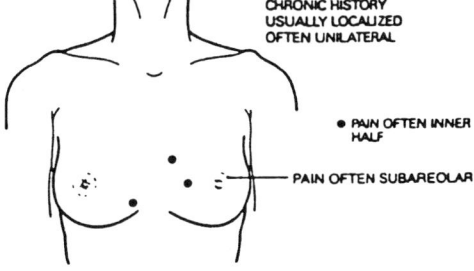

Figure 15.3. Clinical features of noncyclic mastalgia. It is premenopausal or postmenopausal: mean age 43 years. Descriptive terms are "drawing" and "burning." It is not relieved by reproductive events. (From Hughes et al.,[1] with permission.)

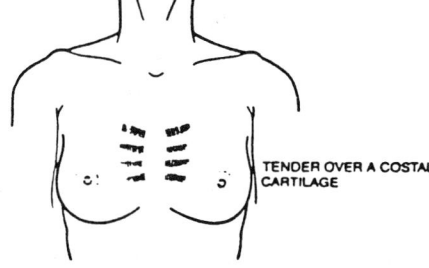

Figure 15.4. Clinical features of Tietze syndrome. It is often unilateral. It may occur at any age, with no time pattern, no palpable abnormality, and a chronic course. (From Hughes et al.,[1] with permission.)

Other Causes of Mastalgia

Other causes of anterior chest pain that patients often confuse with mastalgia include achalasia, cervical radiculitis, cervical rib, cholelithiasis (especially in women who are on oral contraceptives), and coronary artery disease/angina. Others are hiatal hernia, myalgia, neuralgia, phantom pain, pleurisy, and psychological pain. Table 15.2 lists nonbreast etiologies of anterior chest wall pain the patient may perceive as "breast pain" and so present for evaluation of mastalgia. A cyst in the breast, pregnancy and lactation, and mastitis with or without an associated abscess can present as mastalgia as well. Even trauma and tuberculosis may present as mastalgia. Mastalgia consistent with trauma or sclerosing adenosis is usually persistent and noncyclic, or it may be localized to a previous biopsy site. This situation is more common if the previous biopsy was complicated by an infection or a hematoma. Some painful scars have been noted across Langer's lines of tension. Patients with clinical depression may complain of breast pain and when treated with antidepressants note alleviation of the pain.

Musculoskeletal pain can mimic mastalgia but may be differentiated by some simple principles. Usually musculoskeletal pain is present along the lateral chest wall or can be localized to the costochondral junctions (as with Tietze syndrome). It is unilateral in more than 90% of cases, and radiation of the pain occurs to the axilla or arm in 60% of patients. The duration of musculoskeletal pain is usually shorter with Tietze syndrome than in mastalgia patients.

Table 15.2. Nonbreast etiologies of anterior chest wall pain

Achalasia

Angina

Cervical radiculitis

Cholecystitis

Cholelithiasis

Coronary artery disease

Costochondritis (Tietze syndrome)

Fibromyositis

Hiatal hernia

Myalgia

Neuralgia

Osteomalacia

Phantom pain

Pleurisy

Psychological pain

Pulmonary embolus

Pulmonary infarct

Rib fracture

Sickle cell disease

Trauma

Tuberculosis

Mastalgia Due to Breast Cancer

As previously stated, breast carcinoma does not typically present with mastalgia. When it does, the painful cancers are typically more locally advanced, with invasion of the surrounding structures. One study reported that only 7% of patients with operable cancer presented with mastalgia as the only complaint. Another 8% present with pain plus a palpable mass. The mean age of patients with mastalgia is 34 years, and patients in this age range have a low incidence of invasive breast cancer. Thus the possibility of cancer is remote in young women with mastalgia. Nevertheless, the potential of carcinoma as the cause of symptoms or findings must be pursued even in the youngest patient. One must pay particular attention to women in the cancer age group, however, who present for the first time with noncyclic mastalgia of some duration. Even after a negative workup, return appointments are scheduled for these patients to ensure that a small cancer has not been missed.

Mastalgia due to breast cancer is usually well localized, persistent, and constant. It is more commonly unilateral and noncyclic, and patients describe the pain as intensely sharp. What differentiates these cases from the cyclic and noncyclic types of mastalgia is that the pain is localized and persistent in one particular spot in one breast over a long period of time. This picture signals the need for a high suspicion for cancer. Because more than 40% of women have complaints of breast pain, some cancers are diagnosed in these patients, although cancer is probably not the etiology of the pain. The type of breast cancer most likely to be associated with breast pain is lobular carcinoma, which is difficult to detect on mammography until the cancer reaches an advanced stage. Mammography is the most sensitive diagnostic test to detect such cancers. FNA performed at the site of the pain is usually inconclusive. Occasionally, mastalgia is an initial symptom of subclinical cancer, which is another reason why both clinical and mammographic follow-up are necessary in patients with persistent mastalgia.

Etiology of Mastalgia

Most conclusions as to why mastalgia occurs are purely speculation. A hormonal etiology for cyclic mastalgia seems likely given its close temporal relation to the menstrual cycle and its response to hormonal manipulation. The exact pathogenesis remains unclear. Other theories include edema secondary to water retention; psychoneurosis; endocrine causes such as the cyclic increase in estrogen, decrease in progesterone production by the corpus luteum, and the relative unopposed estrogen activity thereafter; or possibly hyperprolactinemia. Still others include overstimulation of breast cells due to interference with ATP degradation by methylxanthines (caffeine) and an abnormality of prostaglandin synthesis secondary to a deficiency of essential fatty acids leading to an amplification of prolactin effects on breast cells because of deficient production of prostaglandin E_1 (PGE_1). The role of prolactin in the pathogenesis of mastalgia is unclear, but a statistically significant increase in basal prolactin levels has been noted in women with painful

---

KEY PRACTICE POINTS

Breast pain history: Is the pain cyclic or noncyclic? If noncyclic, is it constant or intermittent? Is the pain diffuse or localized? Is the pain of recent onset or long-standing? Is the pain actually in the breast?

Breast pain treatment: Following reassurance that there is no clinical evidence of breast cancer, most women with breast pain do not require prescription medication.

---

breast nodules. Many therapies have been directed toward this theory of hyperprolactinemia.

Mastalgia due to caffeine intake has repeatedly been disproved by well controlled and double-blind studies. The patient's weight may also be a contributing factor to breast pain, especially if obesity is present. Breast clinics that have followed their patients for a period of time have found that the patient's weight and pain are not closely related.

MANAGEMENT

A careful history and physical examination are absolutely necessary for any patient presenting with mastalgia, even if a recent annual breast examination was found to be normal. Any dominant mass deserves full investigation using the diagnostic triad: clinical breast examination, FNA cytology, mammography. Hormonal tests are of little assistance, with the exception of a routine prolactin level in patients with simultaneous complaints of galactorrhea and amenorrhea (to rule out a prolactinoma). Remember that for patients with simultaneous complaints of mastalgia and amenorrhea, pregnancy must be excluded.

The first and most successful treatment for all mastalgia patients whose breast examinations are normal is reassurance that their symptoms are not due to cancer. Reassurance is sufficient treatment in more than 80% of patients. Banishment of the patient's suspicion and fear of the dreaded disease is important. Reassurance does not cure the pain, but it often alters the patient's attitude toward it.

To be successful, reassurance should include an explanation of what mastalgia is and why it is not usually related to cancer. It should be pointed out to the patient that there is no documented evidence that cyclic mastalgia is a risk factor for the development of breast cancer. The patient should be told that mastalgia is common in the general population. Attempting to explain the pain as psychological or nonexistent is counterproductive and destroys the patient's confidence in her doctor.

One of the difficulties with active reassurance is that many doctors dislike using the term "cancer" and therefore resort to euphemisms, which are open to misinterpretation. One doctor said, "You have something in your breast, but there's no need to worry." Another said, "You have fibroadenosis. Although the cause is unknown, it is harmless." Both assured the patient that she need not return. Yet what the patient heard was, "I have cancer. It is incurable and the doctor is abandoning me." As you can see, sympathetic, detailed reassurance is necessary.

More than 80% of patients can be treated by reassurance alone and do not require additional therapy. About 5–15% of patients have pain severe enough to cause considerable interference in their lives, such as sleep loss, work disturbance, or marital discord. Even hugging a child can be painful for some of these patients. For such patients additional treatment may be of some benefit. Among those who require therapy, studies have shown favorable treatment response rates in approximately 77% of patients with cyclic mastalgia and but in only 44% of those with noncyclic mastalgia.

Hormonal Therapy

Bromocriptine

With the discovery of a small elevation of basal prolactin in patients with benign breast disease, bromocriptine (Parlodel) 2.5 mg bid has been suggested. It acts by decreasing prolactin stimulation of breast stroma and parenchyma. The dose is started at 1.25 mg at night and then increased by 1.25-mg increments over a period of 2 weeks (longer if side effects become a problem) until a dose of 2.5 mg twice daily is reached. A controlled study showed that this drug was effective in relieving breast symptoms associated with premenstrual syndrome. Another study showed that the symptoms associated with cyclic mastalgia were reduced with bromocriptine compared to a placebo, but not those with noncyclic mastalgia. However, most women experience severe side effects with bromocriptine; nausea, vomiting , dizziness, headache, abdominal pain, light-headedness (secondary to postural hypotension), and nasal congestion are common. Therefore most gynecologists prefer not to use this drug. Some of these side effects can be avoided by introducing the drug slowly and incrementally, avoiding doses higher than 5 mg/day. The side effects seem to be less if the drug is taken with meals.

Progesterone

The use of progesterone (medroxyprogesterone acetate 20 mg/day on days 10–26 of the menstrual cycle) has been investigated but found to be no more effective than placebo when given orally or as a cream. This therapy was suggested based on the theory that a deficiency of progesterone relative to estrogen during the luteal phase of ovarian secretion causes cyclic mastalgia. However, several investigators have failed to find a lower serum progesterone during the luteal phase in mastalgia patients, which may explain why its supplementation has not proved useful.

Danazol

The only hormonal drug approved by the U.S. Food and Drug Administration (FDA) and the drug most commonly used for treatment of mastalgia is danazol, a synthetic derivative of testosterone and an antigonadotropic agent, introduced in

1971. Danazol acts on the pituitary-ovarian axis, binding both progesterone and androgen receptors; it is thought therefore to have a local tissue effect at the level of the breast. It has also been shown to bind directly to human breast cells, which may be the mechanism of action.

The dose starts at 200 mg/day starting on day 2 of the menstrual cycle. If a clinical response, measured by a decrease in symptoms and nodularity, is obtained after 2 months of therapy, the dose is decreased to 100 mg/day for 2 months. If the clinical response is maintained, the dose is further decreased to 100 mg/day for the last 2 weeks of the menstrual cycle (e.g., days 14–28), or 100 mg every other day if the patient has amenorrhea. This schedule induces a clinical response in more than 80% of cyclic mastalgia patients.

Unfortunately, danazol has a high rate of dose-related side effects associated with the increased androgenic and hypoestrogenic state. The androgenic side effects include weight gain, acne, edema, muscle aches, hirsutism, and lowered voice pitch. Side effects associated with decreased estrogen include hot flashes, decreased breast size, vaginal dryness, dyspareunia, nervousness, vaginal bleeding or amenorrhea, and emotional instability. If it is possible to decrease the dose and still have a clinical response, the side effects can be minimized. Exercise may increase the tolerance of these side effects. It is important to stress the need for mechanical/barrier contraception for patients who could become pregnant, as danazol may be teratogenic.

For noncyclic mastalgia, danazol has been shown to be of some benefit. The overall response in this group is much lower, however, as it is with all other known medications. Thus treatment for noncyclic mastalgia is difficult.

Tamoxifen

Tamoxifen is an antiestrogen drug that was originally formulated as an oral contraceptive, for which it was determined to be ineffective. Later it was found to be of value and without serious toxicity in the adjuvant control of patients with advanced breast cancer and in the nonsurgical treatment and management of early breast cancer. Its mode of action is complicated. It inhibits the uptake of tritiated estradiol in target tissues but has estrogen agonist activity as well. It later increases the synthesis of sex hormone-binding globulin, mimicking estrogen administration.

At a dose of 10 mg/day tamoxifen has been reported by an Italian study to be 80% effective for treating severe cyclic mastalgia, but the drug has not been approved by the FDA for this purpose. It has been reported to reduce serum prolactin levels, which might explain its therapeutic action.

The initial side effects—hot flashes, vaginal discharge, occasional menorrhagia, nausea, and bloating—are reportedly minimal, but the safety of the drug needs to be confirmed. Another study revealed that the problem recurred in approximately one-third of patients after 3 months of follow-up; long-term use is probably necessary. Long-term side effects associated with a decrease in estradiol and the risk of accelerated loss of bone mineral content, with its enhanced risk of pathologic fractures due to osteoporosis and its effect on high density lipoprotein metabolism, may be severe. Some patients on tamoxifen with advanced breast cancer have also been noted to have thromboembolisms, but it is unknown if they are due to the cancer or the drug. Studies are under way to examine the clotting and lipoprotein profiles in patients receiving tamoxifen. It has also been discovered that high doses of tamoxifen have produced hepatocellular carcinoma in rats.

More detailed studies must be performed to determine the appropriate dosage, duration of therapy, and long-term safety. Its use for the treatment of mastalgia is still considered experimental. Note also that the administration of tamoxifen to a patient with an undiagnosed malignancy might lead to the emergence of an endocrine-unresponsive tumor.

Oral Contraceptives

Although not approved by the FDA for mastalgia, oral contraceptives can be helpful and may be considered prior to initiating danazol, as the side effects are much less in the average patient. The best oral contraceptives to use are the ones with decreased estrogen and increased progesterone formulas: ethinyl estradiol $20\,\mu g$ plus norethindrone acetate $1.0\,mg$ (Loestrin 1/20), ethinyl estradiol $0.03\,mg$ plus levonorgestrel $0.15\,mg$ (Levlen), or ethinyl estradiol $0.03\,mg$ plus norgestrel $0.3\,mg$ (Lo/Ovral).

Luteinizing Hormone-Releasing Hormone Agonist

Within 72 hours of use, goserelin acetate (Zoladex, a luteinizing hormone-releasing hormone (LHRH) agonist, induces reversible ovarian suppression with castrate levels of hormones produced by the premenopausal ovary. It has been shown to be of therapeutic benefit in some cancers that are hormone-dependent. This drug is currently under investigation for its potential role in treating mastalgia. It acts by decreasing the estrogen drive to breast tissue. A monthly injection of $3.6\,mg$ goserelin acetate in the form of a biodegradable rod is placed in the subcutaneous tissue of the anterior abdominal wall and replaced every 28 days for a total of six implants. Initial studies show some promise in both cyclic and noncyclic mastalgia patients, but these results require confirmation in larger randomized trials. The significant menopausal side effects may be limiting.

Nonhormonal Therapy

Mechanical Measures

Mechanical measures are suggested as an initial step toward pain relief. They include the use of a well fitting, supportive brassiere without wires and pressure points. Sometimes the patient has recently changed to an irritating brassiere or breast-supporting garment. A heating pad or hot towels may be helpful, and massage can be useful. If obesity is present, weight reduction should be considered. Psychological assistance may prove useful for alleviating any acute stress that may be contributing to the problem.

Dietary Therapy

Dietary therapy for mastalgia has been suggested, including the withdrawal of caffeine, supplements of vitamin E (α-tocopherol) and vitamin B_6, and implementing a low-fat/high-fiber diet. These approaches to treatment are largely unsubstantiated, but many investigators claim large response rates. There is no evidence that caffeine restriction changes any symptoms. One study showed promising results with vitamin E, but when a double-blind placebo study was done to confirm it, no effectiveness was noted over a placebo effect.

Vitamin B_6 (pyridoxine) at a dose of 200 mg/day has been suggested, as this vitamin enhances the decarboxylation of dopa to dopamine and thereby inhibits prolactin levels. It helps the liver detoxify the estrogens. Previously vitamin B_6 has been used to help patients with premenstrual syndrome. It was noted coincidentally to relieve the associated breast discomfort. For this reason vitamin B_6 was studied in mastalgia patients. However, published studies have not confirmed a therapeutic benefit when compared to the placebo effect.

Evening primrose oil has been used based on the theory of a deficiency of essential fatty acids, and some studies show that it may be helpful in mild cases of cyclic mastalgia. Evening primrose oil contains the richest source of essential fatty acids. A dose of 1000 mg, containing 240 mg of γ-linolenic acid, can be given three times daily for at least three months before review. It costs approximately $2.00 per day. The rare side effects of evening primrose oil are nausea and bloating. Because it is a more natural product, patients may prefer to try this therapy before resorting to hormonal therapy. Limiting factors are its high relapse rate and cost of treatment. This therapy is widely used in Europe, especially in the United Kingdom, where it is the first medication of choice prescribed by many physicians for mastalgia.

Fish oil supplementation has been recommended and is currently being used in patients with ischemic heart disease, as it is known to alter plasma lipids. Most of the agents proved effective for cyclic mastalgia alter plasma lipids to some degree.

Analgesics

Various analgesics, particularly nonsteroidal analgesics taken when symptoms occur, are often palliative for many patients.

Diuretics

In the past diuretics were used as the first line of treatment, although there is no physiologic basis for this use. A low-salt diet is probably just as effective. Measurement of total body water early and late during the menstrual cycles of patients with and without mastalgia showed no difference in water level.

Local Injections

Injection of 1% lidocaine (1 cc) and methylprednisone (40 mg) have been used for "trigger points" in noncyclic mastalgia, (e.g., treatment for Tietze syndrome). One study revealed a 90% response rate, but approximately 50% of patients require a second injection, usually 2–3 months later. When no palpable abnormality exists, surgical excision of these "trigger points" in noncyclic mastalgia has been attempted by removing the breast tissue at the site of the pain. Surgical therapy should not be considered unless pressure over the specific area reproduces the pain and a minimum of three clinic visits reveals that the site of pain is constant. The response to surgical treatment is unpredictable.

Individualizing Therapy

The 15% of mastalgia patients not helped by reassurance alone should be evaluated by a pain chart (Fig. 15.2) to define the pain pattern present and to provide a baseline by which to judge the effectiveness of any therapy given. Patients use these charts like calendars, each day shading a box to reflect the quality of her pain for that day. Any association between the occurrence of her mastalgia and her menstrual cycle is then obvious. At least two cycles are needed to establish the pattern of pain present.

All patient therapy should be individualized. For example, a patient with pain severe enough to interfere with her livelihood but who is not interested in overt hormonal therapy might be interested in trying evening primrose oil first. For another patient whose pain is strongly influencing her life style and who is unable to cope, danazol would be an appropriate first therapeutic choice. When danazol is contraindicated or a patient is unwilling to experience its side effects, particularly the weight gain and menstrual irregularity, bromocriptine might be used first. Regardless of which treatment is used, mastalgia symptoms tend to return a few months after cessation of treatment, so long-term treatment is likely to be necessary. Therefore pharmacologic therapy should be reserved for those women who absolutely require it.

The failure of one drug to work does not predict the failure of others, and no factors have been found to indicate which patients will or will not respond to a particular drug. It is likely that more than one drug must be tried to relieve a patient's pain, and simple trial and error is all that can be relied upon. Failure of a response to danazol, however, often leads to failure of other drugs to provide relief. Evening primrose oil should not be recommended as a second-line therapy because studies have shown its response rate in this capacity is no better than would be expected from placebo or spontaneous resolution, which is reported in more than 20% of cyclic mastalgia patients.

Sample Management Scheme for Severe Cyclic Mastalgia

1. *Evening primrose oil.* Try this product first, as it is more natural, with no side effects. No prescription is necessary. If there is clinical improvement after 3 months of treatment, the therapy can be continued for another 2 months before withdrawal. If there is no response after the initial 3 months, another drug should be tried. Recommend a well fitting support brassiere and caffeine restriction if the patient drinks in excess of 5 cups per day.

2. *Danazol.* This drug has been confirmed as the most effective whether given as the first or second line of treatment. Try Danazol 100 mg twice daily with a review at 2 months. If a response is noted, decrease the dose to 100 mg/day for 2 months. If the patient is pain-free after the initial 2 months of treatment, further decrease the dose to 100 mg on alternate days for an additional 2 months before withdrawal. Remember that side effects are less with the lower-dose regimens. If no response is noted, try a different drug.

3. *Bromocriptine.* If used, this drug should be introduced slowly to avoid nausea. Start with 1.25 mg each night and increase gradually, if effective, to the full

dose of 2.5 mg twice daily. Have the patient take the medication with food to reduce nausea. If a response is noted after 2 months of therapy, give an additional 3 months of treatment before considering withdrawal.

Studies show that after a failed treatment with either evening primrose oil or bromocriptine the use of danazol as second-line therapy has an approximately same response rate as when used as first-line therapy. On the other hand, the second-line response of both evening primrose oil and bromocriptine is poor when used after a treatment failure with danazol; yet they each produce response rates equal to that expected with first-line therapy when used to follow the failure of each other. With the exception of danazol, the response rate to third-line therapy is poor. Studies have compared patients with refractory mastalgia to those who achieve a response to first-line therapy and have failed to identify any factors in the reproductive history, presenting complaints, family history of benign or malignant breast disease, or need for subsequent breast surgery that could reliably identify those patients who would achieve a response to drug therapy.

The overall response to these drugs in patients with severe noncyclic mastalgia is lower than in patients with severe cyclic mastalgia, and the refractory nature of noncyclic mastalgia is well known. An optimum response is seldom achieved with the initial treatment. Because the response to hormonal manipulation is so much lower and only small improvements have been noted over placebo, our lack of understanding as to the etiology of this disorder is apparent. Patients should be warned that there is usually a low response rate.

In patients with either type of mastalgia who obtain a clinical response, the drug is usually given for 6 months and then stopped. Relapses are treated by resuming the drug that was previously effective. With danazol, the relapse symptoms may become obvious when attempting to wean the patient from the dose or when the patient is on the maintenance dose. If the relapse symptoms are mild, simply increase the dose to that previously given. If the relapse symptoms are severe, the dose should be returned to the initial twice-daily schedule of 100 mg. When the pain is controlled, the dose can be reduced monthly or at 6-week intervals until the maintenance dose appropriate for that specific patient is found. Remember that the symptoms of mastalgia may be exacerbated by emotional upsets, but contrary to previous beliefs the basis for the symptoms in most cases is not psychological.

Overall, danazol has been shown to produce the best response rate in both the cyclic and noncyclic patterns of mastalgia. The side effects of danazol therapy compared to other hormonal drug treatments are modest (i.e., 22%). It is the most expensive of the drugs available and has the highest reported relapse rate. Bromocriptine and evening primrose oil have similar response rates (45–47%). Bromocriptine is probably the least expensive drug available (other than oral contraceptives), but approximately 33% of patients experience bothersome side effects. Side effects are severe in approximately 12–15% of patients.

Adequate contraceptive advice must be given to treated patients, as hormonal drug treatment may interfere with the effectiveness of the contraceptive pill. The fertility of some patients is enhanced with the use of bromocriptine. If pregnancy occurs during therapy with any of these medications, treatment should be discontinued immediately.

As mentioned previously, surgery has a limited role in the treatment of mastalgia and is rarely indicated. If the pain is persistently localized to a small area, excision may be curative in an exceptional case; but the response is totally unpredictable. If the pain is less localized, surgery is usually contraindicated and is not clinically helpful. Repeated excisions can result in disfigurement and deformity of the breast, often without relief of the breast symptoms: replacing a painful area with a painful scar is not helpful. This option should be reserved for the most refractory of cases. Bilateral or unilateral mastectomy for patients with severe intractable mastalgia should be used with extreme caution and with full awareness by the patient of the complications of prostheses. Psychosexual consultation is advised before considering mastectomy for breast pain.

CONCLUSIONS

Overall, 92% of patients with cyclic mastalgia and 64% of patients with noncyclic mastalgia can obtain relief from their symptoms with the judicious use of the therapies described. This level of successful treatment should be emphasized to the mastalgia patient. Many health care providers have thought that specific treatment of mastalgia is not effective and that breast pain did not merit therapy. Wrong! Times have changed!

Reference

1. Hughes LE, Mansel RE, Webster DJT. Breast pain and nodularity. In: Benign Disorders and Diseases of the Breast: Concepts and Clinical Management. London, Baillière, 1989

16   NIPPLE DISCHARGE

William H. Hindle
Raquel D. Arias

Nipple discharge is the presenting complaint of about 4% of women at their initial visit to the Breast Diagnostic Center (BDC). Among these patients, 75% had elicited nipple discharge (which usually can be effectively treated simply by discontinuing the nipple stimulation and squeezing). Thus fewer than 1% of the BDC new patient population presented with spontaneous nipple discharge. The field was further narrowed at the time of examination when about half of these women were no longer having nipple discharge and no discharge could be elicited. This resulted in only about 0.5% of the BDC new patient population presenting with a history of spontaneous nipple discharge that was demonstrable at the time of their BDC examination.

Several breast clinics in Europe have reported the incidence of nipple discharge (elicited and spontaneous) as the chief complaint to be in the neighborhood of 5%. Other studies from Europe have reported that as many as 80% of women having regular menstrual cycles can elicit (or have elicited) nipple discharge.

HISTORY

A detailed, clinically pertinent history of nipple discharge usually leads to the diagnosis. The critical question is whether the discharge is elicited or spontaneous. Elicited discharge is usually physiologic. Is the discharge unilateral or bilateral? Bilateral discharge is often physiologic and rarely related to neoplasms. Is the discharge milky or bloody? Milky discharge is not due to intrinsic breast pathology and, except for galactorrhea, is physiologic. Pregnancy and lactation-related nipple discharge (almost always milky) is physiologic and not galactorrhea by definition. Is the discharge coming from a single or multiple duct openings? Spontaneous bloody nipple discharge from a single duct has the highest index of suspicion for malignancy.

The patient should be questioned about any medications she is taking. Antihypertensives, estrogen, methyldopa, opiates, oral contraceptives, phenothiazine, reserpine, and tranquilizers can stimulate milky or serous nipple discharge (spontaneous or elicited).

Physical Examination

The primary care physician should perform a complete bilateral clinical breast examination (CBE) of a woman presenting with nipple discharge. In addition, both areolae should be concentrically massaged as described in Chapter 4 (see Fig. 4.12). Although the patient may be aware of exactly where on the nipple the discharge originates, it is imperative that the examiner, with magnification if necessary, determine if the discharge is present and whether it is coming from a single or multiple duct openings.

Women may interpret as "nipple discharge" the secretion or exudate from an abrasion, dermatitis, eczema, excoriation, dermatitis, laceration, Paget's disease, ulceration, or maceration secondary to inversion of the nipple. Careful examination of the nipple should reveal such skin entities as the source of the problem.

Paget's disease usually starts on the top of the nipple as a moist erythematous lesion with a serosanguineous secretion. Over time this changes to a dry, white, scaly "discharge" that may spread down the sides of the nipple and onto the areola. A skin punch biopsy (or incision biopsy), which reveals typical Paget's cells within the epidermis of the nipple, is diagnostic. These malignant cells are thought to spread from underlying ductal carcinoma in situ (DCIS). However, invasive ductal carcinoma can occur by infiltrating malignant transformation. If an invasive component is present, it may grow to a size that is palpable, otherwise there is usually no associated palpable mass with Paget's disease.

The color of spontaneous nipple discharge is useful for the clinical evaluation. Frankly bloody discharge suggests a neoplasm. Milky discharge alerts the clinician to the possibility of galactorrhea, but milky discharge is not associated with intrinsic breast pathology. Dark green, dark brownish, or blackish discharge (particularly from multiple duct openings on the nipple) is usually from periductal mastitis (mammary duct ectasia) and occurs most commonly during the years shortly before menopause. Although the color of spontaneous nipple discharge, from clear watery to cloudy serosanguineous, is usually related to a benign intraductal papilloma, occasionally the source is an intraductal papillary carcinoma. One report from the United Kingdom cited more than a 5% incidence of DCIS with unilateral spontaneous nipple discharge that was serous to bloody. All the intraductal lesions should be excised for definitive histologic diagnosis. Smears of nipple discharge to look for red blood cells are not cost-effective or efficient.

Hemastix, Hematest, or other dipstick test for blood can be used to verify blood in a dark or otherwise suspicious nipple discharge. Some clinicians prefer to blot the nipple with white gauze, which tends to show the precise coloration of the discharge. This procedure can be helpful when looking for bloody discharge.

Milky nipple discharge is physiologic or galactorrhea (see Chapter 17) and not due to intrinsic breast pathology. Unless the patient has menstrual abnormalities or copious spontaneous discharge (usually milky but occasionally yellow or greenish), there is no need for endocrine tests such as prolactin or thyroid-stimulating hormone assays.

In the past, frankly bloody nipple discharge was often accompanied by gross palpable breast cancers. Even Hippocrates once wrote of bloody nipple discharge when describing what surely must have been an advanced breast cancer. Fortunately, with today's increased awareness of breast health and with current standards of care, this malignant etiology of frankly bloody discharge is not frequently seen. However, if a dominant palpable mass is found, a definitive diagnosis becomes urgent and paramount.

CYTOLOGY

Cytologic evaluation of nipple discharge for blood and abnormal cells has not proved useful in clinical practice. "Screening" nipple secretions as an early detection procedure for breast cancer was attempted by Papanicolaou and others using a pumping device. The procedure was not successful owing to the low sensitivity for cancer and the difficulty in obtaining adequate cellular samples from all women to be screened.

Cytologic studies of nipple discharge, particularly elicited discharge, is not cost-effective. Well preserved cells (other than histocytic foam cells) are rarely seen in nipple discharge smears. Only obviously malignant cells would be clinically significant, and they would occur most often in frankly bloody discharge. Furthermore, in all cases an identified intraductal lesion should be excised. Histologic verification is the only method that definitively diagnoses the rare intraductal papillary carcinoma.

Also, although it may satisfy curiosity, the microscopic evaluation of milky discharge does not assist in the medical evaluation and is of no pertinent clinical value. A smear of milky discharge examined for refractile lipid (fat) droplets on an unfixed slide (or on a slide fixed and stained with oil red O fat stain) adds nothing to the diagnostic evaluation. Proteinaceous debris, fat globules, and uninterpretable cell forms are the rule; if such a specimen is submitted, the cytopathologist may feel compelled to write an ambiguous report, which increases physician and patient anxiety.

MAMMOGRAPHY AND ULTRASONOGRAPHY

Diagnostic mammography is an essential component in the evaluation of spontaneous nipple discharge, although the etiology of the discharge is usually not apparent in the mammogram. Microcalcifications consistent with DCIS can be seen by mammography. Sometimes a mass is seen in the nipple or below the areola. Ultrasonography can detect dilated ducts below the nipple–areola complex but does not establish a definitive diagnosis and is not routinely indicated.

GALACTOGRAPHY

Galactography (ductography) can be useful for identifying an intraductal lesion, although a "negative" galactogram does not guarantee that there is no pathology

---

KEY PRACTICE POINTS

Nipple discharge history: Is the discharge pregnancy-related? Is the discharge elicited or spontaneous? Is the discharge unilateral or bilateral? It is milky? Is it bloody? Does it come from a single duct opening on the nipple?

Nipple discharge examination: Is there an associated palpable mass? Are there skin changes on the nipple/areola? Can the nipple discharge be reproduced? Is it reproducible bilaterally? What is the color of the discharge? Is the discharge milky? Is the discharge bloody? Does it come from a single duct opening?

---

in the duct. When the lesion is clearly outlined by contrast medium, it can reveal exactly where in the duct the lesion is located, which allows the surgeon to excise precisely the portion of the duct involved. Thus the area of pathology can be excised, and normal tissue need not be removed. Galactography is particularly useful for peripheral lesions such as those with papillomatosis, which might be missed if only the central portion of the duct system were to be excised.

Many surgeons prefer to place a lacrimal duct probe in the duct before surgery to excise the involved duct. However, the length of duct to be excised to remove the entire lesion is then a surgical estimate, and lesions (e.g., papillomatosis) may be left in the segment of the duct that is not excised.

The patient scheduled for galactography should be informed that she should reschedule the procedure if her nipple discharge stops. The discharge must be present for the mammographer to cannulate the duct from which the discharge is coming.

PHYSIOLOGIC NIPPLE DISCHARGE

Nipple discharge can be squeezed or pumped from the breasts of more than 75% of women during their reproductive years. After menopause, the number falls to 50% and less with advancing age. Elicited discharge is usually milky but can be clear, serous, or serosanguineous. During pregnancy and lactation, frankly bloody discharge can be elicited. This physiologic bloody nipple discharge associated with pregnancy and lactation is thought to be related to the increased vascularity and engorgement around the collecting ducts and the ducts leading to the openings on the nipple. Pregnancy-related nipple discharge does not interfere with breast feeding or harm the infant.

PATHOLOGIC NIPPLE DISCHARGE

Suspicious nipple discharge occurs spontaneously without squeezing the nipple; it is unilateral, comes from a single duct opening on the nipple, and is serous or bloody. This type of discharge is most commonly associated with a benign intraductal papilloma.

Pathologic nipple discharge is nonlactational and persistent. Inspection of the nipple reveals secretion from one or more duct openings on the nipple, in contrast to the weepy skin lesions on the nipple and areola. Pathologic nipple discharge is almost always spontaneous.

In a Swedish study, cancer was found to be the etiology in 6% of women with spontaneous serous or clear watery nipple discharge and in 13% of those with frankly bloody nipple discharge. The specific pathology of spontaneous (nonpregnancy) nipple discharge is age-related. In the general population the histologic diagnoses, in order of frequency, are (1) intraductal papilloma (and papillomatosis), (2) fibrocystic changes, (3) mammary duct ectasia, and (4) cancer. Cancer and duct ectasia are increasingly frequent in the postmenopausal age group.

Mammary duct ectasia (periductal mastitis or plasma cell mastitis) usually occurs during the perimenopausal years. The discharge is often bilateral, and it may be spontaneous or elicited. Typically the discharge comes from multiple duct openings on the nipple. Duct ectasia is self-limited and not related to neoplasms. Antibiotics are of no value even though the term periductal mastitis implies an infection. The histologic appearance is of dilated ducts filled with necrotic proteinaceous debris and aggregates of plasma cells around the dilated ducts. Treatment is not necessary unless the patient insists, and then the only effective treatment is surgical removal of all the involved ducts. The patient may be reassured that the symptoms usually subside after menopause.

Treatment

Excision of the involved duct or ducts (microdochectomy) is therapeutic and provides the definitive histologic diagnosis. Painting the nipple with collodion prior to surgery can assist in identifying the duct or ducts to be excised. This same collodion technique can be used when evaluating a patient who continues to complain of a spontaneous nipple discharge that cannot be expressed (identified) at the time of examination. The incision is usually circumareolar and hardly visible when healed. Breastfeeding is possible after single (selected) duct excision.

17   GALACTORRHEA

Richard J. Paulson

Galactorrhea refers to the secretion of milk from the breast. It is considered normal during pregnancy and the postpartum period, when elevated levels of prolactin act on the mammary glands to produce milk. At other times galactorrhea is nonphysiologic and requires evaluation. As a general guideline, galactorrhea should be evaluated in any nulliparous woman and in any parous woman if a year or more has passed since her last delivery or cessation of breast-feeding.

EVALUATION

The first steps in the evaluation of any nipple discharge, including galactorrhea, are specific, gross, and microscopic* evaluations of the secretion. The galactorrhea is classified according to whether it is spontaneous or must be elicited by local pressure around the nipple. Because a small amount of nipple discharge may be elicited with sufficient pressure on the breast in virtually any woman, the amount of effort required to obtain the nipple discharge may provide a significant clue as to its ultimate clinical significance. When evaluating the galactorrhea, it is worth observing whether the fluid comes from multiple duct openings, as occurs during hormonally stimulated milk secretion, or from a single duct opening, which usually is an indication of a pathologic discharge.

Gross examination can reveal the character of the fluid. Galactorrhea is usually white or clear and watery, though it may be yellowish or even green. Red fluid may be indicative of blood, which is an indication for further evaluation to rule out an intraductal lesion.

The droplet of fluid that accumulates over the nipple can be collected by touching it directly to a microscope slide, topped with a coverslip, and examined under a microscope.* Galactorrhea has a characteristic appearance (Fig. 17.1),

---

* *Editor's note*: On an endocrine-infertility service, microscopic evaluation of milky nipple discharge may be useful. However, in general primary care practice, microscopic evaluation of nipple discharge is not cost-effective and rarely alters clinical management.

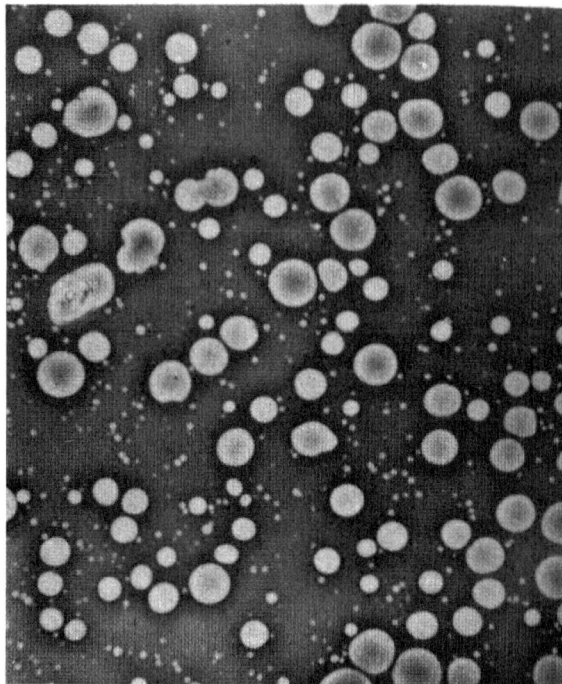

Figure 17.1. Fat droplets seen under the microscope from a patient with galactorrhea. (From Kletzky and Davajan,[1] with permission.)

consisting of round, fat globules of varying sizes. The presence of red blood cells is suspicious for intraductal lesions and necessitates further evaluation (e.g., mammography) of the breast.

LABORATORY EVALUATION

When galactorrhea is confirmed, measurement of serum prolactin levels is indicated. If hyperprolactinemia is suspected, prolactin is best measured before noon, as afternoon levels are normally higher than morning levels. Normal prolactin levels are indicative of idiopathic galactorrhea, and the patient may be reassured that there is no endocrine evidence of a pituitary neoplasm.

Elevated serum prolactin levels require further evaluation. Serum prolactin levels may be elevated by a variety of pharmacologic or pathologic conditions. Table 17.1 lists the pharmacologic agents and Table 17.2 the pathologic factors that affect prolactin concentrations.

The patient's history may provide important clues to the underlying cause of hyperprolactinemia, such as prior chest surgery or the use of phenothiazines. Hypothyroidism should be ruled out by measuring serum levels of thyroid-stimulating hormone (TSH). With hypothyroidism, feedback from thyroid hormone (T_3 and T_4) is diminished. As a consequence, the hypothalamus increases its secretion of thyroid-releasing hormone (TRH), which in turn increases pituitary secretion of TSH. Because TRH acts as a prolactin-releasing factor, prolactin secretion is usually augmented and galactorrhea is common.

Table 17.1. Pharmacologic agents affecting prolactin concentration

Stimulators
    Anesthetics
    Antiemetics
        Metoclopramide (dopamine antagonist)
        Sulpiride
    Antihypertensives
        α-Methyldopa
        Reserpine
    Hormones
        Estrogen
        Thyrotropin-releasing hormone
    Psychotropics
        Opiates
        Phenothiazines
        Tricyclic antidepressants
Inhibitor
    Dopamine agonists
        Dopamine
        L-Dopamine
        Bromocriptine
        Cabergoline
        Quinagolide

Source: Modified from Kletzky and Davajan,[1] with permission.

Patients with prolactin levels of 50 ng/ml or higher are referred for magnetic resonance imaging (MRI) of the sella turcica. The purpose of the MRI is to rule out a macroadenoma, defined as a pituitary adenoma 10 mm or more in diameter. A microadenoma (a pituitary adenoma 9 mm or less in diameter) is managed in the same way as idiopathic hyperprolactinemia (i.e., hyperprolactinemia without a detectable pituitary lesion). Treatment is symptomatic, and no further MRI scans are indicated. If a macroadenoma is found, treatment is also pharmacologic. However, serial MRI imaging must be done to rule out progression of the lesion or pituitary impingement on the remainder of the central nervous system. Surgical intervention is rarely needed.

TREATMENT

Pharmacologic treatment of galactorrhea focuses on the reduction of circulating prolactin levels. Because dopamine acts as a prolactin-inhibiting factor, suppression of prolactin secretion is best achieved by stimulation of dopaminergic receptors by a dopamine agonist. The most commonly used medication is bromocriptine (e.g., Parlodel), which acts directly on pituitary lactotrophs to

Table 17.2. Pathologic factors affecting prolactin concentrations

Brain and pituitary disorders
 Hypothalamic
  Destructive (tumor, encephalitis)
  Idiopathic (functional or biochemical)
  Infiltrative (histiocytosis, sarcoid)
 Pituitary
  Adenoma (micro, macro)
  Empty sella syndrome
  Pituitary stalk section
Chest lesions
 Breast implants
 Herpes zoster
 Thoracotomy scars
Hypothyroidism
Malignant tumors with ectopic production of prolactin
Renal failure

Source: Modified from Kletzky and Davajan,[1] with permission.

diminish prolactin secretion. Because of the common side effect hypotension, which diminishes over time, therapy is usually begun with low doses of medication at bedtime and then gradually augmented. We begin with one-half tablet (1.25 mg) at bedtime for 1 week and then increase the dose to 2.5 mg at bedtime for an additional week. Prolactin secretion is maximal during the sleeping hours, so this regimen also serves well to block the circadian augmentation of prolactin secretion during the night. The dose is then titrated until normal prolactin levels are reached. Idiopathic hyperprolactinemia and microadenomas with relatively low levels (<100 ng/ml) of prolactin usually respond to dosages ranging from 2.5 mg at bedtime to 5.0 mg twice daily. Doses of more than 5.0 mg/day are usually divided into two equal parts given twice daily. Macroadenomas with high levels of prolactin may require substantially higher doses. A maximum dose for bromocriptine has not been established.

A macroadenoma requires treatment regardless of the precise degree or extent of symptoms because these large adenomas may continue to grow, cause erosion of the sella turcica, and impinge on the optic chiasm. We prefer pharmacologic treatment as a first approach for all macroadenomas. The dose of bromocriptine is titrated until a normal level of prolactin is achieved. A repeat MRI scan is performed within 3 months to ensure that the tumor has stopped growing. The dose of medication is then maintained at the minimum level necessary to maintain serum prolactin levels in the normal range. Once therapeutic levels are achieved and the tumor is stabilized, the patient may be monitored with twice-yearly prolactin levels only. If the macroadenoma continues to grow or if the patient cannot tolerate the oral pharmacologic therapy, surgical extirpation of the adenoma may be required.

Treatment of idiopathic hyperprolactinemia and pituitary microadenoma are the same. Long-term studies of microadenomas have not demonstrated progression, growth, or other sequelae that would demand a therapeutic approach different from that for idiopathic hyperprolactinemia. If fertility is not an issue, treatment focuses on reduction of the quantity of breast secretion and reestablishment of normal menses. Bromocriptine effectively reduces the quantity of galactorrhea and eliminates hyperprolactinemia-associated menstrual irregularity. As an alternative, if galactorrhea is not a concern, regular menses may be induced by cyclic progestin withdrawal therapy or with oral contraceptives. Whereas estrogen is known to increase prolactin secretion during pregnancy, there is no evidence that the estrogen in oral contraceptives induces additional growth of pituitary microadenomas. During the long-term follow-up of these patients annual checks of prolactin levels are sufficient to monitor the progress of the hyperprolactinemia. If a sudden increase in prolactin is noted, a repeat evaluation of the pituitary by MRI is indicated.

In a hyperprolactinemic anovulatory patient attempting conception, pharmacologic therapy is indicated to induce ovulation. In an ovulatory patient with hyperprolactinemia, the use of bromocriptine is controversial, as prospective studies have not confirmed its efficacy in hastening conception. Studies have not addressed the issue of hyperprolactinemia and superovulation. In the absence of direct evidence to the contrary, we have utilized concurrent bromocriptine in a dose sufficient to normalize prolactin levels along with clomiphene or exogenous gonadotropins for treatment of hyperprolactinemic patients with otherwise unexplained infertility. In these cases, pharmacologic therapy is maintained until pregnancy is established. At this point, bromocriptine is discontinued. No further therapy is necessary unless the patient has a macroadenoma. In the case of macroadenoma in a patient wishing to conceive, bromocriptine must be continued throughout the pregnancy.

The vaginal route of administration may substantially increase compliance in patients who experience nausea and vomiting with oral bromocriptine therapy. Because of the small size of the bromocriptine molecule, absorption through the vaginal mucosa is excellent. Doses and results are similar to those attained with oral therapy.

A long-acting dopamine agonist, cabergoline, has recently been introduced in the United States.[2] This new medication has the advantage of a long half-life, requiring only twice-weekly dosing, and it appears to be well tolerated.

OTHER FORMS OF THERAPY

Pituitary tumors may be removed by surgical excision via the transsphenoidal approach. This approach, although relatively safe and successful, is associated with a high rate of recurrence. Surgery is reserved for patients with macroadenomas that do not respond to pharmacologic treatment or are symptomatic, or in instances when the patient cannot tolerate the side effects of the oral medication.

Radiation therapy was at one time advised to stop the progression of adenomas. A relatively large dose (4500 rad) was required. Side effects of radiation included damage to the surrounding pituitary gland, resulting in hypopituitarism. This form of therapy is no longer advised.

References

1. Kletzky OA, Davajan V. Hyperprolactinemia: diagnosis and treatment. In: Mishell DR Jr, Davajan V, Lobo RA (eds) Infertility, Contraception and Reproductive Endocrinology (3rd ed). Cambridge, MA, Blackwell Scientific, 1991, pp 396–421
2. Webster J, Piscitelli G, Polli A, et al. A comparison of cabergoline and bromocriptine in the treatment of hyperprolactinemic amenorrhea. N Engl J Med 1994;331:904–909

Recommended Reading

Kletzky OA, Vermesh M. Effectiveness of vaginal bromocriptine in treating women with hyperprolactinemia. Fertil Steril 1989;51:269–292

Klibanski A, Neer RM, Beitins IZ, et al. Decreased bone density in hyperprolactinemic women. N Engl J Med 1980;303:1511–1514

Soules MR, Hansen LW, Tucker KR, Buehler PK. Prolactin secretion in women after plastic breast augmentation and reduction. Ann Plast Surg 1986;17:335–338

Stein AL, Levenick MN, Kletzky OA. Computed tomography versus magnetic resonance imaging for the evaluation of suspected pituitary adenomas. Obstet Gynecol 1989; 73:996–999

18   MASTITIS

Diana E. Ramos
Subir Roy

M astitis is defined as inflammation of the mammary gland, or breast. The most common breast infection—that which accompanies pregnancy or nursing—is called lactational mastitis or puerperal mastitis. Non-puerperal breast infection has been viewed as a minor clinical problem with a low overall incidence.

PUERPERAL MASTITIS

Puerperal mastitis usually begins during the second to fourth week after delivery, but it may occur from as early as 4 days after childbirth to as late as 1 year afterward. The incidence ranges from 0.8% to as high as 20% during hospital epidemics. Patients may complain of a sensation of breast engorgement of the affected breast, significant fever (often 103°F or more), chills, anorexia, headache, and malaise. A diffuse edematous, erythematous, warm area is typically noted on examination. A central palpable mass is suggestive of abscess formation. Enlarged axillary lymph nodes may be tender. If the entire breast is involved, inflammatory carcinoma should be suspected. Urgent antibiotic treatment and frequent reevaluation are critical.

The infection is virtually always unilateral. In more than half of the cases, *Staphylococcus aureus* is cultured from breast milk. The origin of the infection is the infant, who may harbor the organism on the skin, umbilical stump, anus, or nasopharynx. During his or her stay in the nursery, the infant becomes colonized with coagulase-positive *S. aureus* that is penicillin-resistant. The baby in turn colonizes the mother and provides the bacterial nidus for the infection when there is a break in the surface integrity of the nipple. Other common organisms are group A (*S. pyogenes*) or group B (*S. agalactiae*) streptococci, *Hemophilus* species, or *Peptostreptococcus magnus.*

Prevention of peuperal mastitis requires meticulous breast hygiene. Breast milk provides a good culture medium. Clinical infection seldom supervenes, however, unless the flow of milk is interrupted, which may be caused by inspissation of the secretions or by stasis of milk if nursing by the mother is discontinued. Nursing

---

KEY PRACTICE POINTS

Mastitis: Treat as soon as clinically suspected. Reevaluate every 3 days until completely cleared. Change the antibiotic prescription if no response after 1 week. Consider skin punch biopsy if not responding to second antibiotic therapy. Cultures are *not* indicated.

Abscess: Aspirate and drain with 18-gauge needle and local anesthesia. Ultrasonography can confirm the presence of a small abscess. Reevaluate every 3 days until completely cleared. Repeat aspiration/drainage is usually necessary. Treat with antibiotics if there are systemic symptoms or cellulitis. Cultures are *not* necessary, unless there is no response to treatment. Surgical incision and drainage are rarely necessary.

---

should therefore be continued, particularly if milk stasis is a factor in the pathogenesis of infection. If nursing must be discontinued, the milk should be expressed using a breast pump. Only a purulent exudate from the nipple or an abscess should stop nursing.

Dicloxacillin (e.g., Dynapen) 500 mg PO q6h for 7 days or a cephalosporin such as cephalexin (e.g., Keflex) 500 mg PO q6h for 7 days is the best treatment. Another alternative is clindamycin (e.g., Cleocin) 300 mg PO q6h for 7 days. Erythromycin 500 mg PO four times a day for 7 days is an alternative for the penicillin-allergic patient. Antibiotics should be given empirically and the patient reevaluated every 3 days until the inflammation resolves completely. If the infection does not respond to treatment, the antibiotics should be changed and the diagnosis of inflammatory carcinoma considered. Cultures of the infected areas are reserved for infections and abscesses that do not respond to initial antibiotic treatment. Table 18.1 lists suspected organisms, initial antibiotic of choice, an alternate antibiotic, an antibiotic for a woman who is allergic to penicillin, the duration of therapy, and suggested nonpharmacologic treatment for puerperal breast infections.

If there is localized flocculation, suggesting early abscess formation, the flocculent area should be drained by 18-gauge needle aspiration under local anesthesia. Repeated aspirations may be necessary at 3-day interval checkups. A large abscess should be opened and completely drained under general anesthesia to be certain that all loculi have been broken. If possible, the incision should be circumareolar or at least should follow the natural skin lines as demonstrated in the sitting position. Dependent Penrose-type drains should be placed to facilitate complete drainage of the abscess cavity and left in place for 2–3 days. Antibiotics are given in full therapeutic doses and continued for 7–10 days after adequate drainage has been achieved. Nursing is discontinued at this time. Once the infection has cleared, the prognosis is excellent, although there is a 10% recurrence rate of puerperal mastitis with subsequent pregnancies.

Table 18.1. Bacteria-specific antibiotic therapy for puerperal mastitis

Suspected organism	Drug(s) of choice	Alternative drug(s)	Penicillin allergy	Duration (days)	Nondrug therapy
Aerobes					
Staphylococcus aureus (coagulase-positive) Methicillin-susceptible Mastitits without abscess	Dicloxacillin (Dynapen) 500 mg PO q6h Cefazolin 1 g IV q8h	Cephalexin (Keflex) 500 mg PO q6h Amoxicillin/clavulanate (Augmentin) 500 mg PO q6h Ampicillin/sulbactam (Unasyn) IV 1.5 g q6h	Erythromycin 500 mg PO qid Erythromycin 250–500 mg IV q6h Clindamycin (Cleocin) 300–600 mg PO/IV q6h	7–10	Hot compresses; adequate rest and nutrition; can continue breast feeding; if early, increase breast feeding
Mastitis with abscess	Oxacillin (Prostaphlin) or nafcillin (Nafcil, Unipen) 2 g IV q4h Cefazolin (Ancef, Kefzol) 1 g IV q8h	Ampicillin/sulbactam (Unasyn) IV 1.5 g q6h	Erythromycin 500 mg IV q6h Clindamycin (Cleocin) 600 mg IV q6h or 900 mg IV q8h	7–10	Aspiration or surgical drainage of abscess; subareolar vs. areolar
Methicillin-resistant	Vancomycin (Vancocin) 15 mg/kg/day IV q12h or adjust as needed ± Gentamicin IV ± Rifampin IV	Teicoplanin (Targocid) 12 mg/kg/day IV Quinopristin + dalfopristin (Synercid) 7.5 mg/kg q8h IV	Vancomycin (Vancocin) 15 mg/kg IV q12h or adjust as needed ± Gentamicin IV ± Rifampin IV	7–10	

Table 18.1. *Continued*

Suspected organism	Drug(s) of choice	Alternative drug(s)	Penicillin allergy	Duration (days)	Nondrug therapy
Streptococcus sp. Group A (*S. pyogenes*)	Penicillin VK 500 mg PO qid	Cephalexin (Keflex) 500 mg PO qid	Clindamycin 300 mg PO qid or IV q6h	7–10	Adequate rest and nutrition; can continue breastfeeding; if early, increase breastfeeding
	Penicillin G 2 MU IV q6h	Cefradine (Velosef) 500 mg PO qid	Erythromycin 500 mg PO qid or IV q6h	7–10	
	Penicllin G + clindamycin 300 mg IV q6h	Cefazolin 1 g IV q8h	Clarithromycin 500 mg q12h		
		Vancomycin 15 mg/kg q12h, adjusted	Azithromycin 500 mg × 1 then 250 mg PO pd	5	
			Vancomycin 15 mg/kg q12h, adjusted		
Group B (*S. agalactiae*)	Penicillin VK 500 mg PO qid	Cephalexin (Keflex) 500 mg PO qid	Erythromycin 500 mg PO qid or IV q6h	7–10	
	Penicillin G 2 MU IV q6h	Cefradine (Velosef) 500 mg PO qid	Vancomycin 15 mg/kg q12h, adjusted		
	Ampicillin 500 mg PO qid	Cefazolin 1 g IV q8h			
	Ampicillin 1 g IV q6h	Erythromycin 500 mg PO qid or IV q6h			
		Vancomycin 15 mg/kg q12h, adjusted			

Anaerobes				
Peptostreptococcus magnus	Penicillin VK 500 mg PO qid Penicillin G 2 MU IV q6h	Clindamycin 300 mg PO qid or IV q6h Cephalexin (Keflex) 500 mg PO qid Cefradine (Velosef) 500 mg PO qid Cefazolin 1 g IV q8h Vancomycin 15 mg/kg q12h adjusted	Clindamycin 300 mg PO qid or IV q6h Vancomycin 15 mg/kg q12h, adjusted	7–10
Gram-negative aerobes				
Hemophilus sp. *H. influenzae*	Amoxicillin 500 mg PO tid Ampicillin/sulbactam 1.5 g q6h? Amoxicillin/clavulanate 500 mg PO tid Cefuroxime (Ceftin) 250–500 mg PO bid	Trimethoprim/sufamethoxazole 8–10 mg/kg/day PO divided q12h Cefuroxime 750 IV q8h Ceftriaxone 1 g q24h	Trimethoprim/sufamethoxazole 8–10 mg/kg/day PO divided q12h Clarithromycin 500 mg q12h Azithromycin 500 mg PO qd Chloramphenicol	
H. parainfluenzae	Ampicillin 500 mg PO qid Amoxicillin 500 mg PO tid	Trimethoprim/sufamethoxazole 8–10 mg/kg/day PO divided q12h	Trimethoprim/sufamethoxazole 8–10 mg/kg/day PO divided q12h Chloramphenicol	

Table 18.2. Bacteria-specific antibiotic therapy for nonpuerperal mastitis

Suspected organism	Drug(s) of choice	Alternative drug(s)	Penicillin allergy	Duration (days)	Nondrug therapy
Gram-positive aerobes					
Staphylococcus aureus (coagulase-positive) Methicillin-susceptible Mastitis without abscess: *S. epidermidis* (coagulase negative)	Dicloxacillin (Dynapen) 500 mg PO q6h Cefazolin 1 g IV q8h	Cephalexin (Keflex) 500 mg PO q6h Amoxicillin/clavulanate (Augmentin) 500 mg PO q6h Ampicillin/sulbactam (Unasyn) IV 1.5 g q6h	Erythromycin 500 mg PO qid Erythromycin 250–500 mg IV q6h Clindamycin (Cleocin) 300–600 mg PO/IV q6h	7–10	Hot compresses; adequate rest and nutrition; can continue breast feeding; if early, increase breast feeding
	Same as above	Same as above plus ticarcillin/clavulanate (Timentin) 3.1 g V q6h	Same as above plus ciprofloxacin 300 mg IV q12h Ofloxacin 200–400 mg IV q12h	7–10	
Mastitis with abscess	Oxacillin (Prostaphlin)/nafcillin (Nafcil, Unipen) 2 g IV q4h Cefazolin (Ancef, Kefzol) 1 g IV q8h	Ampicillin/sulbactam (Unasyn) IV 1.5 g q6h Ticarcillin/clavulanate (Timentin) 3.1 g IV q6h	Erythromycin 500 mg IV q6h Clindamycin (Cleocin) 600 mg IV q6h or 900 mg IV q8h	7–10	Aspiration or surgical drainage of abscess; subareolar vs. areolar

Methicillin-resistant	Vancomycin (Vancocin) 15 mg/kg/day IV q12h or adjust as needed ± Gentamicin IV ± Rifampin IV	Teicoplanin (Targocid) 12 mg/kg/day IV Quinopristin + dalfopristin (Synercid) 7.5 mg/kg IV q8h	Vancomycin (Vancocin) 15 mg/kg IV q12h or adjust as needed ± Gentamicin IV ± Rifampin IV	7–10
Gram-positive anaerobes				
Cocci				
Peptostreptococcus magnus	Penicillin VK 500 mg PO qid Penicillin G 2 MU IV q6h	Clindamycin 300 mg PO qid or IV q6h Cephalexin (Keflex) 500 mg PO qid Cefradine (Velosef) 500 mg PO qid Cefazolin 1 g IV q8h Vancomycin 15 mg/kg IV q12h, adjusted	Clindamycin 300 mg PO qid or IV q6h Vancomycin 15 mg/kg IV q12h, adjusted	7–10
Rods				
Propionibacterium sp.	Erythromycin 500 mg PO qid Penicillin VK 500 mg PO qid	Clindamycin 300 mg PO qid	Erythromycin 500 mg PO qid Clindamycin 300 mg PO qid	

Table 18.2. *Continued*

Suspected organism	Drug(s) of choice	Alternative drug(s)	Penicillin allergy	Duration (days)	Nondrug therapy
Gram-negative anaerobes					
Bacteroides sp. (oropharyngeal strains)	Penicillin VK 500 mg PO qid Penicillin G 2 MU IV q6h Clindamycin 300 mg PO qid or IV q6h	Cefoxitin 1 g IV q6h Cefotetan 2 g IV q12h	Clindamycin 300 mg PO qid or IV q6h		
B. fragilis	Metronidazole (Flagyl) 500 mg IV q8h	As above; clindamycin 600–900 mg IV q8h Ampicillin/ sulbactam (Unasyn) 1.5 g IV q6h Ticarcillin/ clavulanate (Timentin) 3.1 g IV q6h	Metronidazole (Flagyl) 500 mg IV q8h Clindamycin 600–900 mg IV q8h Imipenem-cilastatin (Primaxin) 500 mg IV q6h Alatrofloxacin 300 mg IV q24h Clinafloxacin 300 mg IV q12h		Aspiration or surgical drainage

Nonpuerpal Mastitis

Nonpuerperal mastitis, also called squamous metaplasia infection, is clinically distinct from puerperal mastitis. The disease is characterized as partial blockage of the lactiferous ducts by keratotic debris and by squamous metaplasia of the epithelium lining the milk sinus. Almost all cases of the disease are found in premenopausal patients and seem to appear more commonly during the premenstrual phases of their cycles. There is currently no universal agreement as to the etiology of nonpuerperal mastitis, although it has been suggested that these infections occur after manipulative obstetric procedures; other studies have suggested that oral stimulation of the breast during sexual intercourse may be a predisposing factor.

All such patients present with complaints of mild to severe breast pain, localized edema and erythema in the subareolar region, and a firm, tender mass upon palpation with multicolored discharge either through the nipple or near a Montgomery follicle. There are three general presentations.

The first is nonpuerperal mastitis without an abscess, which may be caused by *S. aureus*, *P. magnus*, or *Bacteroides fragilis*. It should be treated empirically with amoxicillin/clavulanate (e.g., Augmentin) 500 mg PO q6h for 7 days. Cephalexin 500 mg PO q6h for 7 days is an alternate choice. Another alternative is clindamycin 300 mg PO q6h for 7 days. For the patient who is allergic to penicillin, erythromycin 500 mg PO q6h is an alternate therapy. Table 18.2 lists the bacteria-specific suspected organism, initial antibiotic of choice, an alternate antibiotic, an antibiotic for a woman who is allergic to penicillin, the duration of therapy, and suggested nonpharmacologic treatment for nonpuerperal breast infections.

The second type of presentation also has inflammation with suppuration, and the preferred therapy is aspiration or surgical drainage and antimicrobial therapy effective against mixed aerobes and anaerobes. The organisms include coagulase-negative *Staphylococcus*, *Bacteroides* sp., *Propionibacterium* sp., and *Peptostreptococcus*. Dicloxacillin 500 mg PO q6h and metronidazole (e.g., Flagyl) 500 mg PO q8h, both for 10 days, are appropriate treatment for chronic mastitis. These chronic infections may lead to disfigurement of the breast, usually secondary to repeated operations (surgical drainage).

The third presentation is characterized by a history of multiple recurrent infections over many years. Suppuration, sinus tracts, fistulas, and subareolar abscesses are usually noted. Aggressive surgical management may require complete duct excision and perioperative antibiotic therapy as for chronic mastitis. *S. aureus* is rarely isolated from those with chronic disease; anaerobic streptococci are the most frequently recovered microbial flora.

19 FIBROCYSTIC CHANGES

William H. Hindle

L ack of dynamic studies of the detailed structure of the normal female breast in its entirety has led to misinterpretation of local histologic variations. Probably all women have some microscopic fibrocystic changes somewhere within their breasts. Especially during the reproductive years of a woman's life, histologic variations in breast anatomy are common and diverse. Although the breast develops from a uniform epithelium that invaginates into the supporting mesenchyme (see Fig. 3.1), the anatomy, histology, pathology, and physiology of the female breast are heterogeneous. The structure and histology of the female breast is dynamic, changing with age and hormonal influences such as pregnancy, the menstrual cycle, and the use of exogenous hormones.

The term "fibrocystic disease" is a misleading catch-all phrase that historically was thought to be a specific entity with premalignant potential. Search of the literature reveals more than 45 terms, entities, and specific histologic diagnoses (Table 19.1) that used to be lumped together under this wastebasket term. In 1985 the College of American Pathologists formally determined that "fibrocystic disease" was medically inappropriate and suggested instead that if a similar terminology was necessary the terms "fibrocystic change" or "fibrocystic condition" should be used. However, a specific histologic diagnosis or description is preferred and is more useful for clinicians. The pertinent clinical aspects of fibrocystic changes are summarized in Table 19.2.

The landmark histologic work of Dupont and Page,[1] published in 1985, established that only atypical proliferative epithelium had clinically meaningful premalignant potential (fivefold relative risk of breast cancer). Having the combination of atypical epithelial hyperplasia and a first-degree relative (mother or sister) with diagnosed invasive breast cancer increased a woman's relative risk to 11-fold. Atypical epithelial hyperplasias accounted for about 4% of all the benign breast biopsies in the Dupont and Page study. Nonatypical epithelial hyperplasia (moderate, florid and solid, or papillary) and papillomas with a fibrovascular core were found to have a "slightly increased" relative risk (twofold or less, "a weak association") of breast cancer. In a later study,[2] sclerosing adenosis was identified as having a similarly low increased relative risk. None of the other specific histologic changes was found to have an increased relative risk. The

Table 19.1. Histologic diagnoses that have appeared in the literature as "fibrocystic disease"

Adenosis
Apocrine change
Apocrine metaplasia
Benign breast disease
Blunt duct adenosis
Chronic cystic mastitis
Chronic indurative mastitis
Chronic mastitis
Cystic disease
Cystic hyperplasia
Ductal atypical hyperplasia
Epitheliosis
Epithelial cyst
Epithelial duct hyperplasia
Epithelial hyperplasia, mild
Fibroadenoma
Fibroadenosis
Fibrosis
Fibrous dysplasia
Fibrous mastopathy
Florid adenosis
Florid hyperplasia
Hyperplasia, moderate
Inflammation
Lobular atypical hyperplasia
Macrocyst
Mammary duct ectasia
Mammary dysplasia
Mastitis
Mastopathy
Mazoplasia
Metaplasia
Microcyst
Papillary hyperplasia
Papilloma with fibrovascular core
Papillomatosis
Periductal mastitis
Sclerosing adenosis
Solid hyperplasia
Squamous metaplasia

KEY PRACTICE POINTS

Fibrocystic changes: The term "fibrocystic disease" is *not* a valid medical diagnosis. Most women have fibrocystic changes in their breasts.

Table 19.2. Characteristics of fibrocystic changes

Fibrocystic changes are most common during a woman's reproductive years.

Fibrocystic changes are often focal (localized) but in a scattered pattern.

Most fibrocystic changes are focal normal variations in microscopic anatomy (histology).

Only proliferative epithelial changes, particularly atypical hyperplasia, have an
associated increased relative risk of invasive breast cancer.

"slightly increased" relative risk group accounted for 24% of the benign breast biopsies. The remaining 70% did not demonstrate an increased relative risk over the 17 years of follow-up.[1]

Unfortunately, there are no characteristic symptoms, physical findings, or mammographic findings that correlate with atypical epithelial hyperplasia. It is a specific histologic tissue diagnosis most often coincidentally noted in a breast biopsy specimen obtained for another indication. Neither fine-needle aspiration nor tissue core-needle biopsy is an effective or reliable procedure for its diagnosis. Multiple permanent tissue sections and microscopic appraisal of the surrounding (nearby) ducts are necessary for the definitive histologic diagnosis of atypical epithelial hyperplasia. Furthermore, there is no known successful treatment. Patient counseling with careful surveillance at annual clinical breast examinations and mammograms is appropriate.

Fibrocystic changes, especially if numerous microcysts are present, may be associated with cyclic mastalgia. The symptoms (diffuse cyclic breast pain) and signs (diffuse tenderness and prominent nodularity, particularly in the upper outer quadrants of the breasts) tend to be estrogen-related and can fluctuate with the hormonal variations of the menstrual cycle, decrease at menopause, and subsequently subside completely; they sometimes recur in estrogen-deficient women when they begin estrogen replacement therapy.

Fibrocystic changes are often found in breast biopsy specimens from a palpable dominant breast mass, particularly in women of reproductive age. In many hospitals and outpatient surgeries, fibrocystic change in all its various forms is the most common histologic diagnosis in breast open surgical biopsy (OSBx) pathology reports. Analysis of the final pathology reports of consecutive breast OSBx performed on the general surgical service of the Los Angeles County and University of Southern California (LAC + USC) Medical Center during 1991–1994 revealed that more than 30% were some variation of fibrocystic change. The frequency of fibrocystic change is inversely correlated with age and is an unusual histologic diagnosis in a postmenopausal woman.

For the primary care clinician and the patient, it is often confusing and misleading to use the term "fibrocystic changes." Although the clinician should think in terms of specific histopathology, any symptoms, physical findings, mammographic findings, and possible etiologies should be clearly described and communicated to the patient in "plain" English. Such explanations allow less chance for confusion, unnecessary worry, and possibly inappropriate action.

Reference

1. Dupont WD, Page DL. Risk factors for breast cancer in women with proliferative breast disease. N Engl J Med 1985;312:146–151
2. Jensen RA, Page DL, Dupont WD, Rogers LW. Invasive breast cancer risk in women with sclerosing adenosis. Cancer 1989;64:1977–1983

20   FIBROADENOMA

William H. Hindle

A fibroadenoma is the most common benign breast neoplasm. Although Hughes et al.[1] suggested that a fibroadenoma is one of the multiple benign breast lesions covered by the generic term "aberrations of normal development and involution" (ANDI), most clinicians and pathologists continue to classify fibroadenoma as a nonmalignant neoplasm (tumor).

In the Breast Diagnostic Center (BDC) experience (July 1988 through June 1995) fibroadenomas accounted for more than 34% of the 3267 fine-needle aspiration (FNA) cytology diagnoses of palpable dominant breast masses. A similar pattern emerged from a 1991–1994 series of consecutive breast open surgical biopsies (OSBx) of a palpable mass at the Los Angeles County and University of Southern California (LAC + USC) Medical Center, for which the final histologic diagnosis was fibroadenoma in more than 30% of the 1269 cases.

Fibroadenoma is most common during the early reproductive years of a woman's life and is the most frequent diagnosis of a palpable dominant breast mass in women in their twenties and thirties. A fibroadenoma per se is not premalignant. However, as with other ductal-type epithelium elsewhere in the breast, malignant transformation of the epithelial cells (parenchyma) is possible. There are published reports of invasive ductal carcinoma within an otherwise benign fibroadenoma, but it is a rare occurrence.

PHYSICAL CHARACTERISTICS

As are all other dominant breast masses, fibroadenomas are usually accidentally found by the woman herself. Physical examination reveals a distinct, firm, rubbery, mobile, well circumscribed mass that may seem oval. Some fibroadenomas are smooth and lobular, and some are tender, particularly when endogenous (or exogenous) estrogen levels are relatively high, such as at ovulation or shortly before the onset of menstruation. Fewer than 20% are multiple (in either breast) by palpation. There are no associated skin changes or axillary adenopathy. Although a strong clinical impression can be gained by palpation, definitive diagnosis of a fibroadenoma is not possible by physical examination.

Mammographic and Ultrasonographic Characteristics

Mammography of a fibroadenoma usually reveals a smooth, longitudinal, mobile, well marginated mass of uniform density. Some fibroadenomas are lobulated. About 20% of fibroadenomas are multiple and can be bilateral. Although a mass that fulfills the mammographic criteria for a fibroadenoma (Table 20.1) can be described in the mammographic impression as "probably," "consistent with," or "suggestive of" a fibroadenoma, a definitive diagnosis of fibroadenoma is not possible by mammography. Ultrasonography of a fibroadenoma shows similar characteristics and a uniform echographic pattern within the mass. Although the imaging impression of a fibroadenoma by ultrasonography may be highly suggestive, a definitive diagnosis of a fibroadenoma is not possible by ultrasonography.

Table 20.1. Mammographic characteristics of a fibroadenoma

Circumscribed (well defined margins)

Fatty halo sign

Low to moderate radiopaque density

Oval or lobulated

Overlying structures not always apparent

Peripheral calcifications may be present (degeneration)

Sharply outlined

Ultrasonography: homogeneous echogenicity

Cytology

Only cytology (with an adequate cell sample obtained by FNA) and tissue histology (the specimen obtained by tissue core-needle biopsy or OSBx) can establish a definitive diagnosis of fibroadenoma. The cytologic and histologic characteristics of a fibroadenoma are listed in Tables 20.2 and 20.3, respectively.

Table 20.2. Cytologic characteristics of a fibroadenoma

Abundant naked (bare) nuclei

Multiple sheets of monolayers of benign ductal cells

Normal stroma (connective tissue)

No adipose tissue (fat)

Usually not bloody

Estrogen Association

Fibroadenomas tend to have an estrogen-related sensitivity. The size and tenderness of a fibroadenoma can increase or decrease in correlation with the estrogen

Table 20.3. Histologic characteristics of a fibroadenoma

Pseudocapsule of compressed surrounding tissue

Multiple long clefts lined with a single layer of benign ductal epithelium

Myoepithelial cells outside (second layer) the ductal epithelium

Bland stroma (often variable patterns) without mitotic figures

No adipose tissue (fat)

levels during the menstrual cycle or with pregnancy. Infarcts can occur spontaneously within a fibroadenoma, causing pain and sometimes an increase in size. When the estrogen levels fall at menopause, fibroadenomas characteristically become smaller and often nonpalpable. Some fibroadenomas calcify during the postmenopausal years and have a characteristic "popcorn" pattern on mammography.

PHYLLODES TUMORS

Some pathologists think that the uncommon phyllodes tumors, with their proliferative changes in the stroma, are a variant of fibroadenoma, but most accept phyllodes tumors as a separate neoplasm. The distinct histologic characteristics of benign phyllodes tumors are listed in Table 20.4. By histologic criteria (Table 20.5) and clinical behavior (which covers a wide spectrum), the stromal component of phyllodes tumors can be malignant (sarcomatous) and can metastasize. In some reviews, clinically evident malignant behavior has been reported in fewer than 10% of phyllodes tumors. Phyllodes tumors often rapidly increase in size, becom-

Table 20.4. Histologic criteria of benign phyllodes tumors

Stromal hypercellularity

Irregular intracanalicular growth pattern: leaf-like pattern of elongated stromal
   protrusions into dilated ducts and bordering breast tissue

Well defined "pushing" margins without infiltration

Fewer than three mitoses per 10 high-power fields

Absence of stromal cellular atypia (pleomorphism)

Table 20.5. Histologic criteria of malignant phyllodes tumors

Stromal hypercellularity

   Overgrowth of fibrosarcomatous stroma

   Rare benign epithelial structures

Stromal infiltration of surrounding tissues

Nuclear atypism and pleomorphism of the stromal cells

Prominent mitotic activity of the stroma

Bizarre giant cells

ing clinically apparent within a matter of months. They are diagnosed most frequently in women in their forties or early fifties, but the age range of occurrence is wide and overlaps that of fibroadenomas.

TREATMENT

In the BDC a woman with a diagnosed fibroadenoma is counseled and given the option of excision (at a time of her convenience) or of being followed. If she elects to be followed, she is seen again in 6 months for reevaluation. Thereafter the follow-up is annual clinical breast examination (CBE) and mammography (if she is 30 years of age or older). In addition, the patient is instructed to examine her breasts regularly. She is to return immediately if the size increases, she notices changes in the fibroadenoma, or she experiences pain.

Many women elect to have their fibroadenomas removed. The BDC protocol is to excise a fibroadenoma by OSBx enucleation, often through a circumareolar incision. Surgical enucleation is a technique distinctly different from the National Surgical Adjuvant Breast and Bowel Project (NSABP) breast cancer lumpectomy protocol. (See Chapters 12, 13, and 22 for detailed descriptions of these surgical procedures.) Fibroadenomas do not have a vascular stalk and are readily separated from the surrounding compressed stroma and adipose and glandular tissue by blunt, sharp dissection. There have been no reports (from 1988 to 1997) of an adverse consequence or outcome of the BDC policy of offering elective removal or continuing follow-up of a fibroadenoma.

Reference

1. Hughes LE, Mansel RE, Webster DJT. Benign Disorders and Diseases of the Breast. London, Baillière, 1989, pp 15–25

21 Multidisciplinary Treatment Planning and Patient Counseling

Angela Demman Treinen

The woman with breast cancer faces a complex journey of decision-making through multifaceted therapies with consequences that affect all aspects of her life. These ongoing complexities are best managed by a team of health care providers committed not only to collaboration but to the involvement and support of the patient and her loved ones throughout the experience. Because teamwork and psychosocial support are paramount, this chapter discusses the essential functioning of the interdisciplinary team in the context of the patient's quality of life.

In many settings the process of diagnosing a breast cancer requires that a woman schedule multiple appointments in different locations over several days or weeks, with each step of the process producing escalating anxiety while she awaits results. The goal of providing timely and accurate diagnoses and efficient referrals is better served by a comprehensive service in one location where multiple specialists work together in caring for women with breast disease. Services should include the clinical breast examination (CBE), diagnostic mammography with a full range of specialized views available, breast ultrasonography, ultrasound-guided fine-needle aspiration (FNA), stereotactic and mammography-guided tissue core-needle biopsies, and on-site cytopathologic interpretation.

INTERDISCIPLINARY TEAM

Studies have shown that delays in diagnosis and initiation of treatment occur more often in settings that lack a dedicated multidisciplinary staff.[1] The importance of a competent cohesive interdisciplinary team is paramount, as it dictates much of a woman's breast cancer experience. Team members come from multiple disciplines within medicine and ancillary services (Table 21.1). Each discipline plays an essential role in determining the treatment plan and providing information necessary for the patient's decision-making. The representation of all the disciplines promotes the process of treating the patient as a whole human being, rather than just a collection of faulty parts.

KEY PRACTICE POINTS

Breast center coordinator: The nurse coordinator/counselor is the indispensable component for the success and growth of a comprehensive breast center.

Essential members of the multidisciplinary treatment planning team: Mammographer, medical oncologist, pathologist, plastic (reconstructive) surgeon, radiation oncologist, surgical oncologist.

Table 21.1. Specialties represented on the USC/ Norris Breast Center interdisciplinary team

Gynecology
Mammography
Medical oncology
Oncologic nursing
Pathology
Plastic surgery
Radiation oncology
Social services
Surgical oncology

The team is as strong as its weakest member or weakest system. Examples of weak team components include a skilled surgeon with an incomplete pathologic picture; a time constraint that prevents the radiation oncologist from meeting with an apprehensive patient; or not having at hand the prognostic indicators, which causes the medical oncologist to delay making systemic therapy recommendations.

CHALLENGES FACING THE INTERDISCIPLINARY TEAM

Patient Communication

The period from the discovery of the cancer to initiation of treatment has been described by many patients as the most stressful and frightening time of their entire cancer experience.[2] The implementation of a comprehensive team approach soon after the initial diagnosis establishes significant sources of support.

Traditionally it has been the surgeon who informed the patient of a cancer diagnosis. With the advent of radiologic diagnostic technology, the diagnostic phase of breast cancer often is now in the hands of radiologists and primary care practitioners, with the patient never seeing a surgeon until after the diagnosis is confirmed. For nonpalpable lesions, multiple biopsy options exist. Unless a radiologist or primary care practitioner is comfortable discussing treatment options, many believe an oncologic surgeon should be involved in the initial biopsy decisions. For palpable solid masses, the primary care provider often performs a diagnostic FNA and refers to an interdisciplinary team for consultation as indicated. However, the patient usually does not have a close personal relationship with the radiologist or the surgeon and may prefer to receive all information from her primary care practitioner.

Team Leadership

Leadership of the team varies based on the progression of the woman's diagnosis and therapies. Conventionally, the team leader has been the oncologic surgeon with a transition to the other disciplines depending on the treatment regimen, for example to radiation oncology or medical oncology following surgery. It must be remembered, however, that the patient ultimately is in the driver's seat, and this basic value should dictate all discussions and team interactions. Given that the patient has the final say, strong medical staff leadership within the breast team is vital. Unfortunately, a breast cancer team's effectiveness is at risk when systems do not support involvement of all team members and when strong personalities rather than scientific findings are allowed to dictate practice.

Interdisciplinary Team Meetings

Leadership is not as critical as the assurance of continuous communication among team members. Working as a team means meeting as a team. The interdisciplinary team should meet regularly to discuss individual patient treatment plans and follow-up care. With the ever-changing data on breast cancer therapies, members must maintain open communication and be able to challenge and discuss pros and cons of new and time-tested diagnostic and therapeutic options.

The initiation of an interdisciplinary team often requires additional conversations until relationships and standards of care are solidified. Team members who meet only once a week may not find this sufficient. Communication must be ongoing. For example, surgeons who practice at multiple institutions and who have busy practices and many hours in surgery often hinder team communication by their unavailability. Open communication, in formal and informal settings, must be established and committed to by each team member.

At the University of Southern California (USC)/Norris Comprehensive Cancer Center, because of our association with the USC School of Medicine, the weekly interdisciplinary conferences of the Breast Center (USC/NBC) are attended not only by specialist team members but also by resident physicians, technologists, technicians, and others who come to learn from the challenging and interesting cases presented. The addition of expert lecturers, status reports of ongoing research, and community outreach programs add a nice boost to educating the team members and validating and supporting basic research efforts and translational research.

There should be regular meetings to discuss operational issues facing the breast cancer team, such as systems problems, the need for new equipment, and the development and evaluation of quality outcome indicators. Offsite strategic planning meetings on an annual or more frequent basis have proved helpful and effective.

Team meetings for pleasure should also be considered. An occasional social gathering can be more helpful in building team cohesiveness than multiple hospital meetings, memos, and policy sessions. Caring for women with breast cancer and their families, although rewarding and exciting, can be taxing. It is vital in cancer care to appreciate and reward ourselves for what we do well.

Requirements for Consultation/Record Retrieval

Accurate histories and verified information are essential for diagnosis and treatment planning. All team members must have access to the mammography films, ultrasound films, pathology slides (including multiple biopsy results), and reports of prognostic indicators. The gathering of these records is often laborious, time-consuming, and frustrating. Past mammograms needed for critical comparison may have been obtained at different sites or stored elsewhere. One should not underestimate the stress experienced by patients and loved ones during what seems like wasted time spent acquiring these records. Many patients fear alienating their physicians by frequent requests for information, reports, and records. Clerical support for obtaining these diverse records can be critical.

When the team is asked to provide second opinion services, it is helpful to have pathology slides and mammography films 2 days in advance to facilitate a streamlined complete consultation, particularly when complex pathologic or mammographic findings are involved. Most hospitals have a policy that slides and films must be reread by physicians in their own pathology and radiology departments before surgery can be performed at their facilities.

The maintenance and return of these records is also challenging. For patients seeking outside opinions, identifying which records are to be kept versus which are to be copied and returned is complicated. This process often requires clinical judgment and necessitates the creation of complex criteria. Even within environments where ambulatory clinics are physically connected to the inpatient setting, maintenance and availability of records can be a challenge. Incomplete dictation, transcription, or filing can stifle the team's productivity. With the advent of computerization in pathology and radiology, these previously nightmarish systems have a hopeful future.

Scheduling Patient Visits

Scheduling multiple team members to see multiple patients is a formidable task. Depending on the complexity of the case and the extent of patient education and support provided, time with each health care provider varies. Keeping all of the physicians on schedule without wasting their and the patient's time is important but complex. Initially breast cancer is a crisis. Women need support and counseling as they assimilate the findings of the diagnostic process and therapeutic considerations. A phone or in-person contact by a specially trained sensitive nurse prior to the multidisciplinary consultation can assess the patient's and family's learning needs as well as help determine which specialists are needed for consultation and the appropriate time frames.

Sharing the patient is important. When patients sense a lack of communication between practitioners, they report feelings of confusion, frustration, vulnerability, and sometimes anger. Multiple opportunities for communication between team members throughout the day enhances efficiency and provides the patient with a sense of security knowing that her team is working together. It is ideally accomplished when the medical staff sees patients in the same setting. When interdisciplinary consultations can not be done in the same location on the same day, a reliable system must be in place to secure timely verbal and written communication of findings, concerns, and recommendations.

Many breast centers struggle with the question of who should be present at an initial consult for a woman newly diagnosed with breast cancer. Some opt for a system where all team members see all patients. Others choose an individualized approach based on the patient's clinical status, psychosocial needs, and financial limitations. There are pros and cons to having medical oncology represented at the initial consult. Medical oncologists provide significant input to discussions of breast conservation versus mastectomy. Futhermore, it is helpful for patients to initiate a relationship with the medical oncologist, although it can be done at a later time. Medical oncology consults are usually time-consuming (and therefore relatively costly) and add one more coordination piece to an already challenging schedule. At USC/NBC we have opted to include medical oncology consultations when appropriate to assess issues of neoadjuvant therapy, evaluation for trials, fertility, or the need for axillary dissection.

Many breast centers include a psychologist or psychiatrist as a regular member of the interdisciplinary team to interface with the patient and family. At USC/NBC we choose to use these professionals on an individual consultant basis as needed after the baseline assessment has been completed. Our experience has been that patients who experience anxiety and depression involving their diagnosis and treatment often do well with the education and support provided by the team, with occasional short-term anxiolytic medications and psychotherapy referral, as needed.

Establishing a Common Language

It is important to establish a common language for team members when dealing with breast disease, both benign and malignant. For example, an anesthesiologist, preoperative nurse, or surgical resident may cause panic by using the terms "partial mastectomy" or "quadrantectomy" for a patient who understands only that she is having a "lumpectomy." Precise terminology is significant for billing insurance companies. Discipline is involved in the accurate identification of billing codes: Resident physicians, physical therapists, operating room nurses, or other coders can easily mislabel procedures, particularly the more complicated reconstructive surgeries. Routine in-house auditing of these practices helps to maintain accuracy and to determine the source of inappropriate information. It is essential that procedures are labeled correctly for each hospital's cancer registry, which collects information on therapies and outcomes for the national databank.

Documentation

With a multidisciplinary consult some physicians like to have the chart present during the examination, rendering it unavailable for preview by other team members or review by specialists wanting their documentation. To solve this problem some centers assign one team member per patient to summarize the consultations. Another option is to have a separate patient schedule with key information. This allows team members to know the status of all patients and appointment times and provides a centralized place for notes.

Patient Dignity

Ideally, the patient is dressed and in a comfortable chair (versus the end of an examining table), when talking with the consultation team about her treatment plans and therapeutic options. This positioning supports her dignity, maintains her identity, and allows her to take notes if she so desires. Each of the interdisciplinary team members should have an opportunity to examine the patient before providing input on the proposed treatment plan. Maintaining the woman's dignity and accomplishing multiple examinations within a reasonable time frame requires strategy and dedication. Most patients do not mind dressing and undressing if the procedures and purpose are explained prior to their visit.

A patient should be encouraged to have a loved one (or ones) accompany her to and during consultations, but some women wish to discuss their diagnosis privately. They may not want to share their personal history, emotions, or concerns with family members or friends. For women who speak another language, a translator should be provided if she does not want to use a family member who can translate for her. Patients should be allowed to tape-record discussions if they wish.

It remains a challenge for a woman to maintain her dignity and privacy while undergoing what seem like dehumanizing procedures, such as prone stereotactic tissue core-needle biopsies, repeated mammograms, and multiple breast examinations. Repeated efforts should be made to explain the necessity and expectations of each procedure.

Continuity of Care

Time spent in the hospital for surgery is minimal compared to that in the variety of ambulatory settings required to assess and treat the breast cancer patient. On average a patient may have five to seven physicians involved in her diagnosis and treatment, many with their own nurses, billing offices, partners, and scheduling secretaries. Even with dedicated team members, it is a challenge to facilitate and coordinate care for these women and their families throughout their cancer experience.

At USC/NBC, coordination of the woman's overall experience is the responsibility of an advanced practice nurse (APN), who is either a clinical nurse specialist or nurse practitioner. The APN provides complex patient education and psychosocial support, schedules appropriate referrals, identifies pertinent clinical research issues, and assists in reducing health care costs without compromising the quality of care delivered. In many other breast centers this essential role is performed by a specifically trained nurse coordinator/counselor.

As the patient progresses with her therapy, it is important that all team members be aware of her current status. Many centers have instituted interdisciplinary practice guidelines that follow the patient throughout her treatment, documenting and measuring her experience with a predetermined care plan. This practice informs all team members of the progress of the patient, past history, teaching to date, and the treatment plan initiated thus far.

The flow of information meets understandable resistance if multiple separate charts are maintained, for example, in physician's offices or the radiation oncology department. Although an immediate solution is to copy all physician input at each patient encounter, the logistics of this practice can be oppressive and even un-workable due to multiple visits with multiple practitioners. Instead, some breast cancer teams have opted for weekly summations (e.g., from radiation oncology and physical therapy) and follow-up reports at multidisciplinary conferences.

The many nurses working with different specialists interact with the patient but may seldom encounter each other. Bringing all these nurses together on a regular basis to discuss their patients is beneficial. Periodic nurse meetings are worthwhile for problem identification, streamlining systems, and consolidation of patient education materials. This type of interaction and periodic meeting process is also valuable for the multitude of secretaries who touch the lives of breast cancer patients.

Numerous follow-up visits and laboratory work scheduled by multiple secretaries can be daunting for patients and ideally is combined into a centralized system. At USC/NBC these efforts have been effectively undertaken by a special secretary who assists the APN coordinator/counselor.

To maintain continuity, communication back to the patient's primary care provider (PCP) is essential. Providers frequently complain of not being informed of the status of their patients or of not receiving the results of the initial or subsequent consultations. It is important to ensure two-way communication, not only to cultivate referral sources but because with the advent of managed care more patients are being followed by PCPs than oncologists after their cancer therapies are completed.

Billing

Clearly all efforts should be made to streamline billing not only to decrease the anxiety the patient already may have but also to decrease the cost of multiple billing services and to increase the rate of collections. For those interdisciplinary team members not in a health maintenance organization (HMO), concerted efforts should be made to combine these systems. It is done in the USC/NBC using the computerized financial services of the Norris Center.

Patient Education

Upon diagnosis, patients often have little or erroneous information about breast cancer. Women and their loved ones differ in the amount, type, and timing of information they desire or require. The team must tailor education and support based on each patient's knowledge base and personal information-seeking strategies. Clinicians must address any fears that may be blocking the absorption or retention of key information critical to the patient's decision-making. Questions such as, "What is your primary concern right now?" or "What is your greatest fear at this time?" often allow the practitioner to address patient misunderstandings or nonapplicable concerns. For example, a woman diagnosed with ductal carcinoma in situ (DCIS) need not worry about the horrific lymphedema her grandmother experienced with a radical mastectomy 30 years ago. Adjuvant chemotherapy for breast cancer is better tolerated with the arrival of selective serotonin-receptor antagonists, and sometimes a brief discussion of this subject relieves fear sufficiently that the woman is able to focus on the issues at hand.

Patients should be offered a copy of their medical records including radiology, surgery, pathology reports, and prognostic indicators. Videotapes, models, photographs of irradiated and reconstructed breasts, printed materials, and computer-assisted instruction are helpful, as a patient's comprehension and assimilation of information can be enhanced by the use of multiple mediums. Numerous books on breast cancer are available in the lay literature, and extensive resources are available on the Internet (see Chapter 30 for a list of resources).

QUALITY OF LIFE

Quality of life (QOL) is defined as distinct areas influenced by a person's experience, beliefs, expectations, and perceptions.[3] QOL is a multidimensional construct generally accepted to include several important domains: functional status, disease- and treatment-related symptoms, psychological and spiritual functioning, and social and economic domain.[4,5] The assessment of QOL is inherently complex, especially for women with breast cancer. Patients with greater confidence in their own social support report less psychosocial distress.[6]

Frequently women with breast cancer experience psychological morbidity, which is demonstrated as affective distress, impaired role functioning in work and family settings, disrupted social integration and support, compromised coping, aversive somatic symptoms, unmet practical needs, financial and insurability issues, or changes in body image, sexuality, and fertility.[7] Studies show that women who experience psychosocial problems do so for at least 1 year after the diagnosis of breast cancer.[8] Understandably, psychological distress is high immediately following diagnosis, especially with advanced breast cancer and recurrent disease.

Sensitive compassionate assessments can help clinicians to intervene and minimize complications, support adaptations, improve QOL, and possibly lengthen survival time.[9] The breast cancer team needs to assess the predictors of a woman's adjustment to her diagnosis of breast cancer and to her treatment. A psychosocial assessment includes cognitive function, body image and self-esteem, social support, coping strategies, stage of disease, previous experiences with cancer, socio-economic status, and cultural, ethnic, and religious influences. These factors are central and influence QOL for breast cancer patients and their loved ones. The findings of the assessment help identify patients at risk for poor psychological adjustment (Table 21.2). For further discussion of psychosocial assessment see Chapters 30 and 31.

Table 21.2. High risk predictors of poor psychosocial adjustment to breast cancer

Experiencing many illness-related demands

Significant life-event stresses before diagnosis

Problems communicating with spouse

Interpersonal tensions with family members/friends

Having little support from others

Not having a partner

Difficulty with body image

Pretreatment psychiatric morbidity

Physical disability

Complications of surgery (postoperative infection, poor wound healing, limited range of motion of arm)

Advanced stage of disease

Side effects of therapy

Source: Based on data adapted from Northouse,[2] Lewis et al.,[10] Maunsell et al.,[11] Schag et al.,[12] and Bloom and Kessler.[13]

Breast cancer and its therapy constantly insults a woman's sexuality, from the invasive diagnostic process and body-altering surgery to systemic adjuvant chemotherapy and hormonal therapy. The impact of systemic therapies on sexuality includes alopecia of eyelashes, eyebrows, and pubic hair; a 10- to 15-pound average weight gain; skin changes; and vaginal changes. Adjuvant therapy-induced premature menopause can result in a negative impact on all phases of the sexual response cycle: desire, arousal, and orgasm.[14]

Shover suggested that factors other than the extent of the breast surgery may play a large role in a woman's sexual satisfaction.[15] Women undergoing breast conservation therapy (BCT) have not been shown to experience significantly better QOL or mood than women having a mastectomy; lumpectomy patients experience fewer problems with clothing and body image.[5] Providing women with the opportunity to participate actively in the treatment-planning process may determine satisfaction as strongly as any specific treatment option.

Previous sexual problems, poor psychological adjustment, unhappy relationships, or the lack of a committed partner at the time of diagnosis may place a woman at higher risk for sexual dysfunction. Depression, pain, or other physical discomforts may interfere with progression of the sexual response. Identifying high risk factors can enable the clinician to intervene earlier. The health care team is responsible for assessing the patient's need for information and intervention surrounding sexual issues. Sexuality interventions include counseling, use of vaginal lubricants, and birth control information and instruction.

The impact of a diagnosis of breast cancer can be as distressing for a partner as it is for the patient, with spouses reporting psychosomatic problems such as sleep disturbances, increased feelings of anxiety, and depression.[16] These spousal symptoms usually begin at the time of diagnosis and continue through the first year after surgery.[17,18] Interestingly, studies show that a breast cancer experience does not negatively effect marital adjustment.[19] Husbands report that one of the most difficult aspects of the breast cancer experience is helping their wives deal with the emotional impact of the disease.

It is estimated that about one-third of couples experience difficulty in the area of sexual problems following a breast cancer diagnosis. Breast cancer-related stress can lead to feelings of powerlessness, fatigue, or anxiety, all of which may disrupt the frequency, pleasure, and importance of sexual activity for either or both partners. Partners are often concerned about how to be physically intimate after breast surgery. The couple's former patterns of intimacy may need adjustment. These intimacy concerns usually respond favorably to pertinent patient education and minimal counseling.

IMPACT OF BREAST CANCER ON FAMILY

Breast cancer touches everyone concerned. It is truly a family disease. In addition to the normal demands of the family, members must now support the relative with breast cancer while simultaneously experiencing their own grief and anxiety brought on by the cancer diagnosis of a loved one.[20]

The impact of the illness is different based on the developmental phase of the family.[21] Women with multiple responsibilities and school-age children may require more assistance.[18] There are practical considerations for cancer patients and their families, including personal care, meal preparation, child care, shopping, housekeeping, transportation, home finances, and medical bills. Although one might believe that these issues affect only young women, many grandparents whose adult children are in the workforce are the primary caretakers for their grandchildren and so may be affected. Additionally, women are opting to have children later in life.

Children are directly affected by the stressful events of their mother's illness when she is diagnosed and treated for breast cancer. Their responses vary depending on their age and developmental stage. In most studies breast cancer does not seem to have had a detrimental impact on a woman's relationships with her children.

Adolescent daughters report significantly more emotional discomfort with their mother's breast cancer illness than daughters who were younger or older at the time of the diagnosis.[22] Adult women experience fears about inheriting the disease. Daughters and siblings cannot help but consider their own mortality. It is valuable to have family members schedule appointments to evaluate risk, have baseline clinical breast examinations and mammography as indicated, provide education and support, and initiate their own individualized breast cancer screening plans.

Addressing QOL issues is a continual process that involves multiple disciplines and numerous potential interventional approaches. Psychosocial interventions should be individualized and tailored to address the specific needs of the family.

Studies suggest positive effects of social support, cognitive-behavioral therapy, and supportive information,[23] which are further reviewed in Chapter 30.

CONCLUSIONS

Clinicians are privileged to assess and treat human responses to illness. The interdisciplinary team faces daily challenges when caring for women with breast cancer and their loved ones. Commitment to enhancing the patient's QOL improves the quality, efficiency, and effectiveness of breast cancer care.

References

1. Bedell MB, Wood ME, Lezotte DC, et al. Delay in diagnosis and treatment of breast cancer: implications for education. J Cancer Educ 1995;70:223–228

2. Northouse LL. The impact of breast cancer on patients and husbands. Cancer Nurs 1989;12:276–284

3. Testa MA, Simonson DC. Assessment of quality-of-life outcomes. N Engl J Med 1996;334:835–840

4. Ferrans CE. Quality of life through the eyes of survivors of breast cancer. Oncol Nurs Forum 1994;21:1645–1651

5. Ganz PA, Schag AC, Lee J, et al. Breast conservation versus mastectomy: is there a difference in psychological adjustment or QOL in the year after surgery? Cancer 1992;69:1729–1738

6. Mor V, Malin M, Allen S. Age differences in the psychosocial problems encountered by breast cancer patients. J Natl Cancer Inst 1994;16:191–197

7. Mor V, Allen SM, Siegel K. Determinants of need and unmet need among cancer patients residing at home. Health Serv Res 1992;27:337–360

8. Irvine D, Crooks D, Browne G. Psychosocial adjustment in women with breast cancer. Cancer 1991;67:1097–1117

9. Spiegel D. Psychosocial intervention in cancer. J Natl Cancer Inst 1993;85:1198–1205

10. Lewis FM, Sahlis EH, Shands ME. The functioning of single women with breast cancer and their school-aged children. Cancer Pract 1996;4:15–24

11. Maunsell E, Brisson J, Deschenes L. Psychological distress after initial treatment of breast cancer. Cancer 1992;70:120–125

12. Schag CC, Ganz PA, Polinsky ML. Characteristics of women at risk for psychological distress in the year after breast cancer. J Clin Oncol 1993;11:783–793

13. Bloom JR, Kessler L. Risk and timing of counseling and support interventions for younger women with breast cancer. J Natl Cancer Inst 1994;16:199–206

14. Kaplan HS. A neglected issue: the sexual side effects of current treatments for breast cancer. J Sex Marital Ther 1992;18:3–19

15. Shover LR. The impact of breast cancer on sexuality, body image, and intimate relationships. CA Cancer J Clin 1991;41:112–120

16. Baider L, Kaplan De-Nour A. Impact of cancer on couples. Cancer Invest 1993;11:706–713

17. Zahlis EH, Shands ME. Breast cancer: demands of the illness on the patient's partner. J Psychosoc Oncol 1991;9:75–93

18. Northouse LL, Peters-Golden H. Cancer and the family: strategies to assist spouses. Semin Oncol Nurs 1993;9:74–82

19. Carter RE, Carter CA, Siliunas M. Marital adaptation and interaction of couples after a mastectomy. J Am Med Wom Assoc 1993;47:194–200

20. Christ GH, Wiegel K, Fruend B. Impact of parental terminal cancer on latency-age children. Am J Orthopsychiatry 1993;63:417–425

21. Northouse LL. Breast cancer in younger women: effects on interpersonal and family relations. J Natl Cancer Inst 1994;16:183–190

22. Casselith BR, Lusk EJ, Cross P. Psychosocial status of cancer patients and next of kin: normative data from the profile of mood states. J Psychosoc Oncol 1985;3:99–105

23. Glanz K, Lerman C. Psychosocial impact of breast cancer: a critical review. Ann Behav Med 1992;14:204–212

22 SURGERY FOR BREAST CANCER

Kristin A. Skinner
Gary Dunnington

The primary care physician is involved in the care of the patient with breast cancer throughout the course of treatment: performing routine examinations that screen for breast cancer, referring the patient to the appropriate specialist, counseling the patient about treatment options, and following the patient to identify potential complications or recurrent disease. It is therefore critical that the primary care physician understand all aspects of the care of the patient with breast cancer. Surgical management begins with a biopsy to make the diagnosis followed by staging, definitive surgery, referral for adjuvant therapy when appropriate, and finally long-term follow-up and management of any recurrence.

DIAGNOSIS

Breast cancer is diagnosed by cytology or histology. The choices of technique include fine-needle aspiration (FNA) for cytology, tissue core-needle biopsy (TCNB) for histology, and open surgical biopsy (OSBx), either incisional or excisional, for tissue histology. FNA involves obtaining a sample of cells by piercing (multiple times) and aspirating the mass with a 19- to 25-gauge needle (Fig. 22.1a,b). Slides are prepared, and the cells are examined cytologically for evidence of malignancy. The specimen may be diagnostic for cancer, suspicious for cancer, or show cellular atypia; diagnostic for a benign condition, such as fibroadenoma; nondiagnostic; or insufficient for diagnosis. If a cancer is diagnosed the patient can proceed to definitive treatment. If the FNA shows atypia or is suspicious for cancer, there are two options: (1) the patient can undergo OSBx and wait for the results of histology on permanent sections before proceeding; or (2) the patient can undergo open biopsy, with frozen section diagnosis. If the frozen section confirms cancer, the patient can proceed to definitive surgery at the same procedure. The choice of options depends on the index of suspicion and on patient preference.

If the FNA is nondiagnostic or insufficient for diagnosis, a repeat FNA can be performed or the patient can undergo another type of biopsy. It is critical that a diagnosis be made. If the FNA is diagnostic for a fibroadenoma, and both mammography and clinical examination correlate with a benign fibroadenoma, no further evaluation is required. If doubt as to the diagnosis persists, further diagnostic procedures are indicated.

The TCNB uses a large needle (usually 14 gauge) to obtain a core of tissue that is then examined histologically (Fig. 22.1c,d). Local anesthesia is usually used for TCNB.

The OSBx involves making a small incision directly over the mass or abnormality and removing either the entire mass (an excisional biopsy) (Fig. 22.2c,d) or a portion of the mass (an incisional biopsy) (Fig. 22.2a,b). Generally, the incisional biopsy is reserved for occasions where the mass is so large that excisional biopsy is impractical. Each of these sampling techniques (FNA, TCNB, excisonal biopsy, incisional biopsy) can be performed with radiologic guidance if no mass is palpable.

The method used to diagnose breast cancer depends on the abnormality. Typically, a patient presents with either a palpable mass in the breast or a nonpalpable mammographic abnormality. In general, the least invasive method is used first.

In a patient with a palpable mass, we perform FNA as the first diagnostic modality. This method is simple, is essentially painless, leaves no scar, and if diagnostic for cancer allows definitive surgery with a single trip to the operating room. FNA should be performed after mammography, as the FNA may cause some distortion of the tissues (e.g., by bleeding or hematoma formation), which

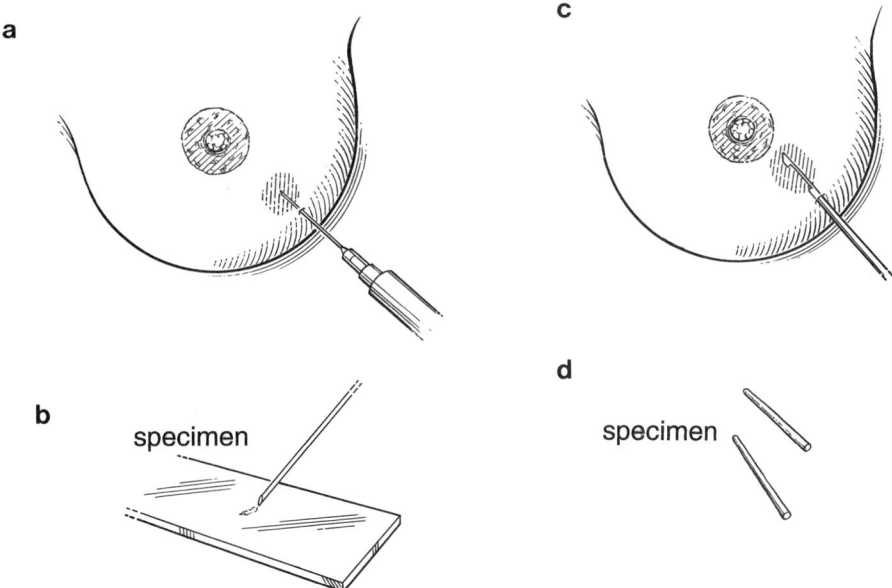

Figure 22.1. (a,b) Fine-needle aspiration. (a) Needle is inserted through the skin directly into the center of the palpable mass. (b) Cellular specimen within the barrel of the needle is ejected onto a slide, smeared, and fixed. Subsequently the slides are stained and sent for cytologic evaluation. (c,d) Tissue core-needle biopsy. (c) Core-needle biopsy device is inserted into the mass and a tissue sample obtained. (d) Tissue "core" samples are fixed in formalin and sent to the pathology laboratory for histologic evaluation.

can make interpretation of the mammogram difficult. Mammography is important not only to visualize the primary lesion but also to rule out the presence of other synchronous breast lesions. The diagnostic accuracy of FNA is dependent, to a large degree, on the experience of the cytologist. At our institution, the University of Southern California/Norris Breast Center (USC/NBC), an FNA diagnostic of cancer can be relied on, so no further confirmation is necessary prior to definitive surgery. In situations where the diagnostic accuracy is not as good or if FNA is suspicious but not diagnostic for cancer, a frozen section can be obtained at the time of definitive surgery to confirm the diagnosis prior to proceeding.

If the FNA is nondiagnostic and the mass is large enough that a good core of tissue would be obtained, TCNB is attempted. This technique is a bit more painful and may leave a small scar, but the benefits include obtaining a larger piece of tissue amenable to histologic examination with a procedure that can be performed easily in the office. Potential complications include hematoma formation and infection. A TCNB is useful only if the mass is sampled; if the needle misses the mass, it is of no use.

Finally, when a diagnosis cannot be made with either of the two techniques described above, we proceed to OSBx. In most cases we prefer excisional biopsy to incisional biopsy. OSBx is performed in an operating room or minor procedure room. Local anesthesia is used, often combined with intravenous sedation, and a small incision is made directly over the mass. For an excisional biopsy, the entire abnormal region is removed along with a rim of normal tissue (clear "negative"

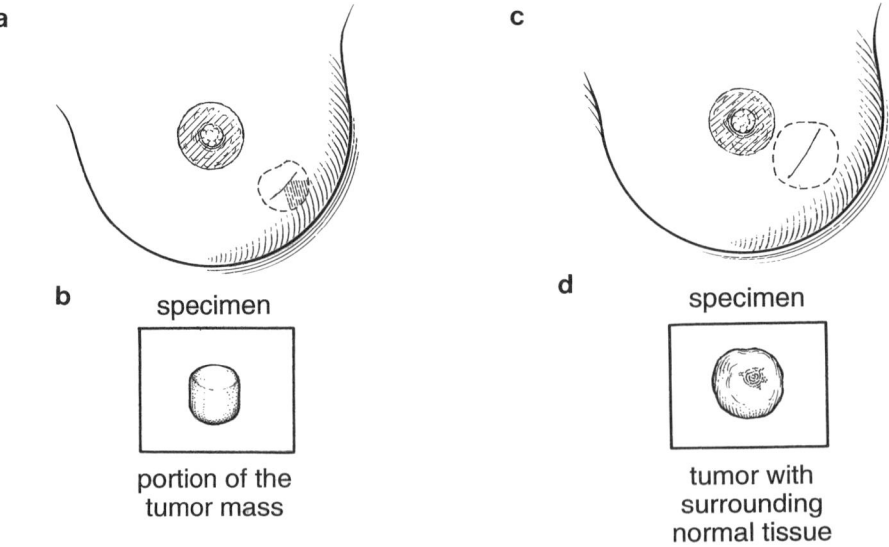

Figure 22.2. (a,b) Incisional biopsy. (a) Incision is made over the mass and a segment of the mass (shaded area) is removed. (b) Specimen is sent to the pathology laboratory for histologic evaluation. (c,d) Excisional biopsy. (c) Incision is large enough to allow removal of the entire tumor and an attached margin of grossly normal surrounding tissue. (d) Specimen is sent to the pathology laboratory for histologic evaluation.

margins). For an incisional biopsy a piece of the abnormal area is removed. Incisional biopsy is performed only when the abnormal region is so large the patient would not have an acceptable cosmetic result with excisional biopsy and FNA and TCNB have failed to confirm the diagnosis, or if neoadjuvant therapy is planned and the biopsy is only for histologic confirmation of malignancy. The benefit of an adequate excisional biopsy is that, assuming clear surgical margins, no further resection of breast tissue is required if the patient elects to undergo breast-conservation therapy.

Diagnosing cancer in a patient with a mammographic abnormality only (i.e., no palpable mass) is more challenging and requires close collaboration between the surgeon and the radiologist. In this case imaging is required to guide the biopsy. The biopsy options include stereotactic- or ultrasound-guided FNA or TCNB (described in Chapters 6 and 7) or needle-directed breast biopsy (NDBB). In the mammography suite, a guidewire (or needle) is placed in the area of concern using mammographic guidance. The patient is taken to the operating room with the wire (or needle) in place (Fig. 22.3a). Using local anesthesia, a small incision is made directly over the area of concern, marked by the tip of the needle. The mammographically abnormal area, including the guidewire, is removed in its entirety along with a rim of grossly normal-appearing tissue (clear surgical margins). A specimen radiograph is obtained to confirm that the mammographic

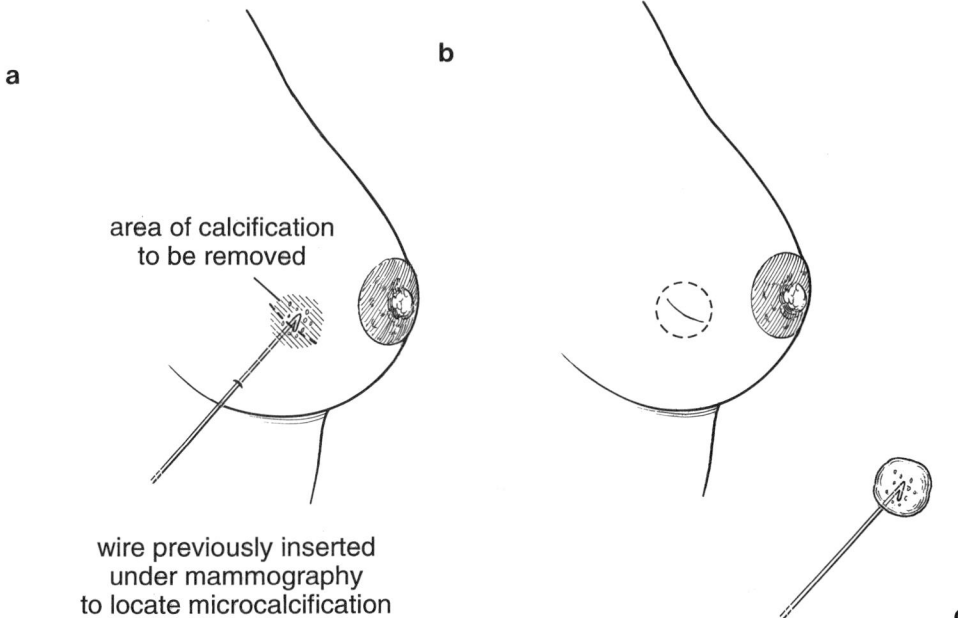

Figure 22.3. Needle-directed breast biopsy. (a) After mammographic placement of a hook-wire (or needle), the patient is taken to the operating room. (b) Incision is made directly over the area of concern, and a specimen, with the wire in place, is removed. (c) Specimen and the wire are sent for a specimen radiograph and then to the pathology laboratory for histologic evaluation.

area of concern has been removed and is in the specimen. The wound is closed with subcuticular absorbable suture stitches (Fig. 22.3b). The tissue specimen (Fig. 22.3c) is submitted to the pathology laboratory for histologic examination.

Our choice of diagnostic approach depends to a great extent on our index of suspicion. If we suspect that the lesion is benign, we prefer FNA or TCNB to save the patient a surgical procedure. If a solid lesion is visualized by ultrasonography, an ultrasound-guided TCNB is simpler and less costly than a stereotactically guided biopsy. Low-suspicion microcalcifications are best biopsied with stereotaxis. However, if we believe that the lesion is malignant, we most often proceed directly to NDBB. In this way the patient need undergo only a single localization procedure, and often a single operative procedure on the breast if the final histologic diagnosis is benign. If cancer is diagnosed, the patient requires axillary lymph node dissection (AxLND).

PATHOLOGY

Once the biopsy has been performed, further management depends on the pathology found. Benign lesions require no further surgical intervention. However, there is a subset of benign lesions associated with an increased risk of breast cancer that signal a need for close clinical follow-up. They are the so-called proliferative lesions, especially if cellular atypia is noted (Table 22.1).

"Malignant" lesions include carcinoma in situ and invasive cancer. Lobular carcinoma in situ (LCIS) is now regarded as a marker for increased risk of cancer in either breast, rather than as a true malignancy. Patients with LCIS have a 20–25% risk of developing cancer over 15 years (a 10-fold higher risk), either ductal or lobular, in either breast.

In contrast to LCIS, ductal carcinoma in situ (DCIS) is a preinvasive form of ductal cancer. It connotes a 25–30% risk over 20 years of developing invasive ductal cancer locally if not treated adequately. Several histologic types of DCIS have been described, including solid, cribriform, micropapillary, and comedotype. Solid DCIS is identified when the lactiferous ducts are filled with solid sheets of neoplastic cells. With cribriform DCIS the neoplastic cells grow into the lumen

Table 22.1. Relative risk of developing breast cancer after diagnosis of benign breast disease

Diagnosis	Relative risk
Nonproliferative lesion: mild hyperplasia, cysts, epithelial-related calcification, fibroadenoma, papillary apocrine change	0.9
Proliferative lesion without atypia: moderate or florid hyperplasia, papillomas, sclerosing adenosis	1.6
Atypical hyperplasia	4.4
All patients	1.5

of the duct, forming lattice-like structures. When the neoplastic cells grow into the ducts, forming papillary structures, the term micropapillary DCIS is used. Finally, when the ducts are filled with malignant cells with areas of central necrosis, the term comedo DCIS is used. Comedo-type DCIS is thought to represent the most aggressive form. DCIS can be further classified, based on the nuclear grade of the cells, into high-grade lesions (nuclear grade 3) and non-high-grade lesions (nuclear grade 1 or 2). Patients with high-grade lesions, comedo-type necrosis, or both are at higher risk of recurrence and invasive cancer than are patients with non-high-grade lesions or other histologic types of DCIS.

Invasive cancer can be ductal (85%), lobular (10%), or medullary (5%). Subtypes of infiltrating ductal carcinoma include tubular (1–2%), colloid or mucinous (2–3%), and papillary (1%). Histologically, lobular carcinomas consist of strands of infiltrating tumor cells, often one cell thick ("Indian file"), loosely dispersed throughout the fibrous matrix, and frequently arranged in concentric rings around normal ducts. Infiltrating ductal carcinoma consists of anaplastic cells in cords, solid nests, tubes, glands, or anastomosing masses, all dispersed in a fibrous stroma. When the malignant cells all form tubules, the tubular carcinoma subtype is said to exist. Colloid carcinoma consists of malignant cells floating in lakes of mucinous material, malignant cells forming glands with abundant intracellular mucin, or a combination of the two. The papillary subtype of infiltrating ductal carcinoma is characterized by malignant cells forming glandular papillae in the stroma. Medullary carcinoma is characterized by solid sheets of large pleomorphic cells, a marked lymphocytic infiltrate, and little fibrous stroma. In general, tubular, colloid, or medullary carcinoma carries the best prognosis, followed by lobular and papillary, and then ductal carcinoma. The surgical approaches to all histologic types of invasive carcinoma are identical.

Invasive cancer can be found in association with DCIS. When there is a microscopic area where the DCIS has broken through the basement membrane, it is referred to as DCIS with microinvasion. It is treated as invasive cancer. When a frankly invasive cancer is composed of more than 25% DCIS and there is a separate focus of DCIS outside the tumor mass, the patient is said to have an extensive intraductal component (EIC). These patients are thought to have an increased risk of local recurrence following breast-conserving therapy unless clear surgical margins are demonstrated both grossly and microscopically.

Patients with Paget's disease present with an eczematous lesion involving the nipple–areolar complex, often with fissures, ulceration, and oozing, and without any gross mass. Biopsy of the lesion shows invasion of the epidermis by malignant cells. Paget's disease of the breast represents an infiltrating ductal carcinoma arising in the main excretory ducts of the breast that has extended to involve the skin of the nipple–areolar complex.

Finally, some patients present with a red, swollen breast with thickened, edematous skin (peau d'orange), with or without a palpable mass. Skin biopsy reveals dermal lymphatics congested with cancer cells. Once cancer is confirmed, the patient is diagnosed as having inflammatory breast cancer. Inflammatory carcinoma of the breast carries a poor prognosis and is generally not treated primarily with surgery.

Staging

Once breast cancer has been diagnosed, the choice of treatment depends on the likelihood of local recurrence and distant spread. Survival following treatment of breast cancer is determined by distant spread. Breast cancer typically spreads to the bone, liver, and lung.

Tumor size and lymph node status are the most important determinants of the risk of tumor spread. Survival is inversely related to tumor size, with the best prognosis in patients with small cancers. Patients with tumors <2 cm in diameter have a low probability of developing metastatic disease and therefore have a high likelihood of surviving. On the other hand, patients with tumors >5 cm are more likely to develop metastases leading to death (Fig. 22.4).

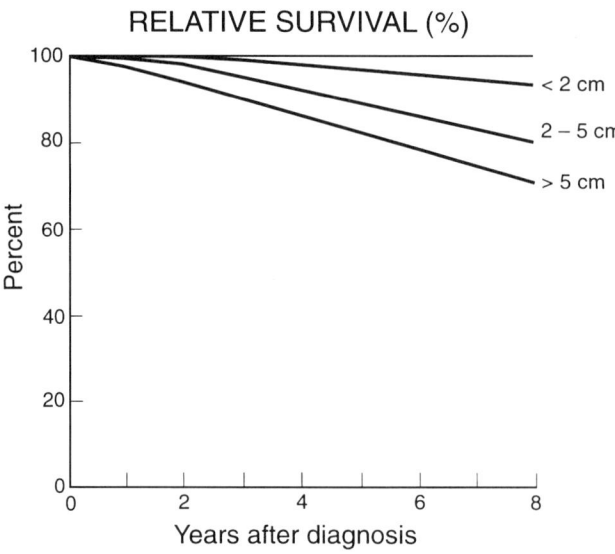

Figure 22.4. Breast cancer survival, after diagnosis and treatment, based on the size of the cancer.

Tumor size is defined as T1 if the tumor is <2 cm, T2 for tumors 2–5 cm, and T3 for tumors >5 cm. T4 designates tumors that involve the skin or the chest wall. Paget's disease of the nipple and inflammatory carcinoma are both considered T4 tumors.

The single most important predictor of outcome following treatment of breast cancer is the presence or absence of lymph node involvement (Fig. 22.5). Patients presenting with distant metastases have the worst prognosis. These three factors—tumor size, nodal status, distant metastases—provide the framework for the TNM staging system for breast cancer.

Nodal status is defined as N0 if there is no involvement of axillary nodes (AxLN), N1 if there are ipsilateral involved nodes that are freely mobile, N2 if the involved ipsilateral nodes are fixed, and N3 if there are involved ipsilateral internal mammary nodes. Patients with involved AxLN are classified N1–2 and have a

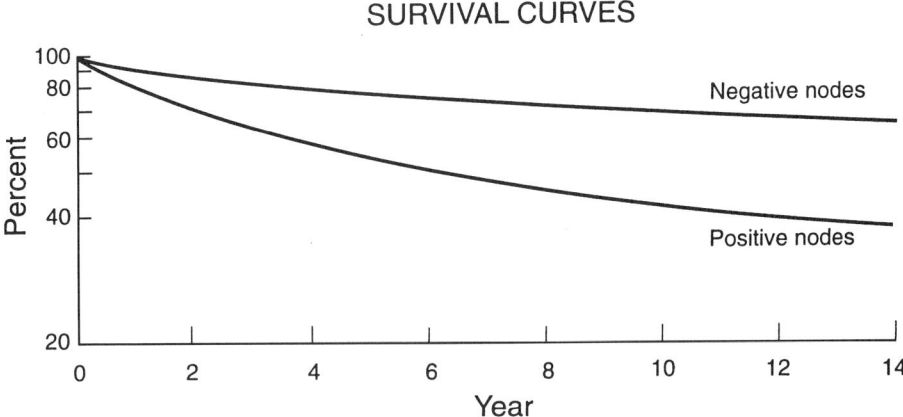

Figure 22.5. Breast cancer survival, after diagnosis and treatment, based on the nodal status of the surgical specimens.

poorer prognosis than patients without AxLN involvement who are designated N0. Distant metastases are either absent (M0) or present (M1). Supraclavicular nodal involvement and contralateral nodal involvement are considered metastatic disease (M1). The TNM status is put together to define a patient's tumor stage (Table 22.2).

Table 22.2. TNM staging system for breast cancer

Stage	Tumor	Nodes	Metastases	Summary
I	T1	N0	M0	Tumor <2 cm without evidence of spread
II	T2 or T3	N0	M0	Tumor >2 cm without spread or
	T1 or T2	N1	M0	tumor <5 cm with mobile ipsilateral nodal involvement
III	T3	N1	M0	Tumor >5 cm with nodal involvement,
	T1–3	N2	M0	any tumor involving the skin or
	T4	Any N	M0	chest wall, any tumor with fixed
	Any T	N3	M0	axillary nodes or internal mammary node involvement
IV	Any T	Any N	M1	Any tumor with evidence of distant metastases, including supraclavicular nodal involvement

Based on the history and physical examination, the patient can be assigned a clinical stage. If the tumor is <5 cm and there is no palpable adenopathy, the risk of distant metastases is so low that routine preoperative staging tests are not indicated. Routinely we order only a complete blood count, liver function tests, and a chest radiograph in these patients prior to definitive surgery. On the other hand, patients with T3 lesions or palpable adenopathy have a significant risk of distant spread. For these patients we obtain chest and abdominal computed tomography (CT) scans as well as bone scans to rule out metastatic disease prior to definitive therapy. A history of bone pain or the finding of hepatomegaly on physical examination warrants a metastatic workup.

TREATMENT

Lobular Carcinoma In Situ

Lobular carcinoma in situ (LCIS) is not a true cancer but, rather, a marker for increased risk (20–25% over 15 years) of invasive cancer. Both breasts are equally affected, and the cancer that develops can be lobular or ductal. Because LCIS is a global marker, the so-called mirror-image biopsy is not useful. The other breast is known to be at increased risk, no one area of either breast carries a higher risk than another, and the finding of LCIS in the contralateral breast does not change subsequent management. Treatment of LCIS should be directed equally at both breasts and is aimed at either prevention or early diagnosis. Treatment options include prophylactic bilateral mastectomy, which few patients elect, or close clinical follow-up with regular mammograms and physical examinations.

Ductal Carcinoma In Situ

In contrast to LCIS, DCIS is a true malignant lesion, a preinvasive form of ductal carcinoma. Because the risk of invasive cancer with DCIS is a local phenomenon, treatment is aimed at adequate local control. Treatment modalities include partial mastectomy alone, partial mastectomy with radiation therapy to the breast, or total mastectomy. The risk of recurrence and invasive cancer is related to the histologic findings (high nuclear grade and comedo-type necrosis) and the size of the lesion. Lesions >2.5 cm have a high incidence of positive margins and residual DCIS on reexcision. Small (<1 cm), lower-risk lesions (noncomedo, non-high-grade) can be adequately treated with partial mastectomy alone, so long as clear surgical margins are ensured. High-risk lesions require treatment of the entire breast to avoid an unacceptable recurrence rate. Treatment options include total mastectomy or partial mastectomy (with clear margins) followed by breast irradiation.

Patients who have had DCIS are at high risk of developing subsequent breast cancer and should be followed closely with mammograms and physical examination. Among the patients who develop recurrence, 50% have recurrent DCIS, and 50% have invasive cancer. As DCIS is noninvasive, no lymph node metastases are expected, and AxLND is not routinely performed. DCIS with microinvasion is treated as invasive breast cancer.

Invasive Breast Cancer

Invasive breast cancer is a spectrum of diseases. With few exceptions, the initial therapy is surgical. Preoperative adjuvant therapy is reserved for patients with locally advanced disease (large T3 or T4 lesions) for whom primary surgery is not possible without major reconstructive measures, patients with metastatic disease, and patients with inflammatory carcinoma. These patients should be referred to a medical oncologist for evaluation prior to surgical intervention. The remaining (most) patients should undergo surgical treatment of the breast and staging of the axillary lymph nodes prior to consideration for adjuvant therapy.

The past decade has brought a major change in the surgical approach to invasive breast cancer. Historically, breast cancer was treated with a modified radical mastectomy (MRM): that is, complete removal of the breast and draining AxLNs (Figs. 22.6, 22.7, 22.8). MRM is performed in the following steps: (1) The incision encompasses the nipple–areolar complex and the skin overlying the cancer, including the biopsy site, and extends from the costosternal junction medially to the axilla laterally. All breast tissue, from the sternum medially, the clavicle superiorly, the insertion of the rectus abdominis muscle inferiorly, and the lateral border of the pectoralis major muscle laterally, is removed in continuity with the AxLNs (Fig. 22.6). (2) The breast tissue is separated from the overlying skin by raising skin flaps superiorly to the clavicle and inferiorly to the insertion of the rectus abdominis muscle (Fig. 22.7a). (3) The breast tissue is lifted off the pectoralis major muscle, which then forms the floor of the wound (Fig. 22.7b). (4) The specimen is sent to the pathology laboratory. It consists of the ellipse of skin that includes the nipple–areolar complex, the biopsy site, the entire breast mound, and the axillary contents, containing the AxLNs (Fig. 22.7c). (5) The skin flaps are brought together over closed-suction drains with subcuticular absorbable suture stitches (Fig. 22.8). The drains are removed 1–2 weeks after surgery.

Treatment by MRM was based on a model of breast cancer growth, first described by William Halsted. It predicts a sequential spread of breast cancer from

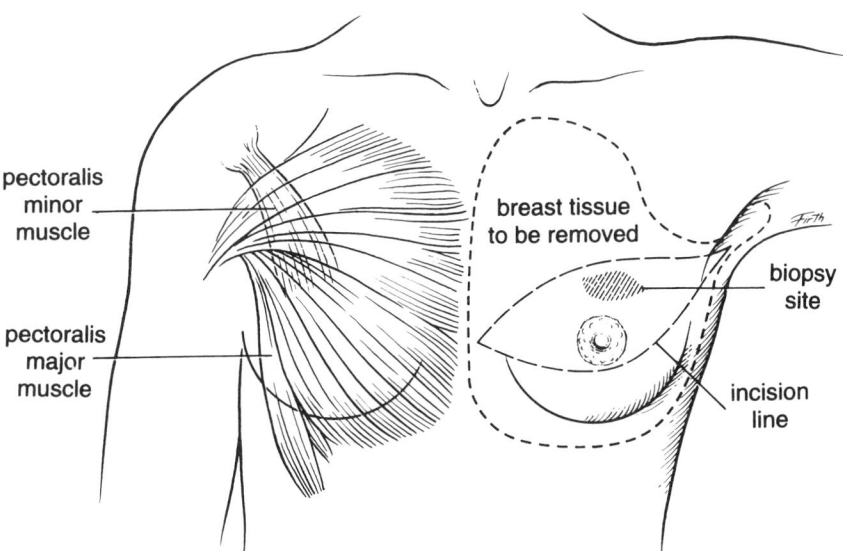

Figure 22.6. Modified radical mastectomy. Left, underlying muscle structure. Right, biopsy site, surgical incision line, and outline of tissue underneath the skin flaps to be removed.

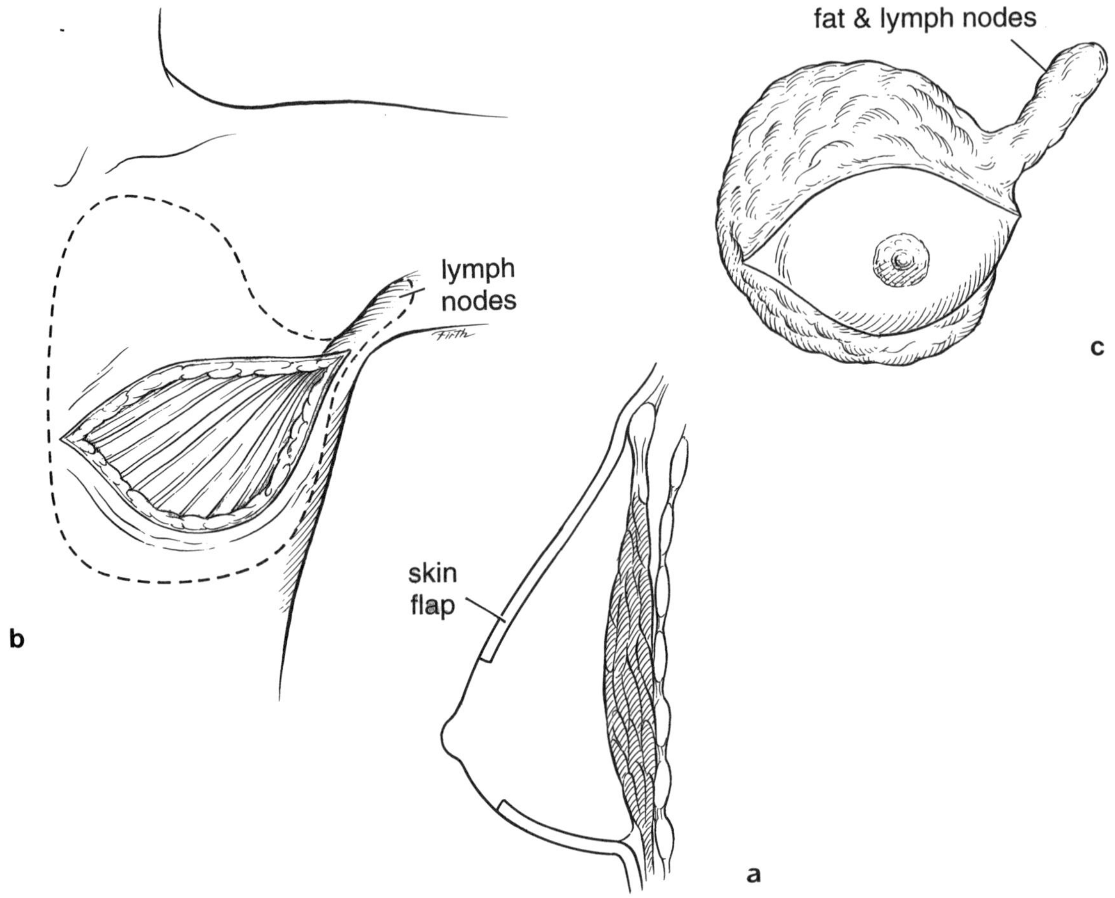

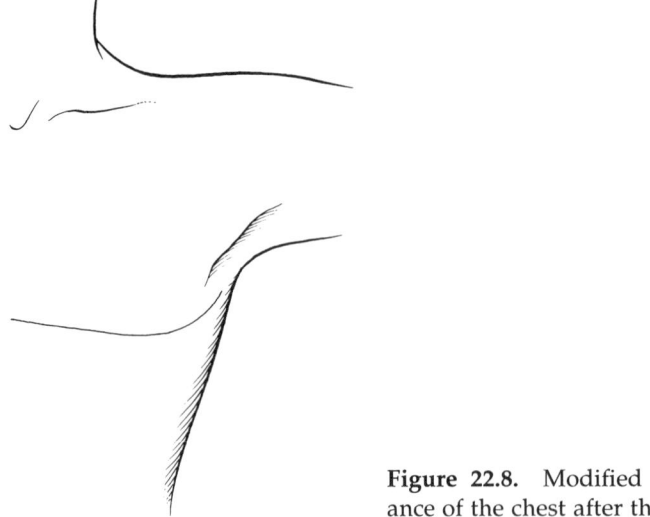

fat & lymph nodes

c

lymph
nodes

Firth

b

skin
flap

a

Figure 22.7. Modified radical mastectomy. (a) Superior and inferior skin flaps. (b) The wound, showing the muscle floor after the breast has been removed. (c) Intact surgical specimen.

Figure 22.8. Modified radical mastectomy: appearance of the chest after the incision has been closed.

the local tumor to the draining lymph nodes and then to distant sites. Theoretically, removing the breast and draining lymph nodes would stop cancer in its progression so long as the disease had not spread beyond the lymph nodes. Eventually, it became clear that breast cancer did not always follow this systematic progression, with some patients developing distant metastases despite having no nodal involvement. This discovery led to the systemic model of breast cancer, proposed by Bernard Fisher, which suggested that breast cancer is a systemic disease from its outset. The implication of this model is that, because breast cancer is a systemic disease, the extent of local treatment for breast cancer does not affect survival. This assumption led to several controlled trials that clearly demonstrated that T1 and T2 breast cancers can be adequately treated with conservation of the breast, with recurrence rates and long-term survival equivalent to those seen following MRM. No prospective trials have yet been performed that prove the effectiveness of breast-conserving therapy (BCT) for T3 or T4 lesions. BCT involves partial mastectomy (wide excision, lumpectomy, or quadrantectomy) to remove the cancer with adequate clear margins, AxLND to stage the draining lymph nodes, and breast irradiation to the remaining breast tissue.

The steps for BCT are as follows: (1) Two skin incisions are made (Fig. 22.9a,b). The first is a small incision that encompasses the biopsy scar directly over the mass. The entire mass with a rim of grossly normal surrounding tissue (clear surgical margins) is removed through this incision. The second incision is small, under the arm, through which the axillary contents are moved. (2) The two specimens, consisting of the tumor with a rim of normal surrounding tissue and the AxLNs embedded in fatty tissue (Fig. 22.9c), are sent to the pathology laboratory for histologic evaluation. (3) The wounds are closed with subcuticular absorbable suture stitches (Fig. 22.10). A closed-suction drain left in the axilla is removed 1–2 weeks after the surgery.

Breast irradiation is essential to successful BCT, as patients who undergo BCT without breast irradiation have an unacceptably high local recurrence rate (35–40% compared to 5–12% with breast irradiation). Both BCT and MRM remove the draining lymph nodes in the axilla.

Axillary lymph nodes are anatomically divided into three levels, based on their position relative to the pectoralis minor muscle: Level I is lateral to the pectoralis minor; level II is underneath the pectoralis minor; and level III is medial to the pectoralis minor on the anterior chest wall. AxLND can be performed removing only level I nodes (up to 10 nodes, also called lymph node sampling), removing both level I and II nodes (usually totaling >20 nodes), or removing all three levels (usually totaling >30 nodes). The major complication of AxLND is lymphedema, which can be debilitating. The risk of lymphedema increases with the extent of dissection and amount of nodal tissue removed. AxLND carries no survival benefit; it is done as a staging maneuver to assist in determining patient prognosis and selecting appropriate therapy, and to prevent axillary recurrence. The presence of involved lymph nodes signals a need for chemotherapy, more than four involved nodes suggests a need for axillary and chest wall radiation, and more than 10 involved nodes qualifies the patient for bone marrow transplant protocols. It is important to remove enough nodes to determine whether the patient falls into any

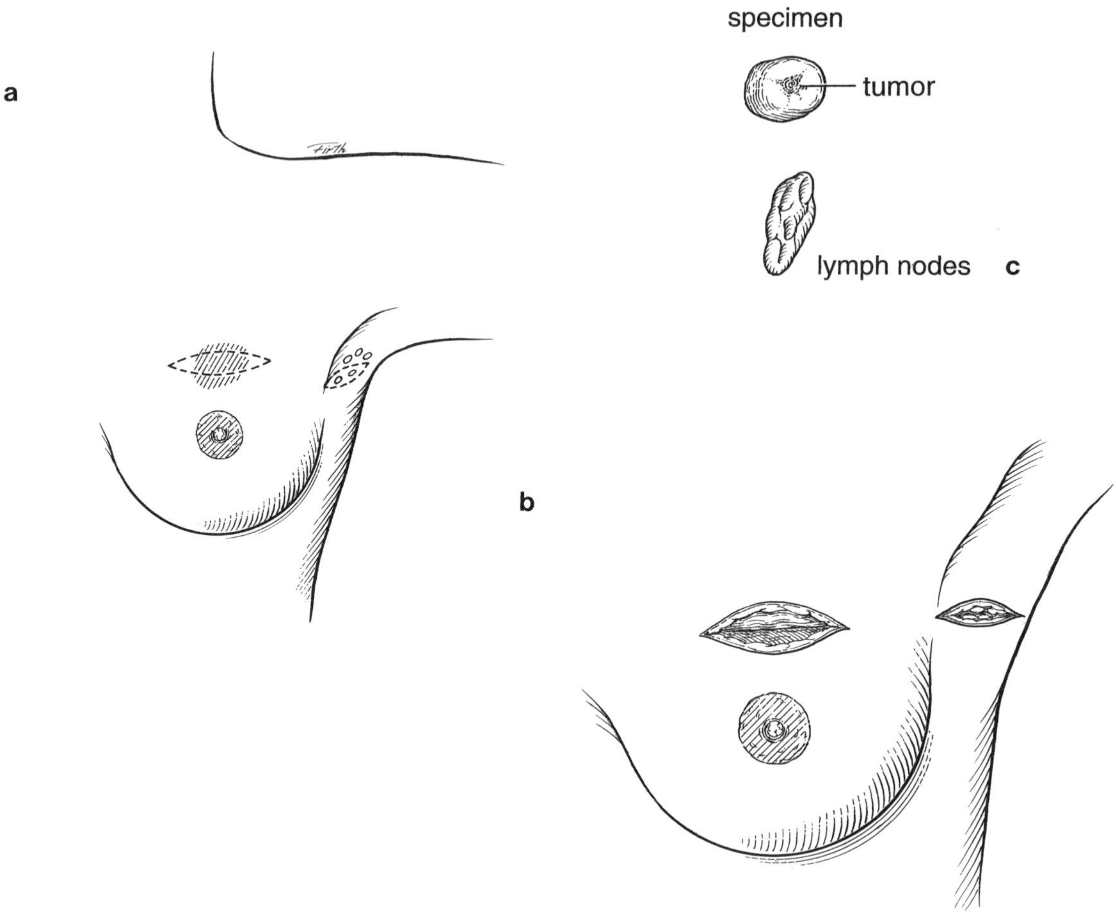

specimen

tumor

lymph nodes   c

a

b

Figure 22.9. Breast-conserving surgery. (a) Location of the incisions over the mass and over the axillary lymph nodes. (b) The two wounds after the tissue has been removed. (c) Both specimens are sent to the pathology laboratory for histologic evaluation.

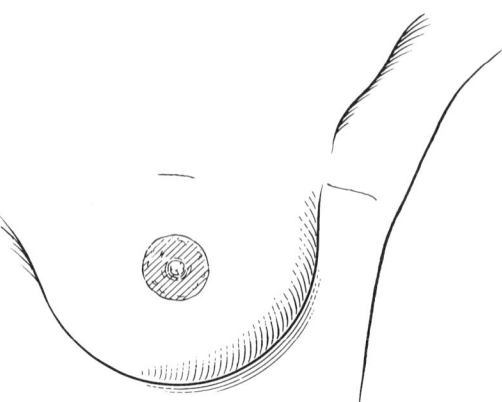

Figure 22.10. Breast-conserving surgery. After healing of the incisions.

of these treatment groups. On the other hand, as AxLND does not improve survival it is important to balance the risk of lymphedema with the presumed benefits of better staging and prevention of recurrence.

We routinely perform a level I–II dissection, which we believe minimizes the risk of lymphedema while removing enough nodes to obtain prognostic information and decrease axillary recurrence rates. Node sampling is considered only in patients with a low risk of nodal involvement: large, high-grade DCIS, DCIS with microinvasion, or small invasive cancers (i.e., <5 mm). Level III dissection is reserved for patients with massive axillary involvement, who may have more than 10 involved nodes, or those with obvious involvement of level III nodes, to minimize the risk of axillary recurrence.

Indications for Breast Conservation Therapy

Indications for BCT include invasive breast cancer that is resectable by partial mastectomy with an acceptable cosmetic result in a patient who is able to complete radiation therapy. Contraindications to BCT are listed in Table 22.3. The only absolute contraindications to BCT are those that preclude the complete regimen of resection with negative margins, axillary dissection, and breast irradiation. Breast irradiation is contraindicated in patients who have collagen-vascular disease and in those who have undergone prior irradiation to the area. A patient who refuses to undergo breast irradiation is not a candidate for BCT. BCT is contraindicated in patients with inflammatory carcinoma and in those whose tumors cannot be resected with a partial mastectomy achieving adequate margins. Pregnancy is a relative contraindication for BCT because breast irradiation must be delayed until the postpartum period. Cosmetic results are considered when determining the suitability of BCT, but care must be taken to remember that it is the patient's assessment of cosmesis that is important, not that of the surgeon. T3 breast cancers are a relative contraindication to BCT because there are no prospective data showing the efficacy of BCT in this patient population, and it is more difficult to perform partial mastectomy in patients with these large tumors.

Table 22.3. Contraindications to breast-conserving therapy

Absolute contraindications
    Collagen-vascular disease
    Prior breast irradiation
    Patient refuses radiation
    T4 tumors
    Inability to achieve negative margins on partial mastectomy
Relative contraindications
    Pregnancy
    Poor cosmesis
    Inability to save the nipple
    T3 tumors
    Recurrence following breast-conserving therapy

However, BCT is being used with increasing frequency in this group of patients, most often in the setting of preoperative chemotherapy, with acceptable results. Patients with T4 cancers, including inflammatory carcinoma and tumors involving the skin and chest wall, should receive neoadjuvant chemotherapy and possibly radiation therapy followed by MRM. Recurrent breast cancer following BCT is a relative contraindication because the patient has already undergone breast irradiation and has failed this form of therapy, although in selected cases BCT is appropriate.

Any patient who is not considered a suitable candidate for BCT is offered MRM, with the option of immediate or delayed reconstruction, after discussing the reasons for this recommendation. Patients who are considered eligible for breast conservation are given the option of either MRM or BCT, with careful explanations of the risks, benefits, and alternatives of each option. The final decision is ultimately that of the patient. It must be made clear that the two treatments are equivalent in terms of survival, and that the decision should be based on the patient's personal preference.

Complications of Surgery for Breast Cancer

The risks, benefits, and alternatives of BCT and MRM are different and should be understood by the patient (Table 22.4). Potential complications of BCT include seroma or hematoma, wound infection/abscess, need for reexcision if margins are involved, risk of local recurrence, and radiation changes in the breast. The major

Table 22.4. Risks and benefits of surgery for breast cancer

Procedure	Risks (incidence)	Benefits
Breast-conserving therapy	Hematoma (0–2%)	Breast preservation
	Seroma (2–5%)	
	Wound infection (2–5%)	
	Local recurrence (5–12%)	
	Radiation changes in the breast (100%)	
	Poor cosmesis (0–2%)	
Modified radical mastectomy	Hematoma (0–2%)	No radiation therapy
	Seroma (2–5%)	No need for
	Wound infection (2–5%)	mammographic
	Flap necrosis (0–2%)	surveillance on
	Local recurrence (5–10%)	involved side
Axillary dissection	Hematoma (0–2%)	Better staging
	Seroma (2–5%)	Better able to select
	Lymphedema (1–3%)	therapy
	Nerve injury (<1%)	Decreased axillary
	Decreased range of motion in shoulder (10–20%)	recurrence

benefit of BCT is breast conservation, but it must be made clear that the breast will not be completely normal.

The potential complications of MRM include seroma or hematoma, wound infection, flap necrosis possibly requiring plastic surgical reconstruction, and risk of local recurrence. Major benefits include avoidance of radiation therapy and no further need for mammographic surveillance on that side. Breast reconstruction can give the patient a cosmetically appealing breast, but there is loss of sensation in the skin of the reconstructed breast.

Regardless of whether the patient chooses MRM or BCT, an AxLND is performed. Potential complications of AxLND include seroma or hematoma formation; lymphedema; or injury to either the long thoracic nerve, causing a "winged" scapula, or to the thoracodorsal nerve with latissimus dorsi paralysis and decreased range of motion in the shoulder. The latter problems are usually temporary and rarely permanent.

Adjuvant Therapy

Once the patient has undergone surgery, the decision is made regarding what, if any, adjuvant therapy is indicated. Another change in the management of breast cancer over the past decade is the understanding that many, but not all, patients benefit from some form of adjuvant therapy.

The Fisher (systemic) model of breast cancer predicts that all patients should benefit from adjuvant systemic therapy. It is clear, though, that there are subsets of patients with breast cancer who do well without adjuvant therapy.

A more accurate model is probably Hellman's spectrum model, which suggests that breast cancer is a spectrum of diseases, with biology that is a blend of the Halsted model and the Fisher model. This model predicts that some cancers are systemic from an early stage, whereas others remain a local disease until the primary tumor is large. This makes decisions regarding systemic therapy a statistical and intuitive exercise based on the presence or absence of prognostic factors. Information obtained about the primary tumor at the time of surgery and pathologic examination includes size, histology, nuclear grade, S-phase, lymphovascular invasion, estrogen (ER) and progesterone (PR) receptor content, and oncogene or tumor suppressor gene expression. The presence and extent of lymph node involvement is determined. Based on all of this information, the patient's risk for developing local recurrence or metastatic disease is estimated. Patients at risk for metastatic disease are referred for hormonal therapy or chemotherapy.

Radiation therapy is a treatment aimed at local control. All patients who elect to undergo BCT are referred for breast irradiation. Patients who have large (T3 or T4) primary tumors are at increased risk of local recurrence and should be considered for chest wall irradiation. Patients with more than four positive axillary nodes are considered candidates for axillary and chest wall irradiation to prevent locoregional recurrence.

Hormonal therapy is a systemic treatment aimed at controlling growth of tumors that are hormonally dependent. ER and PR positivity is a marker of hormonal dependence. Hormonal therapy, as the sole adjuvant treatment, is usually reserved for patients who are postmenopausal with ER$^+$ and PR$^+$ tumors and low risk of recurrence. Hormonal therapy is often initiated after chemotherapy in patients with ER$^+$ and PR$^+$ tumors who have a high risk of distant recurrence.

Systemic chemotherapy, used in patients with an increased risk of distant recurrent disease, is intended to rid the patient of microscopic areas (nests) of tumor cells and so prevent recurrence. With the exception of the elderly (>70 years of age) and those with significant medical problems, all patients with lymph node involvement are referred for chemotherapy. Many patients without lymph node involvement are also considered for chemotherapy, based on their age and the characteristics of their primary tumor. Young patients tend to have more aggressive tumors. Characteristics of the primary tumor that are thought to signal increased risk for metastatic disease include large tumors, tumors with high nuclear grade (high S-phase), tumors with lymphovascular invasion, tumors that exhibit loss of ER and PR expression, and tumors with increased oncogene expression or loss of normal tumor suppressor gene function. Estimating a patient's risk for metastatic disease is complicated, and most patients benefit from referral to a good medical oncologist for consideration of adjuvant therapy.

Follow-up

Follow-up of a patient after surgery for breast cancer is aimed at detecting local or distant recurrence of the cancer and the development of a second primary breast cancer. It should be remembered that, by virtue of their having had breast cancer, these patients are members of a high risk group for the development of breast cancer in their remaining breast tissue. The risk of developing cancer in the contralateral breast is 5–15% over the next 15 years. For this reason these patients should continue to undergo regular annual screening mammography and physical examination of their uninvolved breast.

Follow-up aimed at detecting locally recurrent cancer differs depending on whether the patient underwent MRM or BCT. Following MRM the patient has no significant breast tissue remaining, and so mammography of the involved side is not indicated. Mammography of the contralateral breast continues annually. Local recurrence following MRM is limited to the chest wall and axilla and can be identified by careful physical examination. At the USC/NBC these patients are followed with physical examination every 3–6 months for 3 years and annually thereafter.

The patient who has undergone BCT has remaining breast tissue on the involved side. This breast undergoes significant changes as a result of the treatment: development of postoperative scar tissue, fat necrosis, and radiation changes. We routinely obtain bilateral mammograms 4–6 months after surgery and radiation therapy to establish a new baseline. We then follow these patients with physical examination every 3–6 months for 3 years and annually thereafter. Mammography is performed annually. Follow-up regimens are summarized in Table 22.5.

Follow-up aimed at detection of metastatic disease is individualized to the patient. Patients who are candidates for chemotherapy should undergo metastatic

Table 22.5. Follow-up regimen after surgical treatment for breast cancer

Surgical procedure	Mammography	Physical examination	Metastatic evaluation
Modified radical mastectomy	Contralateral breast annually	Every 3–6 months for 3 years, then annually	Chest radiography annually. Other tests only when indicated by symptoms or physical findings
Breast conservation therapy	Bilateral 4–6 months after completion of radiation therapy, then annually	Every 3–6 months for 3 years, then annually	Chest radiography annually. Other tests only when indicated by symptoms or physical findings

evaluation, including liver function tests, tumor markers, chest radiography, abdominal CT scanning, and bone scans prior to beginning chemotherapy. Thereafter metastatic evaluation should be based on physical findings and symptomatology. We obtain an annual chest radiography, but other routine studies to detect occult metastases are not cost-effective, as they rarely detect abnormalities in the absence of other findings. All patients who have a documented local recurrence should undergo full metastatic evaluation prior to local therapy.

Locally Recurrent Breast Cancer

Local recurrence following mastectomy is detected as a hard subcutaneous nodule on the chest wall. Following a metastatic evaluation that does not reveal evidence of systemic spread of the cancer, these patients are treated with wide excision of the lesion, which may require a chest wall resection and reconstruction. This surgery should be followed by chest wall irradiation.

Local recurrence following BCT is a relative contraindication to another attempt at BCT. With few exceptions, these patients should undergo total mastectomy after metastatic evaluation. As these patients have already undergone breast irradiation, they are not candidates for further chest wall irradiation.

The development of a cancer in the contralateral breast may represent either a second primary tumor or a metastasis from the original tumor (less likely). These patients should therefore undergo a complete metastatic evaluation to rule out disseminated disease. If there is no evidence of other metastases, the second cancer should be treated as any other primary breast cancer. The long-term prognosis of a patient with a second primary breast cancer is determined by the characteristics of the worse of the two primaries.

Once metastatic disease has been diagnosed, the patient is no longer amenable to surgical therapy. Treatment is systemic chemotherapy. Surgery is indicated only for the control of large, fungating tumors and is aimed not at cure but at palliation and wound management.

Conclusions

Surgical management of the patient with breast cancer is a long-term endeavor, beginning with biopsy and extending through lifelong surveillance. It requires close collaboration between the surgeon, patient, radiologist, radiation oncologist, medical oncologist, and the patient's primary care physician.

23 ADJUNCTIVE SYSTEMIC THERAPY FOR BREAST CANCER

Christy A. Russell

Patients with invasive breast cancers require evaluation for two distinct forms of therapy: local and systemic. Although patients and clinicians tend to tie these therapeutic decisions together, optimal management requires that they be evaluated separately. Decisions regarding optimal surgical resection and possible local radiotherapy should not be confused with decisions about optimal systemic management. The sequential timing of local and systemic therapies is best considered upon initial management by the multidisciplinary breast cancer team to ensure the best possible disease-free outcome for the life of the patient.

This chapter discusses the roles of systemic chemotherapy postoperatively and preoperatively (neoadjuvant) and the role of systemic adjuvant hormonal therapy. The indications, choice of agents, dose and duration, and side effects are considered as well.

Several principles guide our use of systemic therapy in the adjuvant setting.

1. The systemic therapy must have substantial activity in the metastatic setting. Some suggest that the greatest benefit might be expected if the individual agent or group of drugs could effect a response in 50% or more patients with metastatic breast cancer. If the drugs are not effective enough to elicit this response in the metastatic setting, it becomes difficult to show any benefit in the adjuvant setting.
2. The drugs must be widely available to clinicians and have a toxicity profile that is clinically acceptable in the long term and the short term.
3. A patient's risk of systemic recurrence must be great enough that the benefits of the therapy with improved survival can be evaluated statistically.

Historically, systemic adjuvant chemotherapy for breast cancer involved trials of surgical oophorectomy and other associated ablative hormonal maneuvers. This era was closely followed during the 1960s with single-agent chemotherapy trials. Although these initial trials are of great historical interest, they provide few useful data because of inadequate numbers of patients and frequently ineffective chemotherapeutic agents. Modern systemic adjuvant chemotherapy for breast cancer can be traced to clinical trials initiated during the 1970s. Since that time we have refined our use of specific drugs and learned more about dose intensity, timing of agents, and indications for certain agents based on well recognized, and until recently some more obscure, prognostic factors.

Prognostic Factors for Breast Cancer

Prognostic factor evaluation of a patient's breast cancer allows the clinician to categorize patients into risk groups for possible systemic recurrence. The two most significant risk factors are lymph node involvement and primary tumor size. It is critical to know the size of the tumor mass as determined by the pathologist. Tumors removed in bits and pieces can never be evaluated for tumor size, an important prognostic factor. Lymph node involvement, evaluated by the number of lymph nodes involved, is likely the single most important prognostic factor for survival after breast cancer. This information guides the oncologist in the choice of agent(s) and the dose intensity of the systemic therapy to be used.

Other commonly used prognostic factors are subclassified as being morphologic or biochemical. These factors are as follows:

Morphologic factors
    Histologic type
    Histologic and nuclear grade
    Lymphovascular invasion
    Proliferative markers such as S-phase or Ki-67
    Occult metastases in lymph nodes or bone marrow
Biochemical factors
    Estrogen and progesterone receptors
    Oncogene expression, such as Her-2/*neu* oncogene
    Tumor suppressor gene mutations, such as *p53*
    Angiogenesis factors

The clinical utility of many of these factors is yet to be determined. In our clinical setting we routinely evaluate patients for the following: tumor size, lymph node involvement (by routine microscopic and micrometastases assays), histologic and nuclear grading, estrogen and progesterone receptors, and Her-2/*neu* gene amplification assay.

Decision-Making for Adjuvant Therapy

Once a patient has been adequately staged, and prognostic factors are available, the medical oncologist must decide on the best choice for adjuvant therapy. Before adjuvant therapy is administered, however, the patient must be educated as to what to expect from the therapy in terms of the expected benefits, risks, and alternatives.

CHEMOTHERAPY

The most extensive data regarding the benefits of systemic adjuvant therapy derive from the Early Breast Cancer Trialists' Collaborative Group (EBCTCG), who conducted a worldwide meta-analysis most recently updated in 1992.[1] This meta-analysis included 133 randomized trials performed worldwide, involving 75,000 women with 31,000 recurrences and 24,000 deaths from breast cancer. The meta-analysis has evaluated the roles of systemic adjuvant chemotherapy, tamoxifen hormonal therapy, and the use of ovarian ablation. Women were subdivided for evaluation by lymph node status, menopausal status, and hormone receptor status.

Benefits for polychemotherapy were the same whether the women were lymph node-positive or node-negative. The absolute benefit is better for women with a larger risk for recurrence. Disease-free survival is improved approximately 28% for women receiving polychemotherapy versus controls, and overall survival was improved by approximately 16%. This was expressed as an increase of disease-free survival from 29.8% to 38.5% and overall survival from 39.8% to 46.6% for lymph node-positive patients; lymph node-negative patients experienced an improvement of disease-free survival from 54.5% to 61.5% and overall survival from 63.2% to 67.2%. The beneficial side effects were seen in all age groups, but the relative reduction in risk of recurrence was 20% in women over age 50 and 37% in women under age 50. This data are summarized in Table 23.1.

To understand the absolute benefit of the chemotherapy being offered, the physician must understand the patient's overall risk of recurrence. For example, if a woman had a 0.5-cm infiltrating ductal cancer removed, had negative lymph nodes, and was found to have a low-grade tumor, her risk of recurrence over the next 20 years is, at most, about 10%; a 25% reduction in her risk of recurrence would only reduce this figure to 7.5% (Table 23.2). A physician and the patient may believe that the use of systemic chemotherapy is this circumstance is not justifiable. If the woman has a 2.5-cm tumor with two positive lymph nodes and her recurrence risk is approximately 60%, however, 4–6 months of chemotherapy makes more sense, as she will reduce her recurrence risk to 45%. It is imperative that the medical oncologist understand the available data using prognostic factors to evaluate a woman's overall risk of recurrence and use that information to educate her about the relative and absolute benefits of the chemotherapy being offered.

Table 23.1. Benefit of polychemotherapy

Patient group, by age	No. randomized	Reduction in annual odds (%)	
		Recurrence	Death
All	18,403	21 ± 2	11 ± 2
<50 Years	6,103	28 ± 4	17 ± 4
>50 Years	12,300	17 ± 3	9 ± 3

Source: Data from the Early Breast Cancer Trialists' Collaborative Group.[1]

Table 23.2. Absolute benefit of therapy based on a 25% reduction in recurrence

Condition	%		
Disease-free after local therapy	50*	75*	90*
Recurred after local therapy	50	25	10
Recurred despite adjuvant therapy	38	49	7.5
Recurrence prevented by adjuvant therapy	12	6	2.5

Source: Data from the Early Breast Cancer Trialists' Collaborative Group.[1]
*Example based on this percentage of disease-free survival after local therapy.

Systemic Chemotherapy Agent Classifications

Antimetabolites

Antimetabolites interfere with normal biochemical reactions within a cell by having structural similarities with existing vital cellular substrates. The end result is interference with the synthesis of DNA precursors. The most common antimetabolites used for breast cancer are methotrexate and 5-fluorouracil (5-FU). They are each used in their parenteral form and can be given as an intravenous push.

Methotrexate

The most common toxicities of methotrexate are myelosuppression and stomatitis. The maximum effect is found between days 5 and 14 after each dose This agent has renal clearance and should not be used in patients with renal insufficiency. Other, less common toxicities include renal tubular injury, hepatotoxicity, and acute pneumonitis. In addition, this drug accumulates in body fluid collections, such as ascites and pleural effusions. Clearance of methotrexate from the body in these circumstances is erratic, and these loculated areas of fluid should be drained prior to the use of this agent.

5-Fluorouracil

Common toxicities of 5-FU, as with methotrexate, are myelosuppression and effects on the intestinal and oral mucosa (stomatitis and diarrhea). The drug is most commonly delivered as an intravenous push. Different toxicities can be expected when this drug is given as a prolonged intravenous infusion.

Alkylating Agents

Alkylating agents interact chemically with DNA by forming a covalent bond with nucleic acid and thus interfere with the function of DNA in the cancer cells. The most commonly used alkylating agent for breast cancer is cyclophosphamide (e.g., Cytoxan).

Cyclophosphamide

An alkylating agent, cyclophosphamide is given either orally in tablet form or by intravenous infusion. Common toxicities include myelosuppression, nausea and vomiting, and alopecia. The hair loss is more severe when the drug is given orally for extended periods. Hemorrhagic cystitis can result from an active metabolite excreted in the urine. This problem can be mitigated by adequate oral intake of fluids and frequent urination or the use of mesna (e.g., Mesnex) intravenously, which inactivates the offending metabolite.

Antitumor Antibiotics

Multiple agents fall under the classification of antitumor antibiotics. A subclassification of these agents are the anthracyclines, of which doxorubicin (Adriamycin) has substantial activity for treatment of breast cancer. It works by multiple mechanisms, including intercalation with DNA, which blocks DNA replication and RNA and protein synthesis. Doxorubicin also inhibits the action of the enzyme topoisomerase II, which functions by maintaining the structure and function of the DNA helix.

Doxorubicin causes myelosuppression and stomatitis. Alopecia is universally seen, and its severity is dose- and schedule-dependent. Doxorubicin is classified as an extravasant, and local extravasation of this drug causes a severe local reaction with tissue necrosis. The most disturbing and life-threatening of the potential side effects of doxorubicin is dose- and schedule-dependent cardiomyopathy. This problem can be delayed by delivering the drug at a lower dose on a more frequent basis, such as a prolonged infusion, or with the use of a cardioprotectant (dexrazoxane, or Zinecard). The drug can be administered only intravenously.

Mitotic Spindle Inhibitors (Taxanes)

The taxanes comprise a new class of agents with a unique mechanism of action. It is the newest group of approved agents for breast cancer. Taxanes shift the equilibrium between tubulin dimers and microtubules, causing assembly and stabilization of microtubules, preventing disassembly, and interfering with the normal function of microtubules in the cell. The two agents with activity in breast cancer are paclitaxel and docetaxel.

Paclitaxel

Paclitaxel (Taxol) causes myelosuppression, alopecia, short-lived arthralgia/myalgia syndrome, peripheral neuropathy, and the possibility of an anaphylactic reaction, which can be prevented or ameliorated by premedication with steroids and histamine-release blockers. This agent is delivered intravenously usually over 1–3 hours, depending on the dose.

Docetaxel

Docetaxel is associated with toxicities similar to those of paclitaxel, with somewhat less arthralgia/myalgia, and less chance of an anaphylactic reaction. It has another unique toxicity, however: the development of peripheral edema and pleural effusions. This reaction is related to cumulative dosing of the docetaxel and can be prevented or delayed by the use of 3–5 days of pre- and postdocetaxel dexamethasone.

Choice of Chemotherapy Regimens

Once the medical oncologist has decided to use chemotherapy, the choice must be made as to the most effective regimen for the individual, taking into account the patient's prognostic factors, menopausal status, and competing health status. Table 23.3 lists many commonly used chemotherapy regimens, each of which has been used in various randomized trials with specific eligibility criteria. Patients who are not entered into clinical trials, which evaluate the difference in benefit among different chemotherapy regimens, can expect to be placed on one of these regimens.

Table 23.3. Effective combination chemotherapy regimens for the treatment of breast cancer

Regimen	Dose (mg/m^2)	Route	Treatment day	Cycle length
CMF				
Cyclophosphamide	100	PO	1–14	4 weeks × 6 cycles
Methotrexate	40	IV	1 and 8	
5-Fluorouracil	600	IV	1 and 8	
CMF				
Cyclophosphamide	600	IV	1	3 weeks × 8 cycles
Methotrexate	40	IV	1	
5-FU	600	IV	1	
CMF				
Cyclophosphamide	600	IV	1 and 8	4 weeks × 4–6 cycles
Methotrexate	40	IV	1 and 8	
5-FU	600	IV	1 and 8	
FAC[a]				
5-Fluorouracil	500	IV	1 and 8	4 weeks × 4–6 cycles
Doxorubicin	50	IV	1	
Cyclophosphamide	500	IV	1	
A to CMF[a]				
Doxorubicin	75	IV	1	A: 3 weeks × 4 then
Cyclophosphamide	600	IV	1	CMF: 3 weeks × 8
Methotrexate	40	IV	1	
5-FU	600	IV	1	
CAF[a]				
Cyclophosphamide	600	IV	1	4 weeks × 4 cycles
Doxorubicin	60	IV	1	
5-Fluorouracil	600	IV	1 and 8	
AC[a]				
Doxorubicin	60	IV	1	3 weeks
Cyclophosphamide	600	IV	1	

[a] A = Adriamycin = doxorubicin.

ONGOING CONTROVERSIES ABOUT THE USE OF SYSTEMIC ADJUVANT CHEMOTHERAPY

So long as our data suggest only a 25–35% reduction in risk of recurrence, the delivery and selection of these agents must continue to improve. It can be undertaken in the context of ongoing and future randomized clinical trials. Some of the current controversies that face medical oncologists today are listed here.

1. *Selection of chemotherapy regimen.* The selection is frequently based on which regimens were most commonly used by their mentors during the training of the medical oncologists. Physician participation in cooperative-group clinical trials likely influences choices of therapy for their patients not participating in the trials. One of the great controversies or areas of dispute continues to be the decision as to when to use an anthracycline-based regimen. Because of the alopecia, the greater propensity for nausea and vomiting, and the risk of cardiac toxicity associated with this agent, most physicians have reserved its use for patients whose disease is considered "high risk" for recurrence. Unless otherwise indicated, it is my policy to use a doxorubicin-based regimen for women with lymph node-positive disease, including all premenopausal women and postmenopausal women with positive estrogen or progesterone receptors (or both), premenopausal females with high-risk lymph node-negative disease, and women whose cancer shows evidence of amplification of the Her-2/*neu* gene.

2. *Combining chemotherapy and hormone therapy.* Clinical trials and the EBCTCG overview have suggested a benefit from the combination of hormone therapy and chemotherapy in multiple clinical situations, including postmenopausal women with negative hormone receptors. Premenopausal women with negative estrogen/progesterone receptors apparently receive no benefit from the addition of hormone therapy to chemotherapy, but treatment of these same women with positive hormone receptors remains an area of controversy.

3. *Dose intensity of chemotherapy.* Multiple trials have suggested the benefit of maintaining the dose intensity of standard chemotherapy regimens. The use of more dose-intensive regimens given sequentially or concurrently, with or without recombinant growth factors, or in the context of autologous stem cell transplantation, continues to be the subject of these ongoing clinical trials. Unless randomized trials show the benefit of these dose-intensive regimens when compared to standard dosing, their use should be considered experimental.

4. *Deciding on which patients should receive chemotherapy.* In February 1995 multiple breast cancer experts met for the Fifth International Conference on Adjuvant Therapy of Primary Breast Cancer in St. Gallen, Switzerland.[2] Tables 23.4 and 23.5 present summaries of the consensus undertaken at this conference. Table 23.4 details the basic recommendations for women with lymph node-positive breast cancer, and Table 23.5 details those for women with lymph node-negative breast cancer.

5. *Sequencing chemotherapy and radiation therapy.* With the growing number of women appropriately selecting segmental mastectomy (lumpectomy) over modified radical mastectomy, the sequence of local radiation therapy to the breast and

Table 23.4. 1995 St. Gallen Consensus Conference: adjuvant therapy for node-positive breast cancer

Estrogen receptor states	Standard therapy	Under consideration
Premenopausal		
ER$^+$	Chemotherapy or ovarian ablation	Addition of tamoxifen
ER$^-$	Chemotherapy	
Postmenopausal		
ER$^+$	Tamoxifen	Addition of doxorubicin-based chemotherapy
ER$^-$	Chemotherapy	Addition of tamoxifen

Source: After 5th International Conference on Adjuvant Therapy of Primary Breast Cancer.[2]

Table 23.5. 1995 St. Gallen Consensus Conference: adjuvant therapy for node-negative breast cancer

Condition	Standard therapy	Under consideration
<1 cm, ER$^+$, low histologic grade	None	Tamoxifen
1–2 cm, ER$^+$, low histologic grade		
Premenopausal	Tamoxifen or chemotherapy	Ovarian ablation
Postmenopausal	Tamoxifen	
>2 cm or ER$^-$		
Premenopausal		
ER$^+$	Chemotherapy	Tamoxifen, ovarian ablation
ER$^-$	Chemotherapy	
Postmenopausal		
ER$^+$	Tamoxifen	Addition of chemotherapy
ER$^-$	Chemotherapy	Addition of tamoxifen

Source: After 5th International Conference on Adjuvant Therapy of Primary Breast Cancer.[2]

the systemic adjuvant therapies have become more problematic. If systemic chemotherapy is to be delivered (especially when using doxorubicin), radiation therapy should be given at the conclusion of the chemotherapy.

NEOADJUVANT CHEMOTHERAPY

Because of the increasing number of women being offered chemotherapy in the adjuvant setting, it is reasonable to evaluate the use of "primary or neoadjuvant" chemotherapy, defined as the use of chemotherapy prior to the definitive local therapy (lumpectomy or mastectomy). Primary chemotherapy prevents the delays caused by local postoperative healing that is frequently seen after a mastectomy or lumpectomy. The origins of primary chemotherapy extend back to 1973 when the investigators at the Milan Cancer Institute designed trials for women with stage III breast cancer. Since that time they and others have undertaken subsequent clinical trials evaluating the local response and eventual disease-free survival of women receiving neoadjuvant chemotherapy. The most recent evaluation of primary chemotherapy has been by the National Surgical Adjuvant Breast and Bowel Project (NSABP), which instituted a randomized clinical trial in 1988 comparing primary to postoperative chemotherapy in women with clinically evident, histologically proved infiltrating breast cancer.[3] They evaluated the results of 1523 women randomized to doxorubicin/cyclophosphamide (AC) chemotherapy preoperatively versus postoperatively in women with primary breast cancer. The conclusion was that preoperative therapy reduced the size of most breast tumors and decreased the incidence of positive nodes. The greatest increase in lumpectomy candidates after preoperative therapy occurred among those women with tumors >5 cm. To this point, preoperative chemotherapy has had no impact on disease-free or overall survival from breast cancer. Outside of clinical trials, the use of primary chemotherapy should be considered only for women whose tumor reduction would alter the decision for local therapy (i.e., lumpectomy versus mastectomy).

Hormonal Therapy

Just as the benefits of systemic adjuvant chemotherapy were evaluated in the EBCTCG meta-analysis, so were the effects of tamoxifen hormone therapy. Tamoxifen was originally developed as an oral contraceptive during the early 1960s but did not in fact prevent ovulation or pregnancy. It subsequently was found to have an effect on advanced breast cancer, initially receiving U.S. Food and Drug Administration (FDA) approval for women with metastatic breast cancer, followed by approval for women in the adjuvant setting. Several other hormonal agents are available for the treatment of breast cancer, but most have shown greater toxicity without any improvement in response or survival.

Tamoxifen has both estrogenic and antiestrogenic properties. It competes with estrogen for estrogen receptor binding in normal and malignant breast tissue. In addition, there is inhibition of both transforming growth factor-alpha (TGFα) and autocrine polypeptide-stimulated proliferation. Other antitumor effects of tamoxifen that inhibit tumor growth are the stimulation of TGFβ and inhibition of protein kinase C.

The EBCTCG results on tamoxifen were evaluated by nodal status, age of the patient, estrogen receptor status, duration of use of the tamoxifen, dosage, and whether given alone or in addition to chemotherapy. Tables 23.6–23.10 give the 10-year outcome comparisons for the 30,081 women entered into the tamoxifen randomized trials.

The tables are more informative than the data with regard to systemic chemotherapy and multiple subtypes of breast cancer presentations. They reveal a 25% reduction in the odds of recurrence and a 17% reduction in the odds of death 10 years after the diagnosis of breast cancer. It is not only the estrogen receptor status

Table 23.6. 10-Year outcome comparisons by nodal status

Group	Recurrence-free survival (%)		Overall survival (%)	
	Tamoxifen	Control	Tamoxifen	Control
All patients	51.2	44.7	58.8	52.6
Positive nodes	41.9	33.1	50.4	42.2
Negative nodes	68.1	63.1	74.5	71

Source: Data from the Early Breast Cancer Trialists' Collaborative Group.[1]

Table 23.7. Annual odds reduction in recurrence and death, by patient age

Age (years)	Recurrence-free survival (%)	Overall survival (%)
All patients	25	17
<50	12	6
>50	29	20
>70	28	21

Source: Data from the Early Breast Cancer Trialists' Collaborative Group.[1]

Table 23.8. Annual odds reduction in recurrence and death by estrogen receptor and duration of tamoxifen

Condition	Recurrence-free survival (%)	Overall survival (%)
Estrogen receptor		
Positive	32	21
Negative	13	11
Duration of tamoxifen		
<2 Years	16	11
>2 Years	38	24

Source: Data from the Early Breast Cancer Trialists' Collaborative Group.[1]

Table 23.9. Percent reduction in odds of recurrence and death in women >50 years by nodal status and estrogen receptor status

Condition	Relapse-free survival (%)	Mortality (%)
Axillary nodes		
Negative	28	16
Positive	33	22
Estrogen receptor		
Negative	16	16
Positive	36	23

Source: Data from the Early Breast Cancer Trialists' Collaborative Group.[1]

Table 23.10. Percent reduction in odds of recurrence and death in women >50 years by dosage and duration of tamoxifen

Tamoxifen	Relapse-free survival (%)	Overall survival (%)
Dosage (mg/day)		
20	31	21
30–40	27	18
Duration (years)		
<1	19	13
2	33	23
3+	38	23

Source: Data from the Early Breast Cancer Trialists' Collaborative Group.[1]

Table 23.11. Percent reduction in the odds of recurrence and death from tamoxifen in patients receiving tamoxifen with or without chemotherapy

Condition	Aged < 50 years	Aged > 50 years	All
Relapse-free survival			
Tam only vs. no tam	27.7	30	29
Tam + chemo vs. same chemo	7	28	24
All Tam vs. no tam	12	29	25
Mortality			
Tam only vs. no Tam	17	19	19
Tam + chemo vs. same chemo	3	20	16
All Tam vs. no tam	6	20	16

Source: Data from the Early Breast Cancer Trialists' Collaborative Group.[1]
Tam = tamoxifen; chemo = chemotherapy.

that plays a role in influencing benefits from tamoxifen; the age of the patient and the duration of tamoxifen use do as well. Although investigators speak of a 25% reduction in the risk of recurrence from breast cancer with the use of tamoxifen, these data include women of all ages, with differing dosages and durations of use. Women who use the drug tamoxifen for more than 3 years have a 38% reduction in the risk of recurrence. Accordingly, women whose tumors are estrogen receptor-positive have a 32% reduction in risk of recurrence even when not taking into account the differing durations of tamoxifen use.

The last table of this group (Table 23.11) suggests that postmenopausal women who receive chemotherapy in addition to tamoxifen obtain the same benefit from tamoxifen as those who receive tamoxifen alone. However, for women younger than age 50 the benefit from tamoxifen is marginal when used with chemotherapy but equals that of postmenopausal women when the drug is used alone.

Combined Chemohormonal Therapy

When tamoxifen and chemotherapy were combined, the EBCTCG meta-analysis overview gave indirect estimates of the benefits anticipated from this combined therapy. It was estimated that combined therapy would reduce the risk of recurrence by 45%, and that this estimate would improve to 50% for patients who had received tamoxifen for more than 2 years.

Indications for Use of Tamoxifen, Dosage, and Duration

The 1995 St. Gallen Consensus Conference data[2] in Tables 23.4 and 23.5 expand our current knowledge about the use of tamoxifen in the adjuvant setting. Currently it is recommended that women receive tamoxifen at a dosage of 20 mg/day administered either as a single daily dose or divided into 10 mg bid. The dosage is not altered by the body surface area or the age of the patient.

Toxicity

The side effect profile of tamoxifen is best considered in the context of randomized, placebo-based, double-blind clinical trials. Just such a trial was performed by the NSABP B-14 during the 1980s. The main reason for the trial was to evaluate the benefit and risks of tamoxifen versus placebo in women with lymph node-negative, estrogen/progesterone receptor-positive breast cancer. Toxicity data were available on 2861 randomized patients, half of whom received placebo. Table 23.12 describes the various toxicities reported in this trial. Note the large number of toxicity complaints in women in the placebo arm. Also note that the statistically significant differences between tamoxifen and placebo were seen with hot flashes, vaginal discharge, and vascular thrombi.

Secondary Malignancies

Alterations in the development of secondary primary malignancies have been associated with the use of tamoxifen for breast and endometrial cancer.

1. *Second primary breast cancers.* Women with breast cancer are at increased risk for a second primary breast cancer developing in the contralateral breast. The use of tamoxifen is associated with 40–65% reduction in the occurrence of contralateral

Table 23.12. Toxicity of tamoxifen in NSABP B-14

Toxicity	Percent of patients reporting the symptom	
	Placebo (n = 1439)	Tamoxifen (n = 1422)
Hot flashes	46.2	62.4*
Fluid retention	28.6	30.9*
Vaginal discharge	14.2	28.4*
Irregular menses	17.6	23.6
Nausea	22.6	23.3
Skin rash	14.3	17.7
Diarrhea	12.9	9.8
Vascular thrombi	0.2	1.5*

Source: Data from Fisher et al.[4]
*Statistically signficant difference.

breast cancer. This benefit lasts well past the time of discontinuance of the drug and is greater for those who take tamoxifen for more than 2 years.

2. *Endometrial cancer.* Cancer of the endometrium is one of the most common invasive gynecologic malignancies in women in the United States. Risk factors for the development of this malignancy include exposure to unopposed estrogen (both endogenous and exogenous). Fifteen studies have been reviewed with regard to the association of tamoxifen and endometrial cancer. Twelve of these studies have shown no relation, two have suggested an increased incidence, and one showed a reduced incidence. Unfortunately, these reports do not take into account the women's history of unopposed estrogen (weight, age, use of exogenous estrogens). There is great concern that because of an increased incidence of vaginal discharge and menstrual irregularities in women on tamoxifen, these women are more likely to be evaluated for their gynecologic complaints, and therefore a greater number of endometrial cancers are being found. There is a potential surveillance and ascertainment bias in tamoxifen-treated patients. To date, a causal relation of tamoxifen and endometrial cancer has not been proved. If such a relation exists, the absolute increased risk is poorly understood and is likely to be overestimated. Current recommendations for gynecologic evaluation for women on tamoxifen include a yearly gynecologic examination for patients with an intact uterus. Special studies (e.g., endometrial biopsy and ultrasonography of the uterus) are not indicated in the asymptomatic breast cancer patient receiving tamoxifen unless she is participating in a clinical trial evaluating the value of these practices.

Other Beneficial Effects of Tamoxifen

Two additional beneficial benefits have been reported from tamoxifen, taking advantage of the estrogen-agonist properties of this hormonal agent.

1. *Bone mineral density.* Adequate data exist to show that tamoxifen helps maintain the bone mineral density of postmenopausal women during the course of their exposure to this drug, similar to the effects of estrogen. This benefit is not seen in premenopausal women, and in fact young women show evidence of a slight bone mineral loss while they are taking tamoxifen.

2. *Serum cholesterol.* Tamoxifen lowers total serum cholesterol levels approximately 20% during the duration of use of this hormonal agent. Two clinical trials have reported a reduction in sudden death from cardiovascular events in women taking tamoxifen versus no therapy for their breast cancer. This finding may be attributed to the improved lipid profile in these women.

Other Hormonal Agents

As stated previously, tamoxifen is not the only hormonal agent available for the treatment of breast cancer. In the metastatic setting other hormonal therapies have been shown to be equally efficacious but with inferior toxicity profiles. The use of combined hormonal therapies when compared to the sequential use of these same drugs has also shown no improvement in the survival of patients. Other hormonal

Table 23.13. Hormone therapy for breast cancer

Class	Dose	Toxicity
Antiestrogen		
Tamoxifen	20 mg/day PO	Vaginal discharge, hot flashes, vascular thrombi
Progestin		
Megestrol	40 mg PO qid	Weight gain, fluid retention, vaginal bleeding
Aromatase inhibitor		
Anastrozole	1 mg/day PO	Asthenia, nausea, headache, hot flashes
Aminoglutethimide	250 mg qid + hydrocortisone or 250 mg bid	Rash, somnolence, asthenia, lightheadedness

therapies that could be considered in the frontline setting for metastatic breast cancer are listed in Table 23.13.

CONCLUSIONS

Breast cancer continues to be the second leading cause of cancer-related death for women in the United States, second only to lung cancer. Mortality rates due to breast cancer have decreased during the last several years. This reduction has been attributed to two factors: (1) the more common use of screening mammography for women in the United States, leading to earlier diagnosis of breast cancer at a time when it is potentially curable; and (2) the more frequent use of systemic adjuvant chemotherapy, tamoxifen, or both for all stages of early breast cancer.

It is only through ongoing clinical trials and enrollment of larger numbers of women in these trials that we can further improve the disease-free and overall survival of women diagnosed with early breast cancer. New agents continue to be developed and investigated in these clinical trials. Finding better agents with improved efficacy and toxicity profiles and learning how best to discover and use molecular prognostic factors remain some of our greatest challenges in our quest to cure all women diagnosed with early breast cancer.

References

1. Early Breast Cancer Trialists' Collaborative Group. Systemic treatment of early breast cancer by hormonal, cytotoxic, or immune therapy. Lancer 1992;339:1–15, 71–85
2. 5th International Conference on Adjuvant Therapy of Primary Breast Cancer. St. Gallen, Switzerland. Anticancer Drugs 1995;6:1–96

3. Fisher B, Brown A, Mamounas E, et al. Effect of preoperative chemotherapy on local-regional disease in women with operable breast cancer: findings from National Surgical Adjuvant Breast and Bowel Project B-18. J Clin Oncol 1997;15:2483–1493

4. Fisher B, Costantino J, Redmond C, et al. A randomized clinical trial evaluating tamoxifen in the treatment of patients with node-negative brest cancer who have estrogen-receptor-positive tumors. N Engl J Med 1989;320:479–484

24 SURVEILLANCE OF WOMEN ON TAMOXIFEN

William H. Hindle

Women on tamoxifen therapy are followed by their medical oncologists for surveillance of their breast cancer. These patients are also followed by their primary care providers for their general medical care and surveillance.

It is estimated that there are more than 2 million breast cancer survivors, or "victors" as they prefer to be called, in the United States. Most of these women are postmenopausal, and most are on tamoxifen. Although the biologic actions of tamoxifen in human females are multiple, complex, and end-organ-specific, in general the effects are antiestrogenic on the breast and estrogenic on the uterus, bones, and vascular system. Thus tamoxifen adjuvant hormonal therapy decreases the incidence and severity of osteoporosis and the adverse cardiovascular changes associated with aging. However, like unopposed estrogen therapy, tamoxifen can stimulate subclinical endometrial carcinoma and increase the incidence of endometrial carcinoma, polyps, and thickening, as well as subendometrial microcystic space formation. Furthermore, women on tamoxifen can have increased uterine length, size, and volume and an increased number and size of clinically apparent uterine myomas.

Women with a uterus and on tamoxifen therapy should be closely monitored for evidence of uterine bleeding and should have annual pelvic examinations and Papanicolaou (Pap) smears (as should all women over the age of 20) as well as annual mammography. A woman on tamoxifen who experiences any vaginal bleeding should see her primary health care provider immediately for evaluation. A bimanual pelvic examination, Pap smear, and endometrial biopsy should then be performed. Further procedures and potential treatments (e.g., stopping the tamoxifen therapy) should await the results of the initial evaluation. The paramount concern is to rule out endometrial carcinoma (or premalignant histologic changes). Saline infusion sonohysterography (fluid-enhanced ultrasound evaluation of the endometrial cavity and uterus) and hysteroscopy are appropriate procedures for further evaluation if the biopsy report is benign. Furthermore, her medical oncologist (or the physician prescribing her tamoxifen) should be notified. If the primary health care provider is not trained and experienced in the evaluation of postmenopausal bleeding, the woman should be referred to a gyne-

KEY PRACTICE POINTS

Women on tamoxifen need: an annual mammogram, an annual Papanicolaou smear, an annual pelvic examination, and evaluation of abnormal uterine bleeding *stat*.

Tamoxifen therapy side effects: hot flashes; vaginal discharge, usually watery; vaginal dryness and associated dyspareunia (paradoxical to vaginal discharge); uterine bleeding.

Table 24.1. Reported side effects of tamoxifen therapy

Deep vein thrombosis

Fluid retention

Hot flashes*

Irregular menses

Nausea

Pulmonary emboli

Superficial phlebitis

Vaginal discharge*

Vaginal dryness

Venous thrombosis

Skin rash

Leukopenia

Retinopathy

*Statistically significant increase in placebo-controlled clinical trials.

cologist. A woman with other bothersome side effects (Table 24.1) or complications of tamoxifen therapy should be referred to the medical specialist appropriate for that side effect.

A preliminary National Cancer Institute report of the NSABP P-1 breast cancer prevention clinical trial indicated a 39% decrease in the occurrence of invasive breast cancer, a 47% decrease in noninvasive (in situ) breast cancer, and a 34% decrease in bone fractures for the women treated with tamoxifen compared to those given placebo. However, there was a 136% increase in endometrial cancer (3:1000) and a 41% increase in blood clotting events in the tamoxifen treatment arm of the study compared to placebo. The decrease in invasive breast cancer for women on tamoxifen was seen in all age groups.

25 BREAST RADIATION THERAPY

Silvia Formenti

RADIATION THERAPY FOR BREAST CONSERVATION

It is now generally agreed that conservative surgery with radiation represents a valid alternative to mastectomy for treatment of stage I and II breast cancer. At present, seven prospective randomized trials have shown the equivalence of mastectomy versus conservative surgery and radiotherapy in terms of local recurrence, 5- and 10-year disease-free survival, and overall survival.[1,2] Postoperative irradiation represents a fundamental component of conservative management and the NSABP-B6 study confirms the high incidence of breast cancer recurrence in patients undergoing wide excision without radiation, with 37% local recurrences in node-negative patients and 43% in node-positive patients. Instead, locoregional recurrence following conservative surgery and irradiation for early breast cancer ranges from 5% to 10% at 5 years and from 10% to 15% at 10 years.[3] These figures are comparable to those achieved with mastectomy.

Local Management: A Patient's Choice

At the University of Southern California Norris Breast Center (USC/NBC), a radiation oncologist usually meets with the patient as part of the initial evaluation after a diagnosis of breast cancer. This encounter before definitive breast surgery is important because: (1) it allows the radiation oncologist to examine the patient before removal of the breast cancer; and (2) it enables the patient to understand the options available and to ask questions about radiation. It is important to address the patient's fears or misinformation about radiation therapy at this session.

Although it is crucial to enable the patient to make informed decisions, the choice of breast preservation or mastectomy is a personal one. Most studies on quality of life have documented that patients are equally satisfied with either option, provided they believe they made a free and informed choice.

Indications and Contraindications for Breast Preservation

Most women with T1–T2 (up to 5 cm in maximum tumor diameter) breast cancers are excellent candidates for breast preservation, that is, lumpectomy (segmental

mastectomy) and irradiation. The following clinical factors have shown no correlation with the incidence of breast cancer recurrence in patients undergoing
lumpectomy: primary tumor size (i.e., T1 versus T2), tumor histology, or tumor
location. Patients with subareolar tumors may be considered candidates for conservative surgery and irradiation if adequate excision can be accomplished with
negative margins and if the tumor is well localized.

A different subset is represented by patients with gross multicentric disease or
diffuse microcalcifications (i.e., with more than one quadrant involved clinically
or mammographically). They have been reported to have up to a 40% breast
cancer recurrence rate following conservative surgery and irradiation. These
patients should be adequately informed and advised to choose mastectomy.[4]

Patients who are good candidates for conservative surgery and radiation have
(1) a primary tumor ≤4–5 cm in diameter as determined clinically, mammographically, or pathologically; (2) a single, discrete, well defined tumor; (3)
microcalcifications, if present, that are focal and not diffuse and that must be
completely resected before the start of radiation therapy. Women with implants
for breast augmentation can safely undergo radiation therapy but with some risk
of developing fibrosis between the capsule and the irradiated skin. In our experience this occurrence has not compromised the cosmetic results, but 15- to 20-year
follow-up data are not available.

Relative contraindications to primary radiation therapy include large tumors in
a small breast where an excisional biopsy would result in significant loss of breast
tissue and have an undesirable cosmetic result. Another relative contraindication
is the coexistence of an autoimmune condition: in such settings, more fibrosis and
inferior cosmetic results can occur. Absolute contraindications to primary radiotherapy include pregnancy, gross multicentric disease or diffuse microcalcifications, and previous radiation therapy to the area where the cancer is located.

Axillary Lymph Nodes

Because palpation of the axilla is associated with a more than 30% incidence
of false-negative and false-positive results, an axillary staging procedure is
recommended prior to radiotherapy. The value of the procedure is both prognostic and therapeutic. There is controversy concerning the optimal staging
procedure. A level I and II axillary dissection minimizes the likelihood of missing
nodal involvement and accurately quantitates the extent of nodal involvement.
With clear level I and II nodes, the risk of a level III involvement is about 1%.
On the other hand, a complete axillary dissection provides minimal additional
information while increasing the risk of arm edema, especially if the axilla is to be
irradiated.

The role of regional node irradiation in both histologically negative and positive axillary node patients had been questioned, especially in patients receiving
adjuvant polychemotherapy. Usually the tangent fields used to irradiate the breast
tissue also treat level I nodes. Supraclavicular and apical axillary irradiation is
necessary to complete therapy to the nodes in this area. This field carries the risk
of other complications, such as matchline fibrosis, fibrosis in the supraclavicular

fossa or pectoral fold, brachial plexopathy, increased incidence of arm and breast edema, and apical lung radiation pneumonia and fibrosis.

The presence of four or more positive axillary nodes, or the lack or inadequacy of nodal dissection, represents an indication for axillary and supraclavicular irradiation.

Interdisciplinary Collaboration

In addition to the interdisciplinary initial evaluation of the patient, we have found that continuous communication among the breast cancer team optimizes the patient's care. For instance, we have established a policy that requires the operating surgeon to place radiopaque clips in the tumor bed at the time of segmental mastectomy. These clips are used during radiation treatment to identify the original tumor bed to direct the final tumor boost precisely. Because most breast cancer recurrences occur at the original tumor site, accurate identification of the area to boost is crucial to ensure optimal local control.[5,6] It is important to have access to the final pathology report that describes the status of the margins of resection (involved or uninvolved, <5mm or >5mm from the tumor) and of the findings from the axillary resection specimen. This information is necessary before starting radiation treatment.

Common Side Effects of Irradiation

Most women tolerate breast irradiation quite well. Usually mild fatigue is reported during the treatment. The skin of the irradiated breast undergoes changes such as dryness, erythema, and rarely desquamation with blistering. We encourage patients to wear cotton lingerie and to use aloe vera cream daily after the radiotherapy session. Long-term common side effects include increased firmness of the treated breast and possibly slight retraction.

In women with large breasts, especially if pendulous, it is common to develop blisters at the inframammary fold. At the USC/NBC we have designed an irradiation table modification that permits these women to be treated prone, completely preventing this complication.

Axillary and supraclavicular area radiation is also tolerated quite well. The same skin changes may occur. Because lymphedema of the ipsilateral arm develops in about 30% of cases, we do not irradiate women who have received a full (levels I, II, and III) dissection.

A rare complication is radiation-induced pneumonia; persistent dry cough or shortness of breath, usually occurring after the completion of treatment, suggests this complication. Radiation pneumonia characteristically displays an infiltration limited to the field of radiation. A protracted course of low-dose oral corticosteroids is usually successful in resolving this condition.

Timing of Radiation Therapy

Radiation treatment should begin within 2–4 weeks after surgery and before chemotherapy. For patients required to receive chemotherapy first, irradiation should start no sooner than 3 weeks from the last chemotherapy treatment.

LOCALLY ADVANCED BREAST CANCER

Treatment Options and Results

Historically, unresectable breast cancers have been treated by radiotherapy. The results of radiotherapy alone have been reported in numerous studies and can be summarized as a 5-year survival that ranges between 10% and 40% with local control maintained in 20–70% of patients depending on the total dose of radiation employed. With locally advanced breast cancer the treatment fields include the breast (or the chest wall if radiation is delivered after mastectomy) and the supraclavicular and axillary fields, but higher radiation doses are usually employed. However, because high doses of radiation (70–100 Gy) are associated with a 20% incidence of severe complications (e.g., soft tissue necrosis or severe breast fibrosis), the use of preoperative radiotherapy with a moderate dose of radiation (45–60 Gy) has been extensively investigated. Local recurrence rates of less than 20% are achieved in most studies, unfortunately with disappointing 5-year survival results.

Adding systemic polychemotherapy to modify the outcome of patients with advanced disease has taken place since the late 1970s with the initial results disappointing. Several prospective randomized trials have failed to demonstrate statistically significant differences in survival by adding chemotherapy to locoregional treatment. However, reports from more recent studies support the role of chemotherapy in this disease setting, with 5-year survival rates in the range of 40–50% when chemotherapy is employed up front to facilitate local control of the disease. For instance, Harris et al.[7] reported 77% local control for patients receiving both chemotherapy and radiation compared with 51% for those receiving only radiotherapy. Most important, the 5-year distant relapse-free survival was 45% from the combined treatment, compared to 22% for radiotherapy alone.

The consensus is that both radiation and chemotherapy are needed for this patient population. The sequence has usually designated radiation to be the last therapy used, which has increased the possibility of radioresistance induced by previous chemotherapy.[8]

Treatment Sequencing

The optimal treatment sequencing has not yet been established. Initial chemotherapy, although it could favorably affect control of micrometastases, may be insufficient because chemotherapy is known to be less efficacious when used on a large tumor. Hypotheses stated to explain this phenomenon include (1) innate drug resistance, (2) rapidly acquired drug resistance, and (3) insufficient drug delivery by the microcirculation in large, necrotic, hypoperfused tumors. Alternatively, radiation alone as a preoperative "induction" treatment is often inadequate because tumoricidal doses predispose to unacceptable complication rates when surgery is performed. In addition, delaying systemic treatment in a patient population at high risk of metastatic spread is worrisome with a disease that can have a long natural history but with which systemic relapse leading to death eventually occurs in most patients.

The synergistic use of chemotherapy and radiation has been explored in several studies with conflicting results.[5,6,9–12] Because of the radiosensitizing effect of doxorubicin, the concomitant administration of this drug with radiation produces severe skin toxicity. Therefore other chemotherapeutic agents, including some with known activity in the treatment of breast cancer, have begun to be combined with radiation therapy for management of patients with various malignancies.

USC/NORRIS BREAST CENTER EXPERIENCE WITH LOCALLY ADVANCED BREAST CANCER

Especially with patients with inoperable breast cancer, moderate doses of preoperative radiation are advisable. A combined regimen of radiation with a concomitant chemotherapeutic agent has been the preferred approach. Our group has piloted the use of continuous-infusion 5-fluorouracil and radiation for locally advanced breast cancer in a study that has so far accrued 37 of the planned 40 patients. Over the last 3 years we have been able to demonstrate the feasibility of this combined regimen; most important, we have pilot-tested a paradigm of translational research on breast cancer.[12,13] In fact, all studied patients undergo sequential tumor biopsies to study biologic correlates of response.

Probably the most prominent finding of this study is the association of *p53* status with pathologic response: among the first 30 evaluable patients, 10 of the 16 patients (62.5%) who had no evidence of *p53* mutation at immunohistochemistry achieved a pathologic response to the combined regimen, compared to 1 of 14 patients (7%) with mutated *p53* ($p = 0.004$). In view of these findings it becomes important to investigate the combination of radiation with drugs that may be differently affected by *p53* status. One of such agents is paclitaxel; we are now exploring the use of weekly paclitaxel during radiation therapy (54 Gy) in this patient population.

Treatment of Internal Mammary Lymph Nodes

There is little evidence that excision of the internal mammary nodes with extended radical mastectomy or that preoperative or postoperative irradiation of the nodes increases survival. Although parasternal recurrences are by no means unknown, clinically they occur much less often than one would predict based on the frequency of pathologic involvement of the internal mammary nodes. However, there might be a small set of patients in whom control of nodal disease makes the difference between cure and further dissemination of disease. The main toxic potential of irradiation of the internal mammary nodes is directed at the heart and lungs. The volume of lung irradiated is increased by the use of the supraclavicular field, and the volume of heart irradiated (for left-sided primary tumors only) is increased by moving the medial border of the tangents farther over the midline. The morbidity of irradiation is enhanced by the use of cardiotoxic drugs in chemotherapy regimens.

We limit treating the internal mammary nodes to patients with locally advanced or recurrent breast cancer who show evidence of involvement at pathology examination or at computed tomography (CT) scan. When the internal mammary nodes are treated, one should use a full supraclavicular and axillary field to ensure adequate treatment of the internal mammary nodes in the first and second intercostal spaces, which are usually not fully included in the tangent field. Whenever more than 3 cm of lung is included within the tangents fields (measured as the mid-diameter of lung on a port film), the benefits of such treatment should be questioned and exclusion of the internal mammary nodes considered.

Radiation Therapy for Palliation of Metastatic Disease

Radiation therapy is utilized for palliation of bone metastases. A median survival of 48 months has been reported among breast cancer patients with metastases confined to the skeletal system. In view of this relatively long potential survival, we prefer to deliver 30 Gy in 10 fractions or 44 Gy over 22 fractions in these patients.[14] These fractionation regimens produce fewer side effects and in our experience have been associated with more persistent control of the irradiated area than the more rapid fractionation regimens.

RADIOTHERAPY TECHNIQUES

Breast and Regional Lymph Nodes

Any technique used for radiation therapy aims to cover adequately the area at risk while minimizing the doses given to normal tissue, especially the lung and heart. Furthermore, the selected technique must deliver a homogeneous dose throughout the target volume and be reproducible from treatment to treatment. To achieve these goals, the following conditions are essential: (1) table rotation, gantry rotation, and beam blocks to match fields together at the junction of the en face supraclavicular/axillary field; (2) breast tangents angled so the posterior borders are coplanar, thereby minimizing lung dose, or use of other available techniques to minimize lung and heart irradiation; and (3) wedges in the beam to compensate for the contour of the breast.

Whenever a patient is treated at the USC/NBC, permanent tattoo dots, usually three altogether, are placed to delineate the field margins and to allow future reconstruction of the irradiated fields. This practice has enabled us to match the contralateral tangent fields safely at the patient's midline if a second breast cancer must be irradiated.

Breast Tangents

Most patients are treated on a 4- or 6-MV linear accelerator. The entire breast is ordinarily included in the tangential fields. Treatment consists of two fields per day, usually with wedges. The borders of the fields are as follows.

Inferior: A 2-cm margin is allowed inferior to the inframammary fold.
Superior: The margin of the breast is determined by palpation and is allowed a 1-cm margin. When the supraclavicular field is treated, placement of the match line depends on the location of the primary tumor in the

breast but is usually at about the second intercostal space (usually at the inferior edge of the sternoclavicular junction radiographically).

Lateral: The lateral exit of the tangents is placed in such a way as to include all breast tissue with a 2-cm margin, which usually places it at the mid-axillary line.

Medial: The medial exit of the tangents is at the midline.

Anterior: A 2-cm margin of light is allowed above the highest point of the breast.

Posterior: The edges of the tangents should be coincident; the medial and lateral borders determine their exact position.

No more than 3 cm of lung (as measured at the central axis of the treatment field on a simulator film) should be included within the tangential field. For left-sided primary tumors, care should be taken to exclude as much of the heart as possible from the tangential fields. Occasionally, a substantial part of the superior portion of the breast is in the supraclavicular and axillary field; in such cases, especially with primary tumors of the upper quadrant, careful attention to the adequacy of the match between fields is necessary. A match line through the primary surgical scar should be avoided.

Regional Lymph Nodes

The axillary and supraclavicular field should not be treated unless one of the following applies: (1) there is extensive nodal involvement (e.g., more than four nodes removed are involved) or gross residual disease is left; or (2) axillary sampling is inadequate, or axillary dissection is not performed because of high surgical risk due to medical conditions or the patient's refusal.

Because of an already substantial risk of arm edema, these guidelines to irradiation of the axilla may have to be modified in patients undergoing full axillary dissection (levels I, II, and III). Therefore it is critical that the radiation oncologist be aware of the extent of surgery, particularly whether the axillary vein was stripped, before deciding whether to treat the full axillary field.

A daily dose at a depth of 3 cm is used to treat the full axillary and supraclavicular fields. No bolus is used. The field is angled approximately 10 degrees from the vertical to avoid treating the cervical spinal cord. The borders of the field are as follows:

Inferior: This border is determined by the match line, usually at the second intercostal space (see the description of the borders of the breast tangents, above).

Superior: Radiologically, this border is usually the most superior aspect of the first rib. Except in unusual situations, it is preferable not to "clear" the skin (or "flash") in the supraclavicular region.

Lateral: This border is usually two-thirds of the medial-to-lateral distance through the humeral head; most of the humeral head should be blocked. In some patients with extensive axillary disease, it may be necessary to open the field to include it and also to treat antero-posteriorly and posteroanteriorly to ensure a sufficient dose at depth.

Medial: This setup is started at the center of the suprasternal notch. It follows the midline, and the gantry is then angled.

Breast Boost Techniques

A boost dose—intended to deliver to the primary site a higher dose than can cosmetically be tolerated by the entire breast—is used to minimize the likelihood of a recurrence at the primary site. It may be applied in several ways, depending on the size of the breast, the location and size of the primary tumor, the available equipment, and the personal preference and experience of the radiation oncologist. Interstitial brachytherapy has been used successfully to deliver the breast boost,[6,15] but because it requires general anesthesia and 2–3 days of partial isolation an external beam boost has been substituted. Nowadays electron boosts are used at most academic institutions. In the absence of radiopaque clips, the preoperative description of the lesion at clinical examination, the findings at mammography, and operative notes are helpful for the radiation oncologist when deciding on how to design the boost.

Electrons

A typical electron beam field is a circle or square 8–12 cm in diameter, defined by a lead cut-out or by collimators, with appropriate attention to fall-off at the field edges. The fields may be rectangular or elliptical. A 6- to 11-MeV electrons setting, depending on the thickness of the volume at risk, is employed. The dose is prescribed at "dmax" on the central axis. Energies exceeding 11 MeV deliver an excessive dose to the skin and can compromise the cosmetic result. The volume covered often includes the nipple.

Photons

For primary tumors initially situated deeply within the breast parenchyma and close to the chest wall, an external beam boost (e.g., an en face or three-field anterior plus wedged pair) may be used. One must try to minimize the exit dose to the underlying lung (e.g., by angling an en face field). The breast tissue outside the desired boost area receives a higher dose with external beam boosts than with electron or implant boosts, and it may adversely affect the cosmetic results. Therefore a plan that decreases irradiation outside the boost volume should be chosen.

Axillary Boost Techniques

Occasionally, it is necessary to administer a dose to the axilla exceeding 4600 cGy. The anterior supraclavicular and axillary field is relatively homogeneous. Irradiation to the field delivers a substantial dose to the pectoralis major muscle. Administering a high dose through this anterior field may result in excessive irradiation with resultant symptomatic fibrosis of the muscle plus telangiectasia and atrophy of the overlying skin. Hence an axillary boost technique should be used for a portion of the treatment.

For a posterior axillary boost, the superior border parallels the clavicle; the inferior border is blocked to match the tangents; the medial border is 1 cm inside and parallel to the thoracic cage; and the lateral border is at the middle of the humeral head. The radiation is directed at mid-depth.

RECOMMENDED RADIATION DOSES

The following doses are in compliance with our active USC/NBC treatment protocols.

Whole Breast Treatment

The purpose of treating the breast outside the immediate vicinity of the primary region is to destroy subclinical foci of carcinoma. The following suggested doses are compatible with this purpose in most patients and are well tolerated by the entire breast.

The recommended *treatment dose* is either (1) 200 cGy/day 5 days per week, to a total dose of 4600 cGy in 4.5 weeks; or (2) 180 cGy/day 5 days per week, to a total dose of 5000 cGy in 5.5 weeks. The dose is calculated at a point two-thirds the distance from the apex of the breast to the baseline (line connecting the posterior edge of the two fields) at the mid-separation of the beams. The variation in dose from the base of the breast to its apex should not exceed 15% as provided on a transverse central axis contour.

The *boost dose* should be such that the combination of external beam treatment and boost delivers a total dose of 6000 cGy to the primary site. In women treated with breast preservation, this is achieved by adding a tumor bed boost with the following doses:

Electrons: 1400 cGy, at 200 cGy per fraction (at the 80% isodose depth)
Photons: 1000–1600 cGy, at 200 cGy per fraction

Axillary Lymph Nodes

If treated, the axillary lymph nodes should receive 4600 cGy in 23 fractions over a period of 4.5 weeks in most cases. When extracapsular disease is present, axillary nodes should be boosted to a total dose of 5000–5400 cGy. For gross residual disease, a boost to a total dose not exceeding 5600 cGy should be used.

References

1. Veronesi U, Saccozzi R, Del Vecchio M, et al. Comparing radical mastectomy with quadrantectomy, axillary dissection, and radiotherapy in patients with small cancers of the breast. N Engl J Med 1981;305:6–11

2. Sarrazin D, Le MG, Arriagada R, et al. Ten-year results of a randomized trial comparing a conservative treatment to mastectomy in early breast cancer. Radiother Oncol 1989;14:177–184

3. Fisher B, Redmond C, Poisson R, et al. Eight-year results of a randomized clinical trial comparing total mastectomy and lumpectomy with or without irradiation in the treatment of breast cancer. N Engl J Med 1989;320:822–828

4. Holland R, Veling SH, Mravunac M, et al. Histologic multifocality of Tis, T1–2 breast carcinomas: implications for clinical trials of breast-conserving surgery. Cancer 1985;56:979–990

5. Liljegren G, Holmberg L, Adami HO, et al. Sector resection with or without radiotherapy for stage I breast cancer; five-year results of a randomized trial. J Natl Cancer Inst 1994;86:717–722

6. Fisher R, Sass R, Fisher B, et al. Pathologic findings from the National Surgical Adjuvant Breast Project (protocol 6). II. Relation of local breast recurrence to multicentricity. Cancer 1986;57:1717–1724

7. Harris JR, Sawicka J, Gelman R. Management of locally advanced carcinoma of the breast by primary radiation therapy. Int J Radiat Oncol Biol Phys 1983;9:345–349

8. Swain SM, Sorace RA, Bagley CS, et al. Neoadjuvant chemotherapy in the combined modality approach of locally advanced nonmetastatic breast cancer. Cancer Res 1987;47:3889–3894

9. Hortobagyi GN, Buzdar AU. Locally advanced breast cancer: a review including the M.D. Anderson experience. In: Ragaz J, Ariel IM (eds) High-Risk Breast Cancer—Therapy. Berlin, Springer, 1991, pp 382–415

10. Sheldon T, Hayes DF, Cady B, et al. Primary radiation therapy for locally advanced breast cancer. Cancer 1987;60:1219–1225

11. Rubens RD, Sexton R, Tong D, et al. Combined chemotherapy and radiotherapy for locally advanced breast cancer. Eur J Cancer 1980;16:351–356

12. Formenti SC, Lenz J, Dunnington G, et al. Initial P53 status as potential predictor for pathological response to the combination of 5FU and radiotherapy in locally advanced breast cancer. ASCO Proc 1996;174

13. Formenti SC, Dunnington G, Lenz H, et al. Original p53 status predicts for pathological response in locally advanced breast cancer patients treated preoperatively with continuous infusion (C.I.) 5-fluorouracil (5-FU) and radiation therapy. Int J Radiat Oncol Biol Phys 1997;39:1059–1068

14. Sherry MM, Greco FA, Johnson DH, et al. Metastatic breast cancer confined to the skeletal system: an indolent disease. Am J Med 1986;81:381–386

15. Formenti SC, Lucas G, Puthawala AA, et al. Initial brachytherapy in the breast conservation approach to breast cancer. Am J Clin Oncol 1995;18:331–336

26 RECONSTRUCTION OF THE BREAST AFTER CANCER SURGERY: OVERVIEW

Randy Sherman

As the treatment of carcinoma of the female breast has evolved over the last 10–15 years, so have the methodology and alternatives for breast reconstruction. Less than a generation ago accepted medical practice offered no chance for a woman to hope, let alone consider options, for restoration of an amputated breast. Then, silicon technology, which gave us implantation material that closely reproduced the feel of breast tissue, heralded the advent of modern postmastectomy breast reconstruction.

Although this advance offered hope to thousands of women who had previously been left to hide their deformities, continuing mechanical and aesthetic problems drove surgeons to explore other means to augment the prosthetic breast reconstruction or completely replace it. This led to the development, utilization, and eventual refinement of autologous tissue transfer. The latissimus dorsi muscle and myocutaneous flaps were the first such composite vascularized transfers, followed by the transverse rectus abdominis myocutaneous (TRAM) flap, and subsequently other free flaps including the gluteus myocutaneous flap, the gracilis myocutaneous flap, and the lateral thigh myocutaneous flaps. Further refinements in breast reconstruction followed, including ingenious combinations of flaps and skin grafts to reproduce the look and feel of the nipple–areolar complex.

TIMING

Initial attempts at breast reconstruction following mastectomy were met with suspicion and condemnation as being superfluous and dangerous to the patient's health. It was held that breast reconstruction would not only place the patient in an additional risk category but also mask any local recurrence and thus compromise the ability of the surgeon to treat these problems in a timely and effective fashion. Consequently, breast reconstruction was delayed until at least 6 months after mastectomy and more commonly 2–5 years to ensure practitioners and patients alike that a "cure" had been achieved prior to undergoing reconstruction. As we have evolved into the common practice of immediate reconstruction, with more than a decade of solid data showing no increased risk of recurrence or inability to monitor for recurrence, the choice between immediate and delayed reconstruction is truly one that can be made between the plastic surgeon and the patient based on the respective advantages and disadvantages of each procedure.

Immediate Reconstruction

Breast reconstruction at the time of mastectomy, whether it be placement of an implant, a tissue expander, or transfer of a myocutaneous flap, is generally thought preferable to delaying the operation until a later date. Specific advantages include one less surgical procedure, hospitalization, and anesthesia; less scar tissue in the mastectomy site; and significant psychological benefits. It has been well substantiated that patients undergoing immediate, in contrast to delayed, breast reconstruction have fewer psychological problems during the course of their care. Some procedures may not require additional postoperative hospitalization days or add significantly to rehabilitation or recovery time. Autologous tissue transfer (i.e., the TRAM flap) can keep the patient in the hospital during the primary treatment phase for an additional 2–4 days. Also, postoperative recovery may be prolonged for rehabilitation depending on donor site requirements.

Disadvantages of immediate reconstruction include possible problems with the flap or donor site healing due to infection, dehiscence, or partial flap loss. Although these problems might arise with delayed reconstruction, they can be more problematic during the immediate postoperative period if chemotherapy or radiation therapy must be delayed. Overall, it has been the overwhelming experience of most reconstructive surgeons that patients fare much better both during the perioperative period and in the long term when the patients have breast reconstruction immediately following mastectomy or lumpectomy.

Delayed Reconstruction

As mentioned above, immediate reconstruction has become by far the preferred method. Circumstances that favor delayed reconstruction include the reluctance of the cancer surgeon to participate in or approve reconstructive surgery, poor health of the patient, or ambivalence of the patient in regard to her desire for breast reconstruction.

Some patients, no matter how much information is made available, feel overwhelmed and unable to process the options and choices for simultaneous breast reconstruction. In those circumstances it is best to reassure the patient that she can always return for breast reconstruction when and if it becomes a desirable alternative.

BREAST RECONSTRUCTION OPTIONS

Mammary Prosthesis

Prior to the advent of autologous tissue transfer and tissue expansion, placement of a silicone gel prosthesis was the standard of care, whether immediate or delayed, for postmastectomy breast reconstruction. When considering the requirements for successful breast reconstruction, the plastic surgeon must consider: (1) The position of the mastectomy incision (Figure 26.1); (2) the volume of tissue lost through mastectomy or lumpectomy; (3) the contour of the breast (base dimension, degree of ptosis, nipple–areolar size and position); (4) the potential for restoration of symmetry with the opposite breast; and (5) the potential for surgery on the opposite breast for aesthetic correction or to achieve symmetry with the constructed breast.

When reconstructive options were limited to placement of a subdermal or submuscular implant, the biggest problem was the lack of an adequate skin envelope. It led to breast reconstructions resulting in small, firm, spherical breast mounds that often appeared and felt unnatural and required subsequent capsulotomy and revision. Also, surgery was frequently required on the opposite breast for reduction or alteration to achieve acceptable symmetry. Presently, placement of a mammary prosthesis, most of which today are saline-filled silicone elastomer shells, is limited to restoration of a small breast after a skin-sparing mastectomy. In this particular situation, this option can result in an acceptable appearance with minimal morbidity. The subpectoral placement of a permanent mammary prosthesis is depicted in Figure 26.2b.

Tissue Expansion

Significant strides were made to restore the skin envelope lost after mastectomy with development of a two-staged breast reconstruction where a submuscular tissue expander is placed immediately after mastectomy. It can be enlarged over the course of a 3- to 6-month postoperative interval with instillation of sterile saline through a distally placed port or, in later tissue expander models, a direct

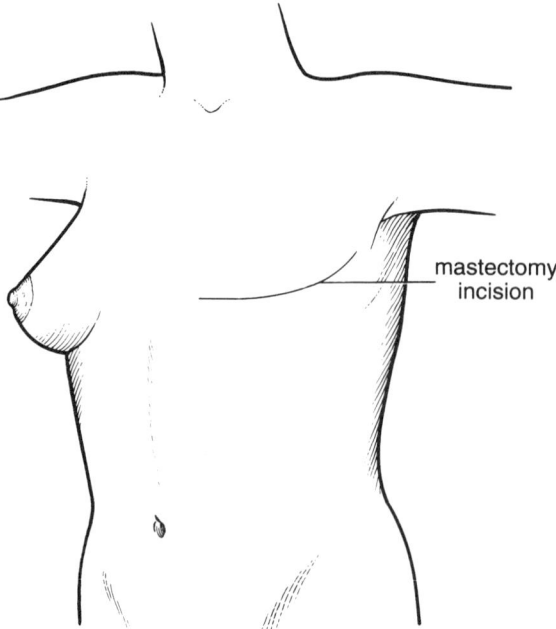

mastectomy incision

Figure 26.1. Usual position of the mastectomy incision.

overhead port. The expanders serve to recruit new skin in addition to stretching and remolding the available skin. Stretch–relaxation curves have been worked out to allow the development of frequency schedules for optimum tissue expansion. Most important when the choosing a tissue expander at the time of surgery is to match the base diameter of the opposite normal breast. The goal of tissue expansion is to enlarge the implant to a volume half again as large as the desired end result. Once that size is achieved, the patient can be taken back to surgery for replacement of the expander with a permanent saline-filled or gel-filled prosthesis. This procedure can be done on an outpatient basis, rarely requiring hospitalization. The final contour and symmetry are planned during this stage of the operation. Ideally, the patient then returns only for a nipple–areolar reconstruction and subsequent tattooing. Problems that may arise include the lack of definition of the inframammary fold and subsequent change in the breast contour and placement due to capsular contracture or rupture and leakage of the implant.

The advantages of this type of procedure are (1) the ease of expander placement; (2) no morbidity or scarring at the donor site; (3) no additional hospitalization; (4) second-stage reconstruction limited to an outpatient surgical procedure; and (5) a single scar at the mastectomy site. The disadvantages of the two-stage expander implant operation include (1) the need for a second operation many months after the initial reconstruction and having to endure a deformity in the interim; and (2) the potential for subsequent problems with the implant, including infection, exposure, rupture, capsular contracture, and a lack of natural feel, as reported by many patients.

The Becker expander prosthesis (Fig. 26.2a) attempted to dispense with the second-stage operation by a procedure that was initially appealing to many reconstructive surgeons, but its complexity and inability to provide consistently superior results limited its usefulness. I have largely abandoned the use of the Becker expander prosthesis, though others in the community and elsewhere continue to use it.

AUTOLOGOUS TISSUE TRANSFER

Latissimus Dorsi Myocutaneous Flap

During the mid-1970s the latissimus dorsi muscle (with its overlying skin) became a viable option for breast reconstruction alone or as a cover for a mammary prosthesis when there is insufficient skin to create a normal-appearing breast. This procedure has the distinct advantages of being able to import well vascularized muscle, subcutaneous tissue, and skin to replace immediately the resected breast mound and overlying skin (Fig. 26.3). In cases where a large breast was removed with a significant loss of volume and substance, the latissimus dorsi has not been found to be adequate but has served handsomely to surround the mammary prosthesis and provide sufficient skin and subcutaneous tissue to restore precisely the skin envelope lost during the resection (Fig. 26.4). The donor site for the latissimus muscle can be hidden by a well positioned oblique or transverse scar on the back, which is covered by the woman's brassiere (Fig. 26.5). If a mammary

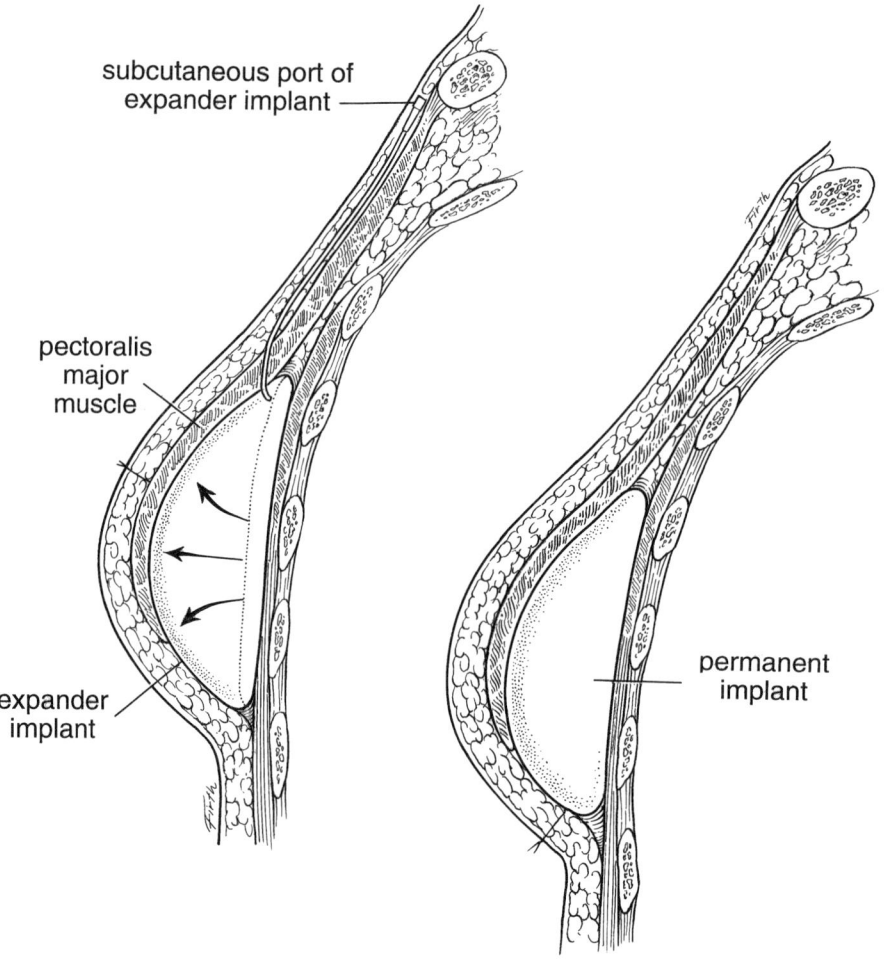

Figure 26.2. a. Becker expander implant with remote port placed subcutaneously. b. Subpectoral placement of the permanent mammary prosthesis.

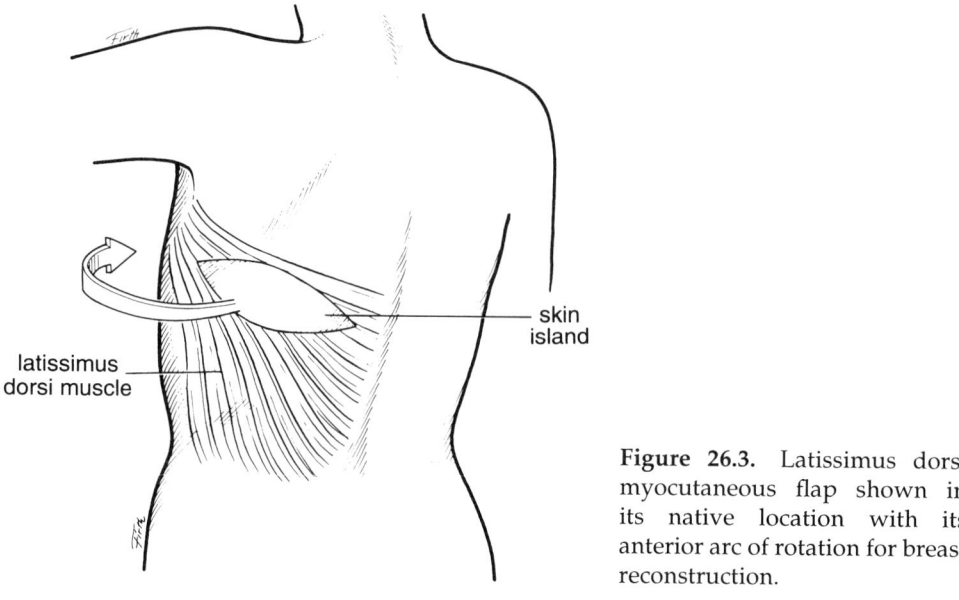

Figure 26.3. Latissimus dorsi myocutaneous flap shown in its native location with its anterior arc of rotation for breast reconstruction.

Figure 26.4. After rotation and inset, the latissimus dorsi myocutaneous flap can help produce a symmetric breast reconstruction.

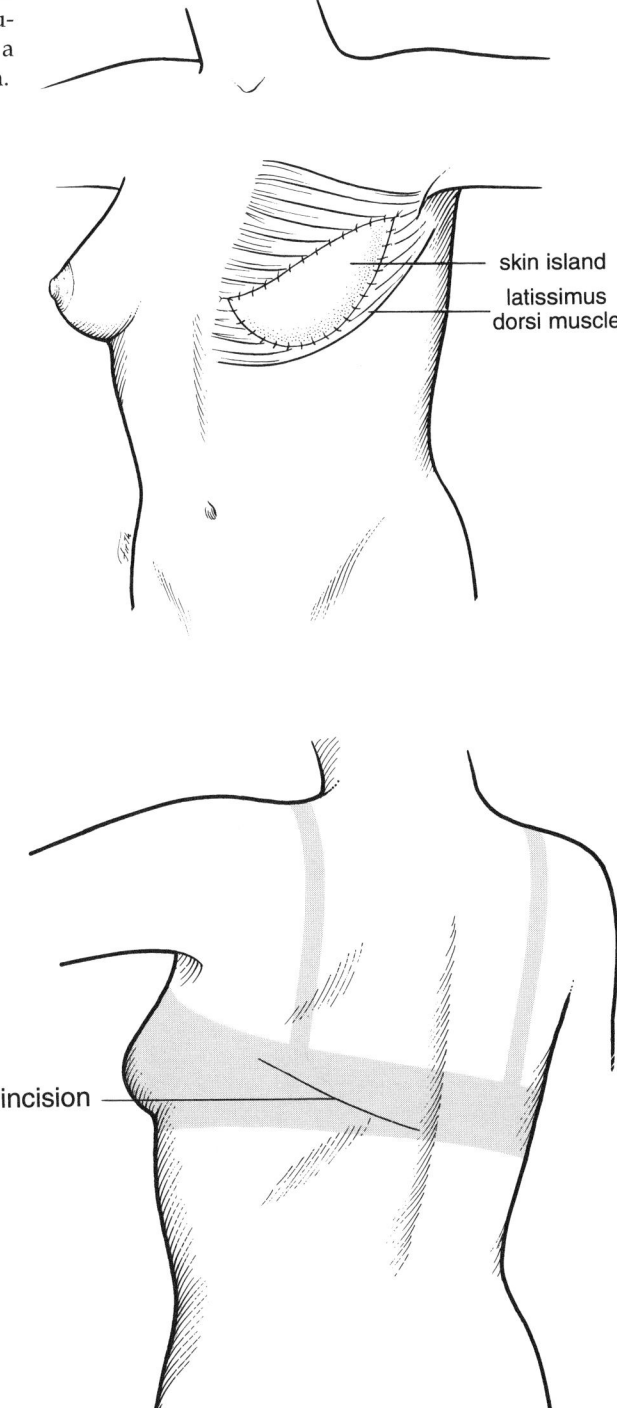

skin island

latissimus dorsi muscle

incision

Figure 26.5. Donor site scar for latissimus dorsi myocutaneous flap can be positioned so it is hidden underneath a brassiere or swimsuit.

prosthesis is used as part of the reconstruction, the broad, flat latissimus muscle can envelope the mammary prosthesis, creating a circumferential submuscular pocket around the implant subjacent to the mastectomy flaps and the skin paddle from the latissimus muscle.

The main problems with the latissimus dorsi myocutaneous flap are the prolonged seromas that tend to form at the donor site. These are easily manageable but may require a JP, Hemovac, or Blake-type drain left in place for up to 2–3 weeks after surgery. Loss of function as a result of harvesting the latissimus dorsi muscle is negligible because of numerous companion muscle groups in the posterior thorax and shoulder girdle, which adequately compensate for loss of latissimus function. In addition to its use for mastectomy reconstruction, the latissimus serves nicely when taken either in whole or in part for partial mastectomy restoration or for those who have had deformities secondary to damage caused by irradiation. This flap has stood the test of time and serves patients well who have small or medium breasts and favor simultaneous or single-stage reconstruction without the desire or ability to utilize the TRAM flap donor site.

Transverse Rectus Abdominis Myocutaneous Flap

The most popular alternative today for autologous tissue transfer in breast reconstruction is the TRAM flap. This tissue transfer utilizes the luxuriant skin and subcutaneous tissue found peri- and infraumbilically in the lower third of the anterior abdominal wall (Fig. 26.6). This flap is supplied either as a superior-based pedicle using the rectus abdominis muscle as a conduit for the superior epigastric

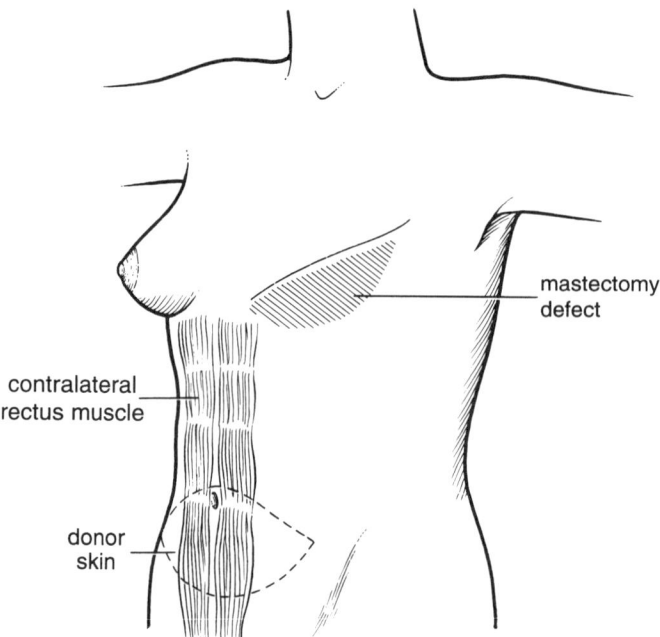

Figure 26.6. TRAM flap allows total breast reconstruction without the use of implants.

artery and vein or as a free tissue transfer based on the deep inferior epigastric artery and vein. If used as an intact pedicle flap, the lower third of the anterior abdominal skin and subcutaneous tissue is isolated most often on the contralateral rectus abdominis muscle, utilizing the periumbilical perforators to vascularize this skin and subcutaneous segment. Three of the four most contiguous quadrants of that skin and subcutaneous tissue construct receive adequate vascularity to be used reliably. The most distant or fourth quadrant is most often thrown away because of its tendency to become ischemic or frankly necrotic during the postoperative period.

The TRAM flap allows women to undergo complete breast reconstruction without the use of any prosthetic materials. It also results in a far superior breast mound and breast contour with a more natural appearing and feeling breast reconstruction. It also has the distinct advantage of giving a woman the opportunity to improve her abdominal contour through an abdominoplasty type of operation. Many women find this distinctly advantageous and are convinced to choose this option mostly because of this aspect of the procedure.

Transfer of the TRAM flap on the deep inferior epigastric vessels requires microvascular expertise (Fig. 26.7) and can be done safely and reliably with anastomoses to the thoracodorsal artery and vein. Most centers that perform this procedure on a regular basis believe that it is safer and more reliable than the pedicled TRAM flap even though the operation takes longer. It is well known that profusion of the third and fourth quadrant of the TRAM flap is superior if taken as a free tissue transfer rather than as a pedicled flap. Repair of the abdominal wall after harvesting the flap is usually accompanied by implantation of Marlex mesh to prevent donor site herniation or laxity.

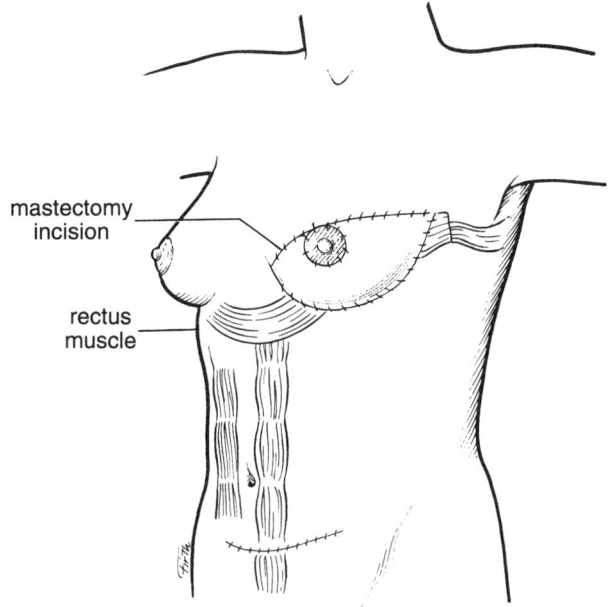

mastectomy incision

rectus muscle

Figure **26.7.** TRAM flap may be transferred using a microvascular technique that allows safe transfer of large volumes of tissue.

Disadvantages of the TRAM flap include (1) significantly more difficult surgery; (2) a donor site scar at the abdomen that approximates an enlarged Pfannensteil wound; (3) potential for herniation or lower abdominal wall laxity at the donor site; (4) potential loss of tissue, either at the donor site in the infraumbilical area or in the TRAM flap itself, requiring revision surgery for removal of any scabbing or fatty necrosis.

Best of all with the TRAM flap is its usual improvement over time, with maturing of the scars and settling of the donor tissue, obviating the need for symmetry surgery on the other breast. Overall, most women having had the TRAM flap rate it high for naturalness in look, feel, contour, and matching of the opposite breast.

Other Autologous Tissue Transfers

When the TRAM flap is unavailable for use and the woman desires autologous tissue transfer, the gluteus maximus myocutaneous flap, Ruben's flap, gracilis myocutaneous flap, and lateral thigh myocutaneous flap serve as potential options for breast reconstruction. Each has the potential to provide adequate volume and additional skin to restore the mastectomy patient to a premorbid appearance. These procedures are rare and beyond the scope of this chapter.

NIPPLE–AREOLAR RECONSTRUCTION

Once the patient is satisfied with the size and placement of her breast reconstruction, she may choose to undergo restoration of the nipple–areolar complex. The nipple is created from a small projecting flap of tissue drawn directly from the underlying skin and subcutaneous tissue. The areola is simulated using a skin graft taken from either a groin locale, the mastectomy scar area, or (in patients who have undergone a TRAM flap operation) the abdominal scar area. Measurements are taken at several points on the opposite nipple–areolar complex to ensure symmetry. This surgery can be done either at an outpatient facility or in the office. Surgery is completed with a bolster tie-over dressing that remains in place for 1 week. Once the nipple and skin-grafted areola are well healed, it is common to finalize the reconstruction using a tattoo-type machine for injections of pigment to achieve a match with the normal areolar color. This also can be an office-based procedure that usually does not require an anesthetic.

CONCLUSION

We have evolved dramatically in our ability to restore the look, feel, and shape of the breast, including nipple–areolar reconstruction that can match nipple size and areolar color and contour close to that of the opposite side. It is imperative that the patient understand from the outset, however, that it is a facsimile breast that does not provide any of the erogenous or tactile function of the former breast. Often the entire reconstruction remains anesthetic for months or even years, although, surprisingly, some women have reported restoration of sensation and, rarely, erogenous sensation in the reconstructed tissues. The patient must be counseled that her relationship with the plastic surgeon will be ongoing and long term because tailoring the breast reconstruction is commonplace to achieve a maximally satisfactory result. If mammary prostheses are used, there may be biomechanical problems that must be addressed over the course of her lifetime.

Breast reconstruction has turned out to be a rewarding procedure that allows a woman to undergo the nightmare of ablative cancer surgery and loss of a significant body part bolstered by the reassurance of normalizing her body image and returning to a fulfilling and wholesome life style. Fortunately, patterns of breast cancer management are turning toward more conservative surgery, with fewer major operations in the future. However, over the next decade or two while the option of modified radical mastectomy continues to be offered, it should be accompanied at all times by an opportunity for a thorough consultation with a plastic surgeon to discuss the possibilities of complete and comprehensive breast reconstruction.

27 PLASTIC SURGERY FOR COMMON BREAST PROBLEMS

Susan E. Downey

PROBLEMS OF THE ADOLESCENT BREAST

Adolescents present to the plastic surgeon for a variety of breast problems, the most common of which are asymmetries secondary to trauma (e.g., burns) and congenital breast asymmetries. Traumatic injury to the developing breast can also result from previous surgeries, can be related to irradiation of the chest wall for treatment of a tumor as an infant, or can result from hemangioma in the surrounding area. Congenital asymmetry should be distinguished from the rare Poland syndrome, which includes not only lack of development of the breast on the affected side but also an associated absence of the pectoralis muscle and occasionally deformities of the hand on the same side. Breast asymmetry is not associated with any anomaly of the reproductive organs.

Treatment should be initiated as soon as the adolescent is identified as having a breast problem. (Teenagers are often ashamed of their anomalies, and their problems are usually discovered by a mother walking in on them while they are dressing.) Significant psychological benefit can be gained from correcting problems early, thereby allowing the child to have normal adolescent development. Teenagers often express increased confidence following corrective surgery.

The primary correction for breast asymmetry is placement of a tissue expander under the affected breast. The tissue expander can then be slowly filled, first to match the size of the opposite breast and then to maintain symmetry as growth proceeds. The process is well tolerated by teenagers in the clinic and does not require an anesthetic. The incision is placed in the inframammary area and is not visible even when the teen wears a bikini or is naked, as it is hidden by the natural overhang of the breast. Most commonly the tissue expander is placed above the pectoralis muscle, just under the breast tissue. If the implant is placed under the pectoralis muscle, it often ends up being too high and the droop of the breast cannot be matched to the opposite side. Once symmetry has been achieved, the teen is seen usually at 3- or 6-month intervals depending on how much the opposite breast is growing. Once the breast growth has stabilized for approximately a year and there is good symmetry between the two breasts, the final saline implant can be placed. Currently, under U.S. Food and Drug Administration

(FDA) guidelines, both silicone and saline implants are available for reconstruction, but only saline implants are available for augmentation.

Adolescents with congenital asymmetry fall into the category of reconstruction, but in general I use only saline implants for teenagers with marked asymmetry. If there is adequate breast tissue over the implant, rippling, which is a problem associated with saline implants, is not seen.

Correction of breast asymmetry has been associated with relatively few complications, the major one being deflation of the tissue expander, which then must be replaced. The saline is absorbed by the body. In some cases if the teen has reached full development, the deflated expander can be replaced with a permanent implant, obviating the need for an extra surgical procedure.

With this type of surgery the scars in general do well, and there is minimal risk of loss of nipple sensation or breastfeeding ability. When the patient has a need for mammography, she should inform the mammographer that she has an implant in place so an additional view can be obtained to maximize visualization of breast tissue.

BREAST AUGMENTATION

Women tend to present for augmentation at either of two times in their lives: (1) during their early twenties because they are dissatisfied with their breast development; or (2) after childbearing, to regain the breast contours lost following pregnancy and breastfeeding.

As stated, under current FDA guidelines only saline implants may be used for breast augmentation; silicone implants are available only for use in breast reconstruction. It is unclear whether silicone will again be available for all types of breast surgery, but several other implant types are being developed. An advantage of the soybean oil implant, currently under clinical study, is that on mammography the breast tissue is more easily visualized through the oil. A disadvantage is that soybean oil implants sometimes can be felt, or rippling is seen (as with saline).

Three surgical incisions are used for breast augmentation (Fig. 27.1): (1) around the nipple area; (2) in the inframammary area; and (3) in the axilla or armpit. Each method has its own risks and benefits. The incision around the nipple area (periareolar) is designed to be a cosmetic scar placed in the area where the skin color changes from the areolar tissue to that of the surrounding breast tissue. It carries with it a slightly higher risk of loss of nipple sensation and loss of ability to breastfeed. The inframammary scar is placed just above the inframammary fold so it is not seen even in a bikini, but it is a scar on the breast mound itself. The axillary approach has a higher risk of complications associated with surgery, including an increased risk of hematoma formation or displacement of the implant. The scar is well hidden, however, and there is no scarring on the breast itself. If a complication should occur with a transaxillary implant, an inframammary approach would be necessary to correct the problem.

Augmentation implants are placed under the breast tissue either above (Fig. 27.2) or under (Fig. 27.3) the pectoralis muscle. Placement above the muscle is

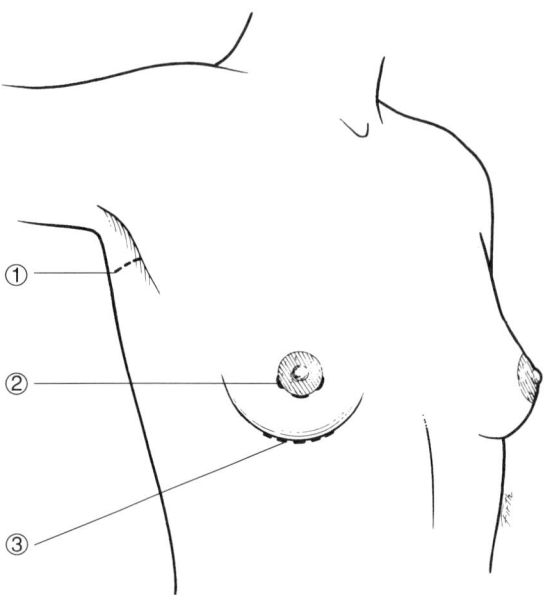

Figure 27.1. Incisions for breast augmentation: 1) in axilla, 2) circumareolar, 3) in inframammary fold.

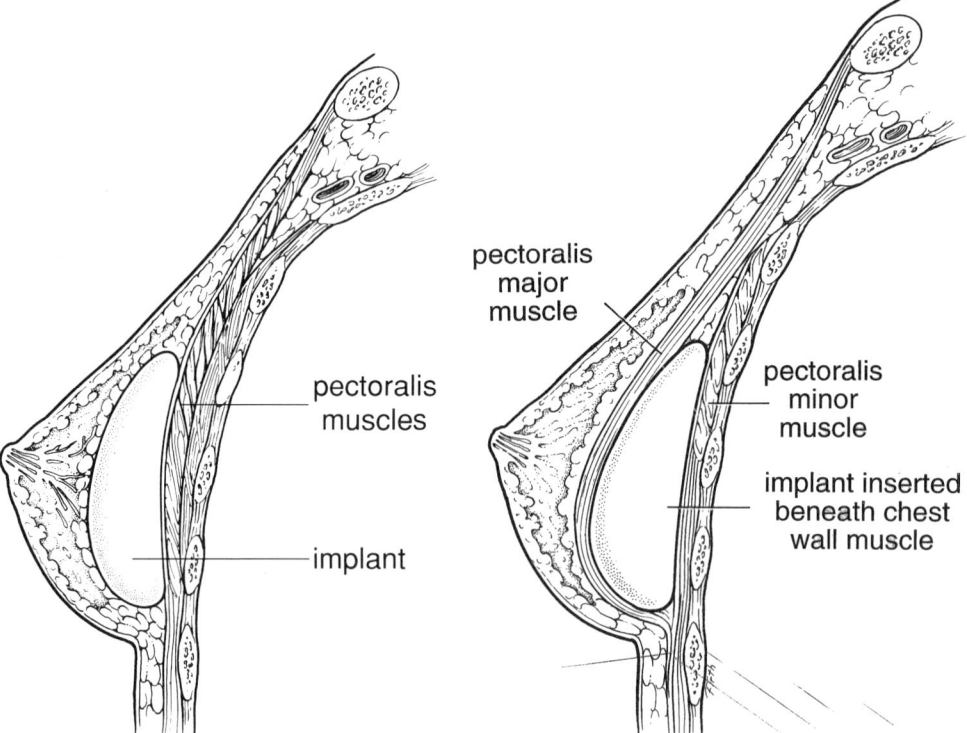

Figure 27.2. Breast augmentation: submammary implant placement.

Figure 27.3. Breast augmentation: subpectoral implant placement.

easier surgery from which to recover and may result in a more natural droop of the breast. The subpectoral approach gives an extra layer of tissue over the breast implant, which is especially important with saline implants or in very thin women, and may give a more natural feel to the implant. It is, however, much more painful surgery that usually requires general anesthesia. There is also a possibility that the implant may ride up too high, requiring surgical revision at a later time. As far as mammography is concerned, it may be an advantage to have the implant behind the pectoralis muscle, as it may be easier to displace the implant posteriorly during filming. All patients with implants should inform the mammographer that they require an extra view (Eklund view) to maximize visualization of their breast tissue. Approximately 5% of the breast tissue may not be seen on mammography once breast implants have been placed.

Saline implants may leak over time but usually do so slowly. The cause is unknown but may be due to a fold that develops within the implant itself. If a leak occurs, the implant must be replaced. Patients should be advised that their implants will probably need to be replaced at some time during their lifetimes.

The major problem associated with breast augmentation is encapsulation of the implant. Scar tissue forms around all implants placed within the body. It is unknown why in some patients this scar tissue continues to contract, leading to a hard scar around the implant and sometimes even to a visible deformity. In severe cases it can be painful, and surgery may be required to replace the capsule. Textured implants have been designed to minimize the risk of encapsulation, but so far they have not solved the problem. Over the years many procedures have been tried to minimize the risk of encapsulation, such as having the patient massage the breast or placing antibiotics or steroids in the pocket. Much is still unknown about the causes of capsular contracture, and it still occurs unpredictably.

Once a woman decides on augmentation, there is the question of what size she would like her breasts to be. Most women do not have a clear idea and need to experiment to find what works best for them. Tie-top plastic bags can be filled with water or rice and used to measure the size needed to fill out brassieres and clothing to the desired proportions. Sometimes sample implants can be tried in different outfits to determine what size best suits an individual woman's frame. The ideal candidate for augmentation is one who wants the surgery to enhance her appearance so she can feel better about herself. Obviously, patients who are acting at another's urging or who believe that changing breast size will make some miraculous change in their lives should be counseled and discouraged from having the surgery.

Breast augmentation is considered a cosmetic operation and therefore is not covered by health insurance. It can be done at an outpatient surgery center or in an operating room in the plastic surgeon's office.

Breast Reduction

Large, pendulous breasts can lead to chronic neck and shoulder pain and can limit a patient's activities. Grooving of the shoulders from brassiere straps may be permanent, even after reduction of the breast tissue. Most women have instant relief of neck and shoulder pain following breast reduction surgery, can more easily buy clothes that fit, and are able to participate in sports they could not enjoy previously.

Women present for breast reductions from the early teenage years until late adulthood. Age is not a contraindication to breast reduction, although because the breasts of a young teenager (e.g., a 14-year-old) may continue to grow, she might need a second procedure at a later time. Nevertheless, if a teenager has extremely large breasts, I recommend that she go ahead with the surgery rather than suffer the physical and psychological consequences of waiting several years. A breast reduction is usually covered by insurance if the breasts are reduced at least two cup sizes, for example, from a DD cup to a C cup.

The most common surgical technique (inferior pedicle) maintains the nipple on a pedicle of breast tissue down to the chest wall (Figs. 27.4, 27.5). This method carries minimal risk of loss of the nipple and a better chance of maintaining nipple sensation. Some women have been able to breastfeed following breast reduction but should be advised that they may not be able to do so. In general the larger the woman before surgery, the greater chance she has of losing some nipple sensation. Some very large-breasted women may not even have nipple sensation prior to surgery. Any risk factors that would adversely affect wound healing, such as smoking or diabetes, would of course increase the risk of problems with nipple viability or nipple sensation following surgery.

The scars from breast reduction are around the nipple–areolar area, straight down from the areola, and then below the breast (Fig. 27.6). The scars are perma-

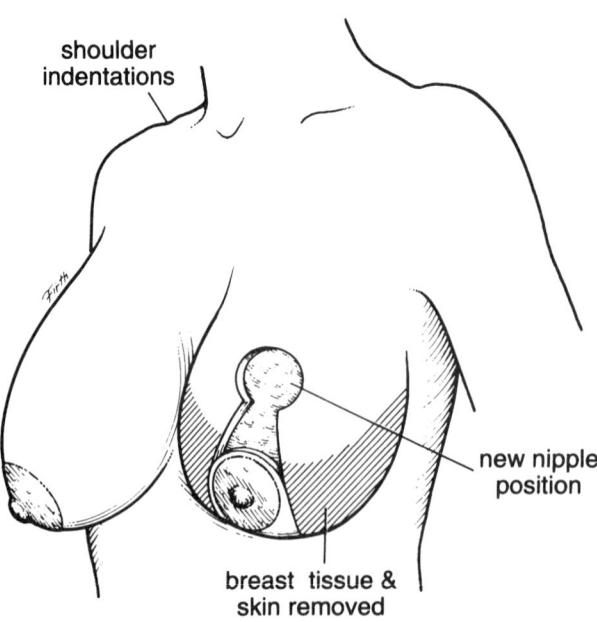

Figure 27.4. Breast reduction: markings and preoperative assessment.

Figure 27.5. Breast reduction: closure of incisions.

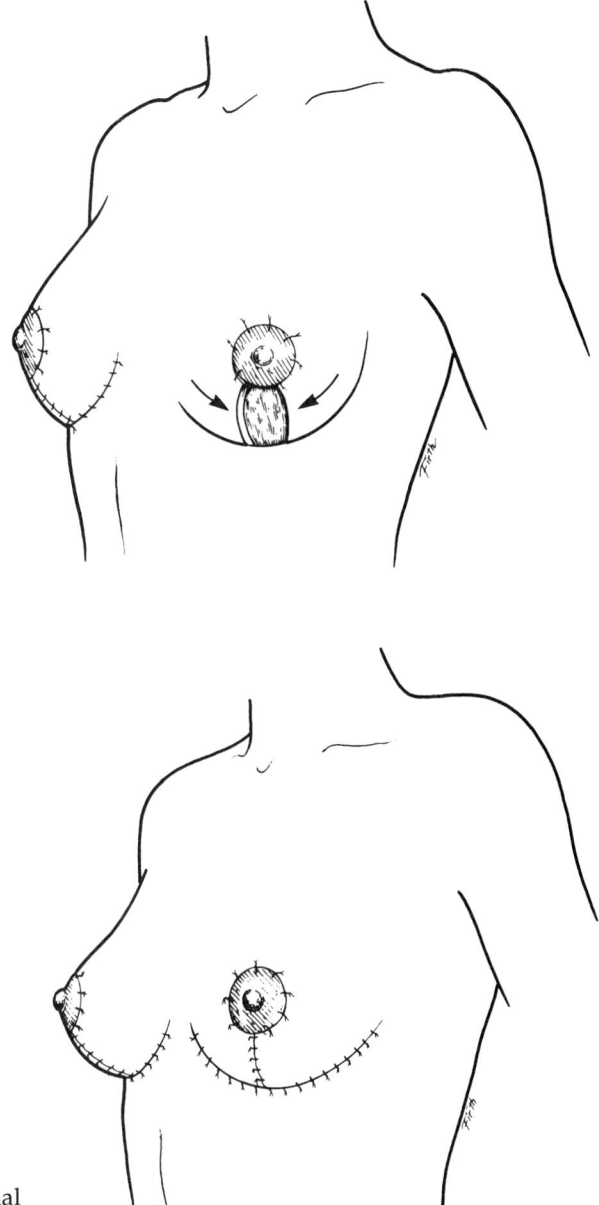

Figure 27.6. Breast reduction: final position of incisions.

nent, but they continue to improve up to a year following the surgery and are not obvious underneath a brassiere and conservatively designed clothes.

Nowadays, only with extremely large-breasted patients is the nipple taken off and replaced at the desired position as a free graft. Disadvantages of a free graft are that the nipple would have no sensation, it would tend to be flat, and there could be pigment changes within the nipple–areolar complex. If at the end of a breast reduction the nipple appears dusky or nonviable, it may be removed and replaced as a skin graft in a salvage operation.

I recommend that all patients over age 35 obtain a mammogram prior to undergoing breast surgery. If there is anything suspicious, surgery should be delayed until a biopsy of the suspicious area is done. Specimens from the reduction mammoplasty of each breast are routinely sent separately to the pathology laboratory so that if an occult problem is found, it is known in which breast the lesion had appeared. If a malignancy is found during the reduction that was not identified prior to surgery, the option of doing a lumpectomy is lost because it would be unclear from which portion of the breast the specimen had come. Patients should obtain a follow-up mammogram 6 months after a reduction to establish a new baseline.

Breast reduction patients are some of the happiest patients plastic surgeons ever see. The relief patients feel from losing the weight around the neck and shoulders certainly outweighs any scars left on the breasts. Patients often note their improved posture and lose weight due to their becoming more active; and they report that they look and feel better in their clothing.

MASTOPEXY (BREAST LIFT)

Over time, especially if there have been large weight fluctuations and pregnancies followed by breastfeeding, all women's breasts droop somewhat. Droop is called ptosis, and for the breast it is defined as the nipple being lower than the inframammary fold (the inframammary fold being directly underneath the desired position of the nipple on the youthful breast). Following pregnancy and

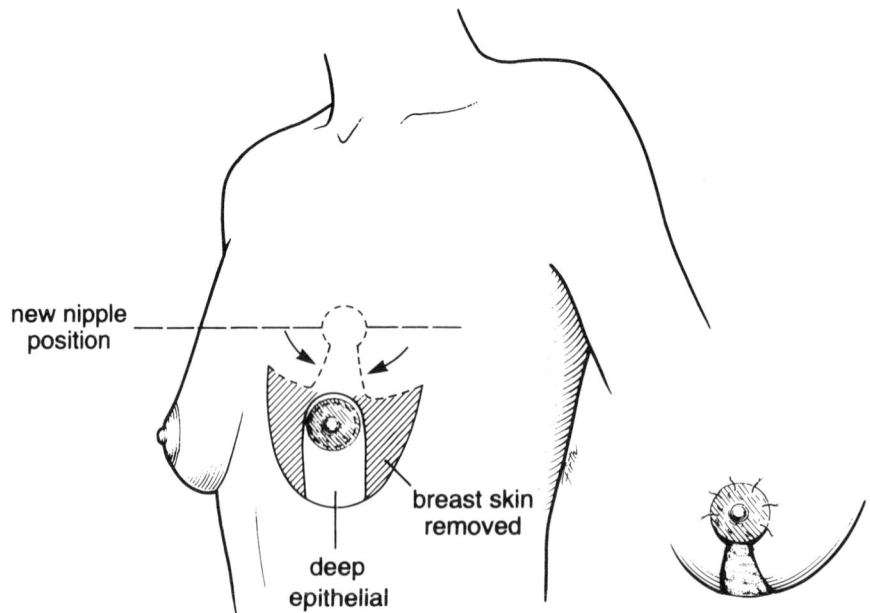

Figure 27.7. Mastopexy or breast lift.

breastfeeding, there is often a loss of fullness in the upper part of the breast, leading to a cosmetically undesirable shape.

Most women present for mastopexy following the birth of their children, and it is advisable to postpone a breast lift if more pregnancies are anticipated. A breast lift reduces the skin envelope of the breast but not the amount of tissue. In some cases an implant may be inserted behind the breast to recreate the fullness of the upper portion.

The major problem associated with breast lifts is scarring. The most common surgical method results in a scar around the nipple–areolar complex, extending straight down to below the breast and then across the inframammary area (Fig. 27.7). Depending on the degree of ptosis, the amount of scarring can be acceptable. Scarring also depends on the patient's healing and skin type.

There is a slight risk of loss of nipple sensation and of the nipple itself, but the major problem associated with breast lift is the scarring. Numerous techniques have been tried over the years to minimize the amount of scarring, including the crescent mastopexy, which elevates the nipple by excising skin above it, but there is little tightening of the remaining breast skin.

Most of these procedures can be performed in the plastic surgeon's office or in a hospital outpatient surgery unit under either local or intravenous sedation. Procedures for breast lift are considered cosmetic and are generally not covered by insurance.

28   BREAST CANCER HEREDITARY RISK ASSESSMENT AND COUNSELING SERVICES

Patricia T. Kelly

As more information about hereditary and nonhereditary breast cancer risk becomes available, conflicting and generalized reports contribute to increased patient questions, concerns, and misconceptions. This chapter discusses some of the more common mistaken beliefs about the relation between breast cancer risk and genetic testing and focuses on ways to talk to patients about these issues.

Mistaken Belief 1: There is an "epidemic" of breast cancer, with incidence rates increasing rapidly in recent years, particularly in young women.

Fact: The incidence of invasive breast cancer diagnosed in women under age 50 has changed little in recent years (Fig. 28.1, 28.2). Even among older women, the increase in diagnoses seen during the 1980s can be explained by greater utilization of early detection techniques and the improved sensitivity of mammography and better training of radiologists. The greater increase in black women is likely due to improved detection in this population in recent years. Incidence rates have been falling since the late 1980s in both black and white women. The increased incidence of in situ breast cancer, particularly ductal carcinoma in situ (DCIS), is probably due primarily to improved mammography techniques, which have resulted in the detection of calcifications.

Mistaken Belief 2: The average woman's breast cancer risk of about 1 : 9 (11%) means that 1 of 9 women at a gathering (in a random group) is likely to have breast cancer.

Fact: Eleven per cent is the average woman's cumulative lifetime risk at age 85. As shown in Figure 28.3, only 2% of the risk occurs by age 50. The risk is 5% at age 50–70 and 4% at age 70–85. As a woman survives each year without a diagnosis of breast cancer, she leaves the risk associated with that age behind. For example, the average woman's lifetime risk at age 50 is 11% minus 2%, or 9%.

Mistaken Belief 3: A woman whose mother has (or had) breast cancer will probably be diagnosed with breast cancer.

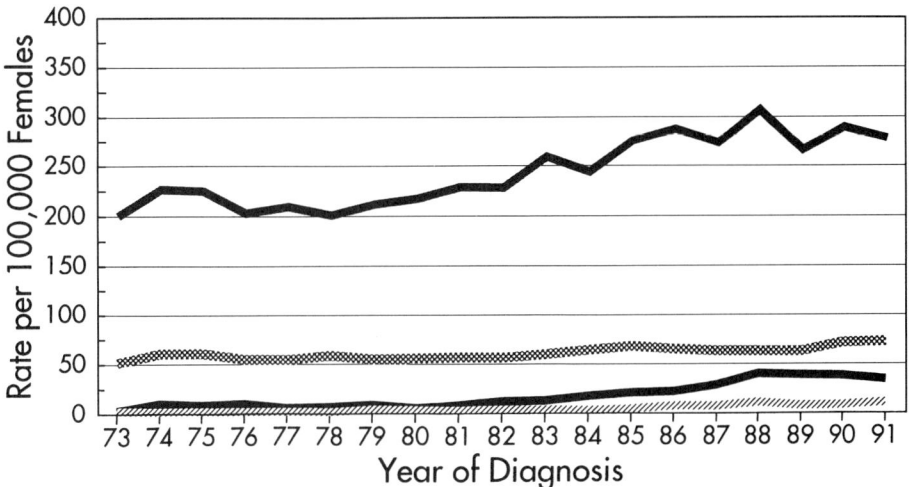

Figure 28.1. Black female age-related breast cancer incidence rates for in situ and malignant (invasive) cancer based on National Cancer Institute (NCI) Surveillance, Epidemiology, and End Results (SEER) data, 1973–1991. From top to bottom: solid curve = malignant, age 50+; hatched curve = malignant, age 20–49; solid curve = in situ, age 50+; hatched curve = in situ, age 20–49.

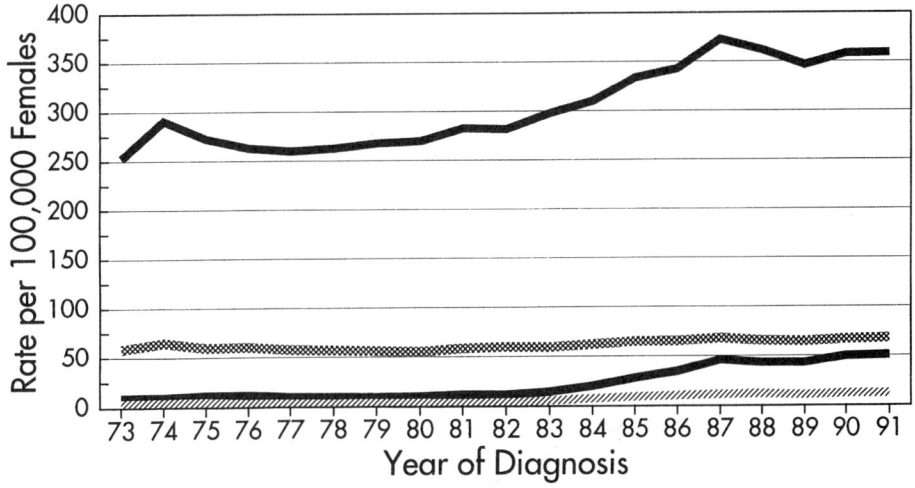

Figure 28.2. White female age-related breast cancer incidence rates for in situ and malignant (invasive) cancer based on NCI SEER data, 1973–1991. See Figure 28.1 for explanation of curves.

Fact: Currently, it is thought that: (1) about 85% of all breast cancers are sporadic, or due largely (or primarily) to nonhereditary factors; (2) about 10% arise from moderately strong hereditary risk factors still to be identified; and (3) only about 5% originate from strong hereditary factors (Fig. 28.4). Thus any three women whose mothers were diagnosed with breast cancer could each have differ-

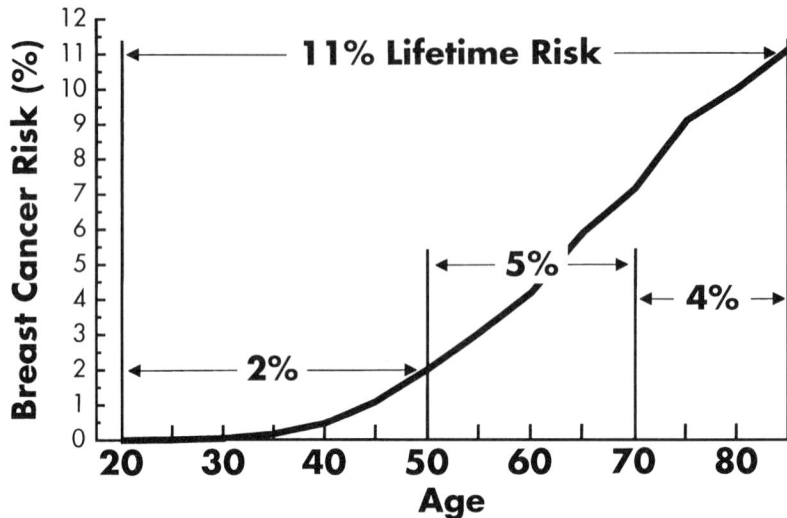

Figure 28.3. Percentage lifetime and age-related risk for invasive breast cancer based on NCI data.

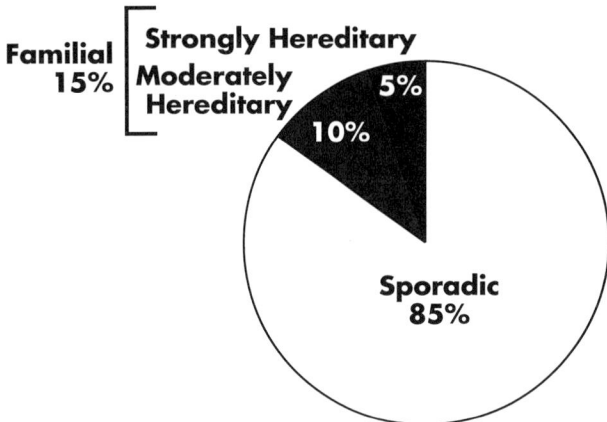

Figure 28.4. Percentages of familial and sporadic (nonhereditary) invasive breast cancer.

ent risks, depending on the origin of their mother's disease. As a group, women with an affected mother and sister have a lifetime breast cancer risk of about 20%.

Mistaken Belief 4: When assessing hereditary risk, only the mother's side of the family need be taken into account.

Fact: An increased hereditary susceptibility to breast cancer can be passed through a woman's father as well as her mother. Therefore when assessing risk due to family history, obtaining information about cancers on the paternal side of the family is essential.

Mistaken Belief 5: Genetic testing for hereditary susceptibility to breast and ovarian cancer can be used to determine accurately whether a woman is or is not at increased risk of breast cancer due to strong hereditary factors.

Fact: At the present time, genetic testing is available to detect mutations in two genes: *BRCA1* on chromosome 17 and *BRCA2* on chromosome 13. Not all of the mutations that increase breast, ovarian, and other cancer risks have been identified in these two genes; nor is it likely that these genes are the only ones in which mutations occur that significantly increase breast cancer risk. Therefore if no mutations in *BRCA1* or *BRCA2* are found in the first individual to be tested in a family where a strong family history of breast or ovarian cancer is present, a negative result is *not* evidence of decreased risk or a lack of hereditary susceptibility. In these cases it is more likely that there is a mutation, but present technology is not yet able to identify it. A strong family history is considered to be one in which at least one of the following is found: two or more affected generations, bilateral breast cancer, breast cancer diagnosed before age 50, or the presence of both breast and ovarian cancer.

Mistaken Belief 6: A woman whose close relatives were diagnosed with breast cancer after menopause is unlikely to have an increased risk of breast cancer due to hereditary factors.

Fact: Women diagnosed with breast cancer at younger ages are more likely to have a hereditary gene mutation that increases cancer risk than are those diagnosed at older ages. However, in one study of women who carried a *BRCA1* mutation, more than one-third of the breast cancer risk and more than one-third of the ovarian cancer risk occurred after age 50. Therefore older age at diagnosis cannot be used as a way to rule out increased hereditary susceptibility.

Mistaken Belief 7: Women who have no family history of cancer or who have only a single relative with breast or ovarian cancer can be assured that they will not benefit from genetic testing.

Fact: A number of studies have now found that women diagnosed with breast or ovarian cancer who have little or no family history of these diseases can have germline mutations in the *BRCA1* gene, particularly if they are diagnosed before age 50.

Mistaken Belief 8: If a woman is found to have a *BRCA1* or *BRCA2* gene mutation, she will be diagnosed with cancer.

Fact: To date, the risks of breast, ovarian, and other cancers associated with a *BRCA1* or *BRCA2* gene mutation have been determined only in special research families that were chosen for the presence of cancers in multiple generations and diagnoses at young ages. These families are heterogeneous; in some families individuals are diagnosed with only breast cancer, in others only ovarian cancer, and in still others a number of different cancers. Because of the special nature of these families and their heterogeneity, the risk of cancer due to mutation carriers may not be relevant to other women who are carriers of a *BRCA1* mutation.

Mistaken Belief 9: Genetic testing results are not clinically useful at the present time.

Fact: Some of my patients with a family history of ovarian or both breast and ovarian cancer have found these tests to be useful. For example, a 38-year-old woman had one sister diagnosed with breast cancer and one with ovarian cancer. Her mother died of breast cancer in her forties. My patient did not want to have her ovaries removed if it could be shown that she did not have a *BRCA1* or *BRCA2* mutation. However, if she were found to have such a mutuation or if no known mutation could be found in her sisters, she wanted a prophylactic oophorectomy. One of her affected sisters was tested and found to have a known mutation in the *BRCA1* gene. My patient was tested, found not to be a carrier of this mutation, and decided not to have her ovaries removed. She understands that she could still be diagnosed with ovarian cancer but believes that she can comfortably live with the average woman's lifetime risk of less than 2%.

Mistaken Belief 10: Prophylactic oophorectomy does not reduce the risk of peritoneal cancer.

Fact: The risk of peritoneal cancer following prophylactic removal of the ovaries appears to be low based on the limited studies now available. Data from the Gilda Radner Tumor Registry show that only 6 of 324 women with a strong family history of ovarian cancer who underwent prophylactic oophorectomy (some followed for 25 years) subsequently developed peritoneal cancer. If these women had not had a prophylactic oophorectomy, an estimated 50–90 ovarian cancers would have been diagnosed in this group.

Mistaken Belief 11: Informed decisions about genetic testing are likely to result when patients are given information about genetics, heredity, and genetic testing procedures.

Fact: Information about genetics, risk, and testing is complex and sophisticated. For patients to understand the ramifications of this information and to make decisions that are truly informed they need information about nonhereditary (Table 28.1), as well as hereditary, risks. Additionally, individuals differ in the ways they learn and make decisions, so this information must be presented at a level and pace that is appropriate for the individual if it is to be understood and appropriately applied.

Patients generally benefit by receiving help when making decisions based on their risks instead of having decisions made for them. Although this approach can be time-consuming initially, it results in improved patient comprehension and compliance, leading to more effective and efficient medical care. Many of the patients who seek genetic testing for cancer risk have special sensitivities and concerns about cancer because of their family and personal histories with the disease. Unless care is taken in the presentation of risk information, emotional reactions can act as barriers to understanding.

Primary care physicians can play an important role in helping patients understand their risk and in making decisions about genetic testing and appropriate follow-up care. The involvement of the primary care physician can help ensure

Table 28.1. Nonhereditary information used for cancer risk assessment and counseling

The following topics are necessary parts of any discussion leading to informed consent for cancer risk assessment, genetic testing, and counseling.

Anatomy
Incidence
Diet and alcohol consumption
Precursor lesions
Cancer etiology
Exogenous hormones
Reproductive history
Environmental exposures
Prognosis and early detection

truly informed consent and appropriate access to and utilization of risk information and genetic testing. Without this help, which requires multiple visits and access to information that encompasses more than genetics and risk, lip service is paid to obtaining informed consent without giving patients an opportunity to learn enough to make it a reality. Without informed consent, of course, these tests have the capability of hurting, not helping, those who could most benefit from the information they provide.

29 Breast Cancer and Exogenous Estrogen in Oral Contraceptives and Postmenopausal Hormone Replacement

Daniel R. Mishell Jr.

Breast Cancer and Oral Contraceptive Use

Because estrogen stimulates the growth of breast tissue there have been concerns that the high dose of exogenous estrogen in oral contraceptives (OCs) can initiate or promote breast cancer in humans. Accordingly, numerous epidemiologic studies have been published in which breast cancer risk among OC users has been reported. In 1991 Thomas published a comprehensive review of the results of all previously published epidemiologic studies of breast cancer risk in relation to use of combined OCs.[1] Both case-control and cohort studies were analyzed, and the summary relative risk was determined using meta-analysis. Fifteen case-control studies were reported between 1974 and 1990; they were conducted in developed countries and included women of all ages at risk for having used OCs. The relative risk of breast cancer with OC use ranged from 0.7 to 1.6 in the individual studies, and only one of these studies reported a significantly increased breast cancer risk. The summary relative risk obtained by combining the data from all the studies was 1.0 (95% confidence interval, or CI, was 1.0–1.1) (Table 29.1).

Results of breast cancer in women who ever used OCs were also analyzed in five cohort studies. None of these studies showed an increased or decreased risk of development of breast cancer with OC use, and the summary relative risk was 1.06 (CI 0.97–1.15) (Table 29.2). The risk of breast cancer in long-term users of OCs was also analyzed in nine case-control and four cohort studies. The summary relative risk of these analyses for the case-control study was 1.1 (CI 0.9–1.2) and for the cohort studies 1.11 (CI 0.91–1.36). Because the confidence invervals overlapped 1.0, the variations in the relative risk are not statistically significant.

Eight case-control and one cohort study analyzed the relative risk of breast cancer in OC users who did and did not have a family history of breast cancer

Table 29.1. Relative risks of breast cancer in women in developed countries who ever used oral contraceptives: case-control studies of women of all ages at risk of exposure

Source, year	Upper age limit of patients	Cases/controls		RR estimate and (95% CI)[a]
		Users	Nonusers	
Henderson, 1974	64	59/69	248/238	0.7 (0.5–1.2)
Paffenbarger, 1977	50	226/398	226/474	1.1 (0.9–1.4)
Sartwell, 1977	74	22/34	262/333	0.9 (0.5–1.5)
Ravnihar, 1979	64	30/65	160/315	0.9 (0.6–1.5)
Kelsey, 1981	74	30/141	300/1207	0.9 (0.6–1.3)
Harris, 1982	54	36/189	73/279	1.0 (0.6–1.4)
Vessey, 1983	50	537/554	639/622	1.0 (0.8–1.2)
Rosenberg, 1984	59	397/2558	794/2468	0.9 (0.8–1.1)
Talamini, 1985	79	15/23	353/351	0.7 (0.4–1.4)
CASH, 1986	54	2743/2802	1870/1774	1.0 (0.9–1.1)
Paul, 1986	54	310/708	123/189	0.9 (0.7–1.3)
La Vecchia, 1986	60	104/178	672/1104	1.1 (0.8–1.5)
Ravnihar, 1988	54	162/467	372/1522	1.6 (1.3–2.1)
Stanford, 1989	>60	481/515	1541/1668	1.0 (0.9–1.2)
WHO, 1990	62	438/1496	716/1888	1.1 (0.9–1.3)
Summary RR[b]	—	—	—	1.0 (1.0–1.1)

Source: After Thomas.[1]
[a] Confidence intervals estimated from published data.
[b] The *p* value of the chi-square test for heterogeneity =0.08.

Table 29.2. Relative risk of breast cancer in women who ever used oral contraceptives: cohort studies

Source, year	Upper age limit of patients (years)	Cases/1000 person-years (no. of cases)		RR estimate (95% CI)[a]
		Ever users	Never users	
Trapido, 1981[b]	>50	0.93 (85)	1.11 (370)	0.84 (0.7, 1.10)
Vessey et al., 1981[c]	45	0.50 (39)	0.52 (33)	0.96 (0.59, 1.63)
Kay et al., 1988[c]	64	0.64 (143)	0.52 (96)	1.22 (0.93, 1.60)
Romieu et al., 1989[d]	65	1.45 (717)	1.76 (1041)	1.07 (0.97, 1.19)
Mills et al., 1989[e]	67	0.93 (29)	1.65 (64)	1.54 (0.94, 2.53)
Summary RR				
Excluding Mills				1.04 (0.96, 1.13)*
Including Mills				1.06 (0.97, 1.15)**

Source: Thomas,[1] with permission.
[a] Numbers in parentheses indicate confidence intervals estimated from published reports.
[b] Boston area.
[c] Britain.
[d] Nurses Health Study (USA).
[e] Seventh Day Adventists (USA).
* The *p* value of the chi-square test for heterogeneity = 0.18.
** The *p* value of the chi-square test for heterogeneity = 0.13.

(Table 29.3). None of the studies showed a significant difference in risk of breast cancer among OC users who did and did not have a family history of breast cancer. Therefore a family history of breast cancer is not a contraindication for OC use. Thirteen case-control studies analyzed the relative risk of diagnosis of breast cancer under the age of 45 associated with OC use. Most of these studies indicated that there was a slightly increased risk of diagnosis of breast cancer under the age of 45 if women used OCs, but this risk was significant in only two of the studies. The summary relative risk for diagnosis of breast cancer under age 45 for OC users was 1.16 (CI 1.05–1.28) indicating that the slight increase was significant. Of these case-control studies, 12 analyzed the relative risk of breast cancer diagnosed under

Table 29.3. Relative risks of breast cancer in relation to use of oral contraceptives in women with and without a family history of breast cancer

Source, year (study design)	Restrictions	Relative with breast cancer	Use of oral contraceptives	RR estimate (95% CI)
Kelsey et al., 1981 (case-control)	None	Any	Any	No increase (data not given)
Vessey et al., 1983 (case-control)	None	Any	None	1.0
			≤48 Months	0.6
			>49 Months	1.1
Hennekens et al., 1984 (case-control)	None	Not mother	Any	1.1 (0.9, 1.2)
		Mother	Any	1.0 (0.6, 1.7)
		Not sister	Any	1.1 (0.9, 1.3)
		Sister	Any	1.4 (0.7, 3.0)
Rosenberg et al., 1984 (case-control)	None	Any	>5 years	0.9 (0.4, 2.1)
CASH, 1986 (case-control)	None	None	Any	1.0 (0.9, 1.2)
		First degree	Any	1.1 (0.8, 1.6)
		Second degree	Any	0.9 (0.7, 1.2)
Lipnick et al., 1986 (cohort)	None	Mother	Any	0.8 (0.4, 1.6)
		Sister	Any	0.9 (0.5, 1.5)
Miller et al., 1989 (case-control)	<45 years old	None	Any	2.0 (includes 1)
		Any	Any	1.9 (includes 1)[a]
Stanford et al., 1989 (case-control)	None	Not mother	Any	1.0 (0.8, 1.2)
		Mother	Any	0.8 (0.5, 1.2)
		Not sister	Any	1.1 (0.9, 1.4)
		Sister	Any	1.2 (0.6, 2.5)
WHO, 1990 (case-control)		None	Any	1.1 (1.01, 1.27)
		Any	Any	1.3 (0.75, 2.16)

Source: Thomas,[1] with permission.
[a] RR = 3.4 in multivariate analysis (95% CI includes 1.0).

age 45 among women who had used OCs for a long time. The summary relative risk was 1.42 (CI 1.25–1.63), a significant increase. This increased risk of breast cancer in women under age 45 if they were using OCs could be due to the fact that these young women taking OCs have greater breast surveillance than women of similar age not using OCs. Alternatively, OCs, like early first-term pregnancy, could stimulate the growth of small, not clinically evident breast cancers so the initial diagnosis is made at an earlier age than occurs in non-OC users. Analysis of results from the largest epidemiologic study, the CASH study, supports this hypothesis. Wingo et al. analyzed data from the CASH study, comparing the risk of developing breast cancer and OC use at different ages.[2] These investigators reported that when breast cancer was diagnosed at ages 20–34 the relative risk was significantly increased in OC users compared with non-OC users (RR = 1.4, CI 1.0–2.1) (Table 29.4). When breast cancer was diagnosed at ages 35–44, the relative risk associated with OC use fell (RR = 1.1, CI 0.9–1.3), and when the breast cancer was diagnosed at ages 45–54 there was a slight decrease in the associated risk with OC use (RR = 0.9, CI 0.8–1.0). In this oldest age group, with the highest incidence of breast cancer among the three age groups, the risk estimate decreased significantly with increasing time since first and last use. The CASH study, like most other studies, found that prior OC use does not increase the risk of diagnosis of breast cancer after age 45, when the disease is most prevalent, and that there is little or no effect on lifetime risk of breast cancer with OC use.

Schlesselman, in 1995, performed a meta-analysis of 25 studies that analyzed the risk of breast cancer associated with different durations of OC use in women between the ages of 45 and 60.[3] In this analysis of nearly 20,000 women with breast cancer, of whom nearly half used OCs, he found there was a nonsignificant trend of slightly increasing breast cancer risk with increasing duration of use (Fig. 29.1).

Table 29.4. Hypothetic annual age-specific breast cancer incidence rates in U.S. women aged 20–54 in 1982

History of OC use	% OC use	RR (95% CI)	Annual incidence per 100,000 women	Rate difference per 100,000 women
Age 20–34				
Never	24.0	Referent	8.5	
Ever	76.0	1.4 (1.0–2.1)	11.9	3.4
All women	100.0		11.1	
Age 35–44				
Never	28.6	Referent	74.8	
Ever	71.4	1.1 (0.9–1.3)	82.2	7.4
All women	100.0		80.1	
Age 45–54				
Never	53.1	Referent	177.5	
Ever	46.9	0.9 (0.8–1.0)	159.8	−17.7
All women	100.0		169.2	

Source: Wingo et al.,[2] with permission.

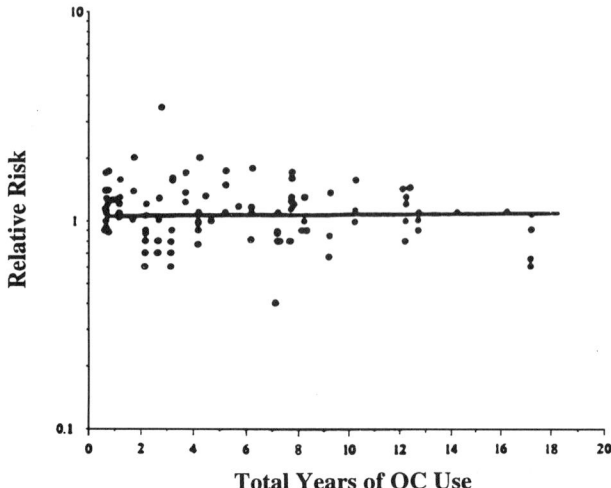

Figure 29.1. Relative risk of breast cancer by total years of oral contraceptive use. (From Schlesselman,[3] with permission.)

The relative risks for 4, 8, and 12 years of OC use were 1.06, 1.068, and 1.072, respectively. Because each of these risk estimates is not significantly increased, the data support the conclusion that there is no adverse effect of prior OC use on the risk of breast cancer between the ages of 45 and 60. The CASH data and these findings are compatible with the hypothesis that OC use, like early first-term pregnancy, increases the risk of the diagnosis of breast cancer at a young age, with no appreciable effect on lifetime risk of breast cancer and possibly a decreased risk during the perimenopausal years when the disease is most common. There are no published data regarding the effect of OC use on the risk of breast cancer in women older than age 60.

In 1996 an international collaborative group reanalyzed the worldwide epidemiologic data relevant to the investigation of the relation between risk of breast cancer and use of OCs.[4] Data from 54 studies performed in 25 countries, involving more than 53,000 women with breast cancer and more than 100,000 controls, were analyzed. The analysis indicated that while women took OCs they had a slightly increased risk of having breast cancer diagnosed (RR = 1.24, CI 1.15–1.30). The magnitude of the risk of having breast cancer diagnosed declined steadily after stopping OC use, so there was no longer a significantly increased risk 10 years or more after stopping their use (RR = 1.01, CI 0.96–1.05) (Fig. 29.2). It is of interest that the cancers diagnosed in women taking OCs were less advanced clinically than those that occurred in the nonusers. The risk of having breast cancer that had spread beyond the breast compared to a localized tumor was significantly reduced (RR = 0.88, CI 0.81–0.95) in OC users compared with nonusers. The Collaborative Group concluded that these results could be explained by the fact that breast cancer is diagnosed earlier in OC users than in nonusers, or that it could be due to biologic effects of the OCs. Furthermore, the collaborative analysis found there was no significant increase in risk of breast

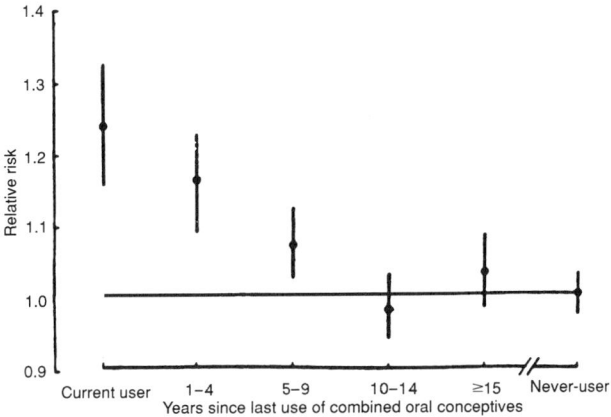

Figure 29.2. Relative risk of breast cancer by time since last use of combined oral contraceptives. (From Collaborative Group on Hormonal Factors in Breast Cancer,[4] with permission.)

cancer with OC use at very young ages, use before a first birth, or use by women with a family history of breast cancer.

The clinical meaning of this vast amount of epidemiologic data with small changes in relative risk is difficult to interpret. It appears that the dose or type of either steroid (estrogen or progestogen) in OC formulations and the duration of OC use are not related to breast cancer risk. Because there is no relation between dose or duration of use of estrogen it is unlikely that the estrogen in OCs initiate breast cancer.

Two findings are important. One is that with current OC use or use within 5 years the risk of breast cancer diagnosis is increased by about 25%. The second is that the increased risk of breast cancer in current OC users is limited to localized disease, as OC users have a significantly reduced incidence of disease that has spread beyond the breast. A decreased risk of advanced disease is also found in older women who had previously used OCs compared with nonusers. Because the increased risk of breast cancer with OC use is confined to current and recent users, if there is an excess in incidence the magnitude of increased incidence is small because breast cancer is uncommon before age 45. Furthermore, the contraceptive steroids probably act to promote the growth or increase the chance of diagnosis of existing cancers but do not initiate breast cancer, as breast cancer has been thought usually to take many years to become clinically evident after the cancer is initiated and there is no increased risk of breast cancer in prior OC users 10 years or more after OC use is discontinued. Overall, the large body of data regarding OC use and breast cancer risk is reassuring.

Neoplastic Effects of Estrogen Replacement Therapy

Much concern has been raised about the neoplastic risks of postmenopausal estrogen replacement therapy, particularly regarding breast and endometrial cancer, as estrogen causes cells in these tissues to proliferate. The possibility exists that exogenous estrogen can stimulate growth of a small nonpalpable breast cancer, and carcinoma of the breast may exist in the preclinical state for as long as 8 years before it is palpable. Therefore it is advisable for all women to undergo mammography to rule out subclinical breast cancer before initiating estrogen therapy and annually thereafter.

Many epidemiologic studies have investigated the relation between exogenous estrogen use and the risk of breast cancer. To date six meta-analyses have been performed in which the data from several published studies are combined to yield a larger database.[5–10] Each of these six analyses concluded that the risk of developing breast cancer among women who had ever used estrogen compared with nonusers was not significantly changed, with most summary results of risks being close to 1.0 (Table 29.5).

There have been several meta-analyses summarizing data from studies of the effect of long-term estrogen replacement therapy and the risk of breast cancer in postmenopausal women.[7–10] These meta-analyses combined data from 5–16 studies of women who had used estrogen replacement for more than 8 years to more than 15 years. Each of the summaries indicated that the relative risk of breast cancer developing with long-term use of estrogen replacement compared with no use was increased about 30%. This degree of increased risk was statistically significant. In the individual studies analyzed, the increased risk with long-term use was mainly observed among European women who had used a high dose of a synthetic estrogen compound not available in the United States. In 1995 Colditz published data from the Nurses' Health Study that showed that current users of estrogen replacement who had been taking mainly conjugated equine estrogen for more than 5 years had a significantly increased risk of developing breast cancer of 1.46 (Table 29.6).[11] Long-term users of estrogen who stopped using it had no increased risk of breast cancer, with the relative risk being approximately 1.0. Because the increased risk was observed only in long-time current users and not long-term past users, it is more likely that the increased risk observed in this study was due to detection bias and not causally related to the ingestion of estrogen. If long-term estrogen use caused an increased risk of cancer, an increased risk should have been observed in all long-term users, not just current users, who would be more likely to have medical surveillance.

Table 29.5. Meta-analysis of overall RR of postmenopausal estrogen and breast cancer in women who had ever used estrogen compared with never users

Author	Year	Studies	Summary RR	CI
Armstrong	1988	23	1.01	0.95–1.08
Dupont & Page	1991	28	1.07	NA
Steinberg	1991	16	1.0	NA
Grady & Ernster	1991	37	1.01	0.98–1.06
Sillero-Arenas	1992	27	1.06	1.00–1.12
Colditz	1993	31	1.02	0.93–1.12

Source: Mishell,[11] with permission.

That same year, a case-control study from Washington State was reported by Stanford et al.[13] These investigators found that long-term use of estrogen replacement for 20 years or more and estrogen-progestin use for 8 years or more did not increase the risk of breast cancer, with the relative risks being 1.0 and 0.4, respectively (Tables 29.7, 29.8). In this study it was found that current use of estrogen or estrogen plus progestin was not associated with an increased risk of breast cancer (RR = 0.9).

Newcomb et al. studied more than 3000 women with breast cancer and more than 3000 controls during 1989–1991 and found no change in the risk of breast cancer with estrogen alone or with estrogen plus progestin, or with all types of hormone replacement therapy with short- or long-term use.[14] The relative risk of breast cancer in women who used these steroids for 4–9 years, 10–14 years, and more than 15 years compared with nonhormone users ranged from 0.90 to 1.11. None of these risks was statistically significant. When the data from this study were restricted to recent users of hormone replacement, no significant increase in the risk of breast cancer was observed with short- or long-term duration of estrogen or estrogen plus progestin therapy (RR = 0.91 and 1.12, respectively) (Table 29.9), similar to the findings of the Stanford et al. study and in contrast to the findings of the Nurse's Health Study.

Another study analyzed the risk of estrogen replacement on breast cancer in nearly 50,000 women studied in the United States between 1973 and 1989.[15] This study found that for both ever-use and long-term use of estrogen there was no significant increase in the risk of developing invasive breast cancer (RR = 1.1) (Table 29.10). However, with long-term (>10 years) use of estrogen replacement, there was an increased risk of developing in situ cancer of the breast with a relative risk of 2.3 (CI 1.1–4.8). Similar rate ratios of risk were observed when the analysis of short- and long-term use was restricted to current users (Table 29.11).

Table 29.6. Duration of current and past postmenopausal hormone therapy and relative risk of breast cancer in the Nurses' Health Study, 1976–1992

Hormone use (months)	Cases of breast cancer (no.)	Person-years of follow-up	Adjusted relative risk (95% CI)[a]
None	972	374,197	1.0
Current			
1–23	82	31,966	1.14 (0.91–1.45)
24–59	140	49,672	1.20 (0.99–1.44)
60–119	150	44,112	1.46 (1.22–1.74)
≥120	141	37,454	1.46 (1.20–1.76)
Past			
1–23	193	81,047	0.90 (0.77–1.05)
24–59	120	54,046	0.86 (0.71–1.05)
60–119	89	34,952	1.00 (0.80–1.26)
≥120	48	18,104	1.03 (0.76–1.41)

Source: Colditz et al.,[12] with permission.
[a] Adjnsted for age, type of menopause, age at menopause, parity, age at first delivery, age at menarche, family history of breast cancer, history of benign breast disease, and time period.

Table 29.7. Relative odds of breast cancer associated with menopausal use of estrogen replacement therapy

Measure of ERT use	No. of cases	No. of controls	Relative odds[b]	95% CI
Duration[c]				
1–3 months	17 (4.2)[a]	13 (3.5)[a]	1.1	0.5–2.4
4 months–2.9 years	39 (9.5)	36 (9.7)	1.0	0.6–1.6
3–4.9 years	16 (3.9)	16 (4.3)	0.9	0.4–1.8
5–7.9 years	29 (7.1)	21 (5.6)	1.2	0.7–2.2
8–11.9 years	22 (5.4)	37 (9.9)	0.5	0.3–0.9
12–14.9 years	20 (4.9)	17 (4.6)	1.0	0.5–2.0
15–19.9 years	18 (4.4)	27 (7.2)	0.5	0.3–1.0
≥20 years	25 (6.1)	19 (5.1)	1.0	0.5–2.0
Years since first use[d]				
<5	36 (8.8)	27 (7.2)	1.2	0.7–2.1
5–9	45 (11.0)	31 (8.3)	1.3	0.8–2.2
10–14	40 (9.8)	38 (10.2)	0.9	0.5–1.5
15–19	28 (6.8)	48 (12.9)	0.5	0.3–0.8
≥20	37 (9.0)	42 (11.3)	0.7	0.4–1.1
Years since last use				
Current[e]	130 (31.7)	122 (32.7)	0.9	0.7–1.3
<5	12 (2.9)	17 (4.6)	0.6	0.3–1.3
≥5	45 (11.0)	47 (12.6)	0.8	0.5–1.3
Type of dose[f]				
Oral conjugated estrogen				
≤0.625 mg/day	66 (16.1)	67 (18.0)	0.8	0.6–1.2
>0.625 mg/day	66 (16.1)	64 (17.2)	0.9	0.6–1.4
Other estrogen	28 (6.8)	32 (8.6)	0.8	0.4–1.3
Unknown type or dose	27 (6.6)	23 (6.2)	1.0	0.6–1.8

Source: Stanford et al.,[13] with permission.
[a] Numbers in parentheses are percents.
[b] Odds relative to nonusers of any menopausal hormone therapy (223 cases, 187 controls), adjusted for age, age at first full-term pregnancy, and family history of breast cancer. Analysis excludes women who used combined estrogen with progestin menopausal hormone therapy.
[c] Analysis excludes one case with unknown duration of use.
[d] Analysis excludes one case with unknown time of first use.
[e] Use within the year before reference date.
[f] Longest used regimen; other estrogen includes nonconjugated oral estrogen and estradiol skin patches.

The Iowa Women's Health Study is a large follow-up study of 36,000 postmenopausal women living in Iowa. Although the study design is similar to the Nurses Health Study, analysis of the Iowa data indicated that current long term users of hormone replacement did not have a significantly elevated risk of diagnosis of breast cancer (RR = 1.13).

Several studies have reported that women who have developed breast cancer postmenopausally while taking estrogen replacement had a significantly greater 5-year survival than women of similar age who developed breast cancer who were not taking estrogen replacement (Fig. 29.3).[16] It is likely that the increased risk of breast cancer observed with long-term use of estrogen, which is found only in current users, is due to detection bias, particularly more frequent diagnosis of

Table 29.8. Relative odds of breast cancer associated with menopausal use of estrogen combined with progestin hormone replacement therapy

Measure of estrogen-progestin HRT use	No. of cases	No. of controls	Relative odds[b]	95% CI
Duration[c]				
1–3 months	15 (4.5)[a]	7 (2.4)[a]	1.9	0.7–4.7
4 months–2.9 years	56 (16.9)	48 (16.6)	1.0	0.7–1.6
3–4.9 years	17 (5.1)	20 (6.9)	0.6	0.3–1.3
5–7.9 years	16 (4.8)	12 (4.2)	1.0	0.4–2.2
≥8 years	8 (2.4)	15 (5.2)	0.4	0.2–1.0
Years since first use[d]				
<5	78 (23.2)	69 (24.0)	1.0	0.7–1.4
5–9	28 (8.4)	19 (6.6)	1.2	0.6–2.2
≥10	6 (1.8)	14 (4.8)	0.3	0.1–0.9
Years since last use				
Current[e]	83 (24.7)	79 (27.3)	0.9	0.6–1.2
<5	26 (7.7)	16 (5.5)	1.4	0.7–2.7
≥5	4 (1.2)	7 (2.4)	0.5	0.1–1.7

Source: Stanford et al.,[13] with permission.
[a] Numbers in parentheses are percents.
[b] Odds relative to nonusers of any menopausal hormone therapy (223 cases, 187 controls), adjusted for age, age at first full-term pregnancy, and family history of breast cancer. Analysis excludes women who used estrogen alone.
[c] Analysis excludes one case with unknown duration of use.
[d] Analysis excludes one case with unknown time of first use.
[e] Use within the year before reference date.

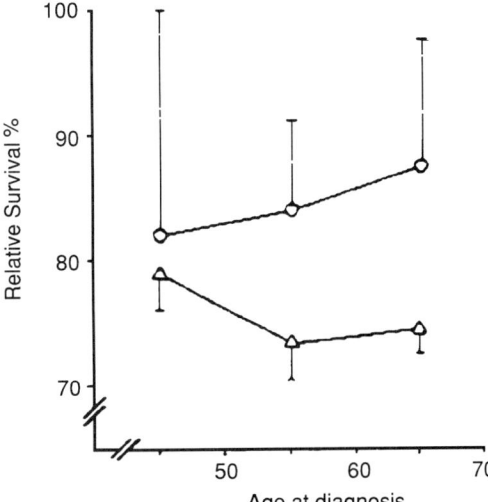

Figure 29.3. Relative 5-year survival with 95% confidence intervals (vertical bars) in breast cancer patients with (circles) and without (triangles) previous estrogen therapy. (From Bergkvist et al.,[16] with permission.)

noninvasive in situ disease. Data from these recent epidemiologic studies do not provide evidence that postmenopausal estrogen use initiates breast cancer by changing normal cells to cancer cells. However, because estrogen can stimulate the growth of a small clinically nonpalpable breast carcinoma, it is important that women receiving estrogen and all women in this age group have a mammogram annually.

Table 29.9. Estimated relative risk of breast cancer according to type of hormone replacement therapy, 1989–1991

Use	All HRT users				Users of estrogen only				Users of estrogen and progestin			
	No. of cases	No. of controls	RR^a (95% CI)	RR^{a,b} (95% CI)	No. of cases	No. of controls	RR^a (95% CI)	RR^{a,b} (95% CI)	No. of cases	No. of controls	RR^a (95% CI)	RR^{a,b} (95% CI)
Never	2207	2574	1.00	1.00	2207	2574	1.00	1.00	2207	2574	1.00	1.00
Ever	923	1124	0.98 (0.88–1.09)	1.05 (0.93–1.18)	587	783	0.90 (0.79–1.02)	0.97 (0.84–1.11)	138	157	0.92 (0.72–1.19)	1.01 (0.78–1.31)
Former	570	665	1.07 (0.94–1.22)	1.12 (0.98–1.29)	339	438	0.98 (0.84–1.15)	1.03 (0.87–1.21)	48	44	1.15 (0.75–1.78)	1.25 (0.81–1.94)
Recent^c	353	459	0.85 (0.72–1.00)	0.92 (0.77–1.09)	248	345	0.80 (0.67–0.96)	0.88 (0.72–1.08)	90	113	0.83 (0.61–1.13)	0.90 (0.66–1.24)
<5 Years	129	171	0.78 (0.60–1.01)	0.82 (0.62–1.07)	74	97	0.78 (0.55–1.10)	0.81 (0.57–1.16)	46	68	0.67 (0.44–1.02)	0.75 (0.49–1.15)
≥5 Years	224	288	0.89 (0.73–1.07)	0.97 (0.79–1.20)	174	248	0.81 (0.65–1.00)	0.91 (0.72–1.14)	44	45	1.06 (0.68–1.64)	1.12 (0.72–1.76)

Source: Stanford et al.,[13] with permission.

HRT = hormone replacement therapy; RR = relative risk; CI = confidence interval.

^{a} Adjusted for age and state.

^{b} Adjusted for type of menopause, time since menopause, age at menarche, age at first full-term pregnancy, history of benign breast disease, body mass index, family history of breast cancer, alcohol consumption, and education.

^{c} HRT use within 2 years of reference date (duration).

Table 29.10. Rate ratios of breast cancer associated with ever-use and duration of estrogen and estrogen-progestin use

Use	Person-years	All cases [c,d]			In situ			Invasive [a]		
		No.	RR	(CI) [b]	No.	RR	(CI) [b]	No.	RR	(CI) [b]
Ever-use [c,d]										
No	145,550	519	1.0	—	54	1.0	—	465	1.0	—
Estrogens only	145,940	566	1.0	0.9–1.2	78	1.4	1.0–2.0	488	1.0	0.9–1.1
Estrogens and progestins	19,969	90	1.2	1.0–1.6	18	2.3	1.3–3.9	72	1.1	0.9–1.4
Duration of estrogen-only use [e,f,g]										
<5 years	73,345	276	1.0	0.9–1.2	30	1.1	0.7–1.7	246	1.0	0.9–1.2
5–9 years	28,780	105	1.0	0.8–1.2	16	1.5	0.8–2.6	89	1.0	0.8–1.2
10–14 years	20,393	76	1.0	0.8–1.3	17	2.1	1.2–3.7	59	0.9	0.6–1.1
15–19 years	8,597	51	1.2	0.9–1.6	8	1.8	0.9–3.9	43	1.1	0.8–1.5
≥20 years	3,978	41	1.2	0.8–1.6	7	2.0	0.9–4.5	34	1.1	0.8–1.5
Duration of estrogen-progestin use [c,e,h]										
<2 years	8,633	47	1.5	1.1–2.1	11	3.3	1.7–6.3	36	1.3	0.9–1.9
2–3 years	3,345	12	1.0	0.6–1.8	5	3.9	1.5–9.7	7	0.7	0.3–1.4
≥4 years	3,805	20	1.4	0.9–2.2	1	0.7	0.1–4.7	19	1.5	0.9–2.4

Source: Schairer et al.,[15] with permission.
[a] Includes cases not confirmed by pathology report.
[b] CI = 95% confidence interval.
[c] Excludes 10 cases (2 in situ, 8 invasive) and 2440 person-years with uncertain hormone use.
[d] Adjusted for attained age and education.
[e] Reference group is no hormone use.
[f] Excludes 17 cases (all invasive) and 3978 person-years with unknown duration of use.
[g] Adjusted for attained age.
[h] Excludes 11 cases (1 in situ, 10 invasive) and 4185 person-years with unknown duration of use.

Table 29.11. Rate ratios of breast cancer associated with current and past duration of estrogen-only use

Estrogen-only use (years)	Person-years	All cases			In situ			Invasive[a]		
		No.	RR[b]	CI[c]	No.	RR[b]	CI	No.	RR[b]	CI
Current duration										
No hormone	145,550	519	1.0	—	54	1.0	—	465	1.0	—
<5	13,786	61	1.4	1.1–1.8	7	1.4	0.6–3.1	54	1.4	1.1–1.9
5–9	10,722	43	1.2	0.9–1.7	5	1.3	0.5–3.2	38	1.2	0.9–1.7
10–14	9,546	40	1.2	0.8–1.6	8	2.3	1.1–4.8	32	1.0	0.7–1.5
≥15	10,885	61	1.4	1.1–1.8	10	2.4	1.2–4.9	51	1.3	1.0–1.7
p for trend						0.04				
Past duration										
No hormone	145,550	519	1.0	—	54	1.0	—	465	1.0	—
<5	56,006	206	1.0	0.8–1.2	21	1.0	0.6–1.6	185	1.0	0.8–1.2
5–9	16,757	56	0.9	0.7–1.2	10	1.5	0.8–3.0	46	0.8	0.6–1.1
10–14	9,753	33	0.9	0.6–1.2	9	2.3	1.1–4.7	24	0.7	0.5–1.1
≥15	7,082	27	0.9	0.6–1.4	5	1.8	0.7–4.4	22	0.8	0.5–1.3
p for trend						0.11				

Source: Schairer et al.,[15] with permission.
[a] Includes cases not confirmed by pathology report.
[b] Adjusted for attained age.
[c] CI = 95% confidence interval.

There have been several meta-analyses of the risk of estrogen replacement and breast cancer in women who had a family history of breast cancer.[5,7,10] Although one of these analyses, by Steinberg et al.,[7] reported that there was a significantly increased risk of breast cancer in women with a family history of breast cancer who took estrogen over nonusers, a more recent comprehensive analysis by Colditz et al.[5] showed that the risk of breast cancer in women with a family history of breast cancer who received estrogen replacement was not significantly increased compared with nonusers (RR = 1.07, CI 0.73–1.56). Data from the Iowa Women's Health Study, in which 12% of 36,000 postmenopausal women reported a family history of breast cancer indicated that the risk of diagnosis of breast cancer was not significantly increased in this group if they received hormone replacement. Furthermore if women with a family history of breast cancer took hormonal replacement their mortality rates was half that of women who did not take hormone replacement. Therefore clinicians can advise postmenopausal women who have a family history of breast cancer that they can take estrogen replacement without increasing their risk of developing this disease.

The effect of administering progestin to postmenopausal women on the risk of breast cancer is not known because of the lack of randomized clinical trials. A retrospective study by Gambrell suggested that a combination estrogen-progestin menopausal hormonal regimen reduced the risk of breast cancer, as it does with endometrial cancer.[17] However, because mitotic activity in breast tissue increases during the luteal phase of the cycle and in vitro studies demonstrate increased mitotic activity in breast tissue with progestin exposure, a deleterious effect of progestin on the human breast is also possible. In support of this hypothesis, Bergkvist et al. reported that postmenopausal women using estrogen and a progestin had a 4.6-fold increased risk of breast cancer, although this increase was not statistically significant.[18] Two meta-analyses of the published epidemiologic data[9,10] concluded that addition of a progestin to estrogen replacement therapy does not alter the risk of breast cancer compared with nonhormonal use (RR = 1.13 and 0.99, respectively). Therefore if a postmenopausal woman has had a hysterectomy, there is no proved benefit for her to take a progestin to decrease her risk of breast cancer. The only reason to take a progestin in addition to an estrogen is to reduce the risk of endometrial cancer. This risk is eliminated by hysterectomy.

CONCLUSIONS

The results of numerous epidemiologic studies published to date do not support the hypothesis that exogenous estrogen in the form of high-dose oral contraceptives or low-dose postmenopausal hormone replacement increases the development of breast cancer by transforming normal cells into cancer cells. The small increased risk of the diagnosis of breast cancer in current but not past OC users and current but not past long-term users of estrogen replacement is most likely due to the confounding factor of increased frequency of surveillance modalities to diagnose breast cancer in current users of estrogen (diagnostic bias). This statement is supported by the facts that the type of breast cancer found in OC users is significantly more likely to be localized to the breast than occurs in nonusers and that the 5-year survival of women with breast cancer taking hormonal replacement is significantly better than occurs in women of similar age who develop breast cancer while not taking estrogen replacement.

References

1. Thomas DB. Oral contraceptives and breast cancer: review of the epidemiologic literature. Contraception 1991;43:597–642

2. Wingo PA, Lee NC, Ory HW, et al. Age-specific differences in the relationship between oral contraceptive use and breast cancer. Obstet Gynecol 1991;78:161–170

3. Schlesselman JJ. Net effect of oral contraceptive use on the risk of cancer in women in the United States. Obstet Gynecol 1995;85:793–801

4. Collaborative Group on Hormonal Factors in Breast Cancer. Breast cancer and hormonal contraceptives: collaborative reanalyses of individual data on 53,297 women with breast cancer and 100,239 women without breast cancer from 54 epidemiological studies. Lancet 1996;347:1713–1727

5. Armstrong BK. Oestrogen therapy after the menopause—boon or bane? Med J Aust 1988;148:213–214

6. Dupont WD, Page DL. Menopausal estrogen replacement therapy and breast cancer. Arch Intern Med 1991;151:67–72

7. Steinberg KK, Thacker SB, Smith J, et al. A meta-analysis of the effect of estrogen replacement therapy on the risk of breast cancer. JAMA 1991;265:1985–1990

8. Grady D, Rubin SM, Petitti DB, et al. Hormone therapy to prevent disease and prolong life in postmenopausal women. Ann Intern Med 1992;117:1016–1037

9. Sillero-Arenas M, Delgado-Rodriguez M. Menopausal hormone replacement therapy and breast cancer: a meta-analysis. Obstet Gynecol 1992;79:286–294

10. Colditz GA, Egan KM, Stampfer MJ. Hormone replacement therapy and risk of breast cancer: results from epidemiologic studies. Am J Obstet Gynecol 1993;168:1473–1480

11. Mishell DR Jr. Menopause. In: Mishell Dr Jr, Stenchever MA, Droegemueller W, Herbst AL (eds) Comprehensive Gynecology (3rd ed). St. Louis, Mosby, 1997, p 1183

12. Colditz GA, Hankinson SE, Hunter DJ, et al. The use of estrogens and progestins and the risk of breast cancer in postmenopausal women. N Engl J Med 1995;332:1589–1593

13. Stanford JL, Weiss MD, Voigt LF, et al. Combined estrogen and progestin hormone replacement therapy in relation to risk of breast cancer in middle-aged women. JAMA 1995;274:137–142

14. Newcomb PA, Longnecker MP, Mittendorf J, et al. Long-term hormone replacement therapy and risk of breast cancer in postmenopausal women. Am J Epidemiol 1995;142:788–795

15. Schairer C, Byrne C, Keyl PM, et al. Menopausal estrogen and estrogen-progestin replacement therapy and risk of breast cancer (United States). Cancer Causes Control 1994;5:491–500

16. Bergkvist L, Adami H-O, Persson I, et al. Prognosis after breast cancer diagnosis in women exposed to estrogen and estrogen-progestogen replacement therapy. Am J Epidemiol 1989;130:221–228

17. Gambrell RD Jr. Use of progestogen therapy. Am J Obstet Gynecol 1987;156:1304–1313

18. Bergkvist L, Adami H-O, Persson I, et al. The risk of breast cancer after estrogen and estrogen-progestin replacement. N Engl J Med 1989;321:293–297

30   Social Work Perspective and Psychosocial Resources

Carol P. Marcusen

The emotions experienced during diagnosis, treatment, and recovery from breast cancer can be extremely stressful for the patient and her loved ones. Breast cancer disrupts a woman's life. It is accompanied by a variety of feelings, such as anger, confusion, depression, and uncertainty. Uncertainty begets fear—fear of treatment and its side effects, fear of changes in one's life, fear of pain, fear of possible death, and fear of cancer's impact on one's relationships. All these feelings are normal, and all are experienced to a greater or lesser extent by the woman with breast cancer. She may find it difficult to resolve these feelings alone or to share them with her spouse, partner, friends, or doctor. It is important that patients, early in the process of treatment, become aware of the psychosocial resources available to them. A referral to a social worker, psychologist, or psychiatrist trained to deal with the psychosocial issues of breast cancer is an important aspect of care that should not be overlooked.

SCREENING

Screening helps the physician determine which patients would benefit from psychosocial assessment and intervention. Rarely in the existing health care environment are all patients routinely evaluated by a social worker, psychologist, or psychiatrist. Screening mechanisms have been developed to assist in the identification of patients at risk or vulnerable to psychological and social problems. These screening mechanisms include routine chart reviews, multidisciplinary rounds, patient self-screening tools, and screening by the physician, nurse, and other caregivers. Issues that would be screened for include (but are not limited to) the following:

1. Physical effects of the treatment plan, i.e., removal of a breast, alopecia, fatigue, nausea, skin reactions, loss of appetite, lymphedema, infection, loss of mobility, pain, and discomfort;
2. Sexual functioning, i.e., concerns with body image, reactions of significant others, fatigue, severity of illness;

3. Social support, i.e., family, friends, colleagues (Friedman et al.[1] found that women who adjusted the best also had the highest levels of family cohesion.);
4. Financial impact of illness: concerns regarding direct costs, indirect costs, and resources;
5. Employment issues, i.e., discrimination, vulnerability, and flexibility;
6. Insurance issues, i.e., coverage or no coverage at all, treatment options, feeling at greater risk to be dropped;
7. Concrete services, i.e., activities of daily living, transportation, shopping, and banking.

ASSESSMENT

Psychosocial assessment is the process by which the social worker evaluates the particular needs of the breast cancer patient and those of the patient's family. Assessment involves obtaining a psychosocial history, devising an initial treatment plan, and communicating the needs of the patient and the treatment plan to other health care team members.[2] The strength of social work lies in the ability of its practitioners to assess people within the context of their environment.

One common method of assessment used by the social worker in a medical setting is the Weisman[3] Seven Questions Assessment Tool.

1. What problems, if any, do you see this illness creating?
2. How do you plan to deal with them?
3. When faced with a problem you must do something about, what happens? What do you do?
4. How does it usually work out?
5. To whom do you turn when you need help?
6. What has happened in the past when you have asked for help?
7. What kinds of problems usually tend to get you down or upset?

The information from the assessment, combined with knowledge of the patient's medical situation and plan of treatment, help the social worker develop an intervention that places the patient at a particular developmental stage, makes a clinical prediction about how the patient and family will fare in this particular system, evaluates the priority that should be given to the patient in the context of many other referrals, evaluates what the particular health care system offers the patient and family, and evaluates the resources available outside of the setting to meet the needs of the patient and family.[4]

An articulate assessment and a clear-cut plan can enhance patient care and satisfaction by enrolling the patient as a partner in her treatment plan, leading to increased compliance. In addition, there is less time spent by the physician dealing with "fallout" from the patient's psychosocial concerns and issues, increased satisfaction by health care providers, and better use of community resources and educational materials.

Interventions

Numerous avenues in the community are available for psychosocial support. Awareness of these resources is an initial step in obtaining help for your patient. A referral to a specialist (e.g., a social worker) knowledgeable in assisting the patient to get the "right" help for her situation is the next step.

Patients may need additional information, education, and friendly advice. They also may need individual, family, or group therapy. Support groups are a source of remarkable strength. Better than many other techniques, participation in a support group helps women share feelings and uncertainties. Not every woman wants or needs a formal support group, but such groups can provide important benefits that are difficult to find elsewhere.

Support Groups

Support groups offer several options to breast cancer patients:

1. An opportunity to learn more about breast cancer and recent breakthroughs in surgical and medical treatments;
2. An opportunity to discuss medical issues with other breast cancer patients who can be a valuable source of additional information and can help sort through difficult or confusing treatment decisions;
3. Networking and friendships that can help one cope with the physical and emotional impact of this disease;
4. Benefits to the person's friends and family members who also learn that they are not alone.

Patients in support groups find that communication with friends and family becomes easier. Research suggests that women with breast cancer who are involved in professional support groups not only benefit psychosocially but also live longer than those who try to cope with the disease alone.[5]

Support groups generally offer open discussion sessions where group members share feelings and talk about their progress. They also offer planned educational sessions that may include visualization and relaxation techniques. Group facilitators are professionals who have expertise in providing resources and answers to questions.

Individual Counseling

Through a variety of therapeutic techniques, the social worker helps the patient focus on specific concerns and set priorities to manage the problems associated with chronic illness.

Family Counseling

Breast cancer affects the entire family.[6] Family members frequently express concerns that include helplessness, confusion, anger, guilt, and worries about financial or physical burdens. Family members may bring dysfunctional coping systems to the cancer experience. Through family counseling the social worker can recognize areas of need and can provide support to the family through a variety of techniques.

Behavioral Interventions

Behavioral interventions include relaxation, guided imagery, hypnosis, meditation, systematic desensitization, and music therapy. Foley[7] explained, "The major goal of these interventions is to promote an increased sense of control by reducing the hopelessness and helplessness that many patients experience."

Bereavement Counseling

It is important to recognize that grieving occurs at many points in the cancer experience. There may be grieving for the loss of predictability in one's life, changes in body image, loss of bodily function, and, of course, death.

Resource Utilization

Breast cancer patients experience a constellation of needs. In studies done in Pennsylvania, Houts et al.[8] estimated that 72% of people who died of cancer in Pennsylvania had at least one unmet need, including activities of daily living, transportation, and obtaining home care. The social worker assists the patient and family in identifying and utilizing existing resources as effectively as possible.

Discharge Planning

Planning the discharge is a clinical social work activity during hospitalization where interventions (psychological, social, medical, concrete) are put together to provide a treatment plan that meets the needs of the individual patient and her family to ensure continuity of care.

Education

Education enhances the personal sense of control and has a direct effect on the patient's and family's ability to cope. Blumberg[9] listed the following goals of cancer patient education:

1. Adjusting to the course of the disease and developing ways to adjust activities and responsibilities of patients and families accordingly;
2. Achieving a sense of participation in and control over the care of one's body;
3. Preventing social isolation caused by the disease condition;
4. Normalizing lifestyle and interactions with others by developing increased coping and communication skills with family, friends, and fellow-workers;
5. Learning about resources to help pay for medical treatments and developing strategies to cope with other economic consequences of the illness.

Program Development

The expertise of social workers in dealing with complex systems and in functioning collaboratively enables them to lead the development of a comprehensive service program for the breast cancer population.[2]

RESOURCES

There are many breast cancer patient support organizations in the community that provide information and support.

American Cancer Society (ACS) has a program called Reach To Recovery. This program uses trained volunteers who have had breast cancer to visit and reach out to share experiences and give support to other women in a time of need. This program is available throughout the United States. Patients are matched with former patients through physician referral. The volunteer provides information and practical tips: She does *not* give medical advice. Other ACS offerings include Special Touch, Early Support, Man to Man, Look Good . . . Feel Better, breast prosthesis and reconstructive surgery information, breast cancer support groups, transportation, and sickroom equipment. National phone number: 800-ACS-2345.

Y-Me is a national breast cancer information and support organization. Y-Me has chapters and volunteer resources in many communities. They offer support groups, advocacy, and patient-to-patient contact. National phone number: 800-221-2141.

National Alliance of Breast Cancer Organizations (NABCO) lists more than 250 other local support organizations. To help find the nearest resource of this kind, call the NABCO national number: 212-719-0154.

Cancer Information Service (CIS) of the National Cancer Institute provides the most up-to-date information on all aspects of cancer in English and Spanish. This service provides referrals to oncologists, medical centers, and clinical trial programs. It also provides written information. Phone: 800-4-CANCER.

Cancer-Fax is a service of the National Cancer Institute. Information similar to that provided by CIS can be obtained by fax. From a fax machine, dial 301-402-5874. Choose English or Spanish. A complete list of titles can be obtained by simply following the voice directions.

Cancer-Net is a service of the National Cancer Institute. To access CancerNet, send an e-mail message to cancernet@icicc.nci.nih.gov with the word *help* (for English) or *Spanish* (for Spanish) in the body of the message. You can include a subject for your message, but the request must be in the body of the message, not in the subject line. The contents list and instructions are sent to you by return e-mail.

National Coalition for Cancer Survivorship is a national network of groups and individuals concerned with survivorship and sources of support for cancer patients and their loved ones. It functions as an information clearing house and advocacy group for cancer survivors. Phone: 301-650-8868.

The Wellness Community is one of the largest support programs in the United States devoted solely to providing free psychological and emotional support to cancer patients and their families. Professionally led support groups, yoga, relaxation training, guided imagery, and tai chi are a few of the many resources available. National phone number: 310-314-2555.

National Lymphedema Association provides information on prevention and treatment of lymphedema. Phone: 800-541-3259.

National Hospice Organization is a nonprofit organization that provides literature and information about hospices to patients and their families. They also provide referrals to local, regional, and national resources. Phone: 703-243-5900.

Cancer Care, Inc. and the **National Cancer Foundation** are voluntary social service agencies that provide professional counseling to cancer patients and their families. These agencies also conduct programs of professional consultation and education, social research, public affairs, and public education. Phone: 212-679-5700.

Association of Oncology Social Work is a national organization dedicated to the enhancement of psychosocial services to people with cancer and their families. It is done through educational programs, advocacy, networking, and research. Phone: 410-614-3990.

Susan G. Komen Breast Cancer Foundation is a national nonprofit organization located in Orange County, California, whose mission is to eradicate breast cancer as a life-threatening disease by advancing research, education, screening, and treatment. Programs include early detection, a friendship network for children of breast cancer patients, a speakers bureau, legislative advocacy, and a resource center. Phone: 800-462-9273.

References

1. Friedman L, Baer P, Nelson D, et al. Women with breast cancer: perception of family functioning and adjustment to illness. Psychosoc Med 1988;50:529–540
2. Stearns N, Lauria M, Herman J, Fogelberg P. Oncology Social Work: A Clinician's Guide. Atlanta, American Cancer Society, 1993
3. Weisman AD. Coping With Cancer. New York, McGraw-Hill, 1979
4. Christ G. A psychosocial assessment framework for cancer patients and their families. Health Soc Work 1983;8:57–63
5. Spiegel D. Effects of psychosocial support on patients with metastatic breast cancer. J Psychosoc Oncol, 1992;10:113–120
6. Abrams RD. Not Alone With Cancer. Springfield, IL, Charles C Thomas, 1974, p 442
7. Foley K. The treatment of cancer pain. N Engl J Med 1985;313:84–95
8. Houts P, Yaske J, Harvey H, et al. Unmet needs of persons with cancer in Pennsylvania during the period of terminal care. Cancer 1988;62:627–634
9. Blumberg B. Adult Patient Education in Cancer. Bethesda, National Cancer Institute, 1983

31   BREAST CARE: A PSYCHOSOCIAL VIEW

Barbara Rabinowitz

Our society has a fascination with breasts, which leads women to conclude that an important part of their worth is measured in breast size and shape. This "mammocentric" view is affirmed and reconfirmed in portrayals of women on magazine covers, in movies, and in popular advertisements. Breast-focused images of women are constant, leaving women with some perhaps less than conscious, yet apparently persistent concerns about their breasts.

There is great variety to the issues that may surface around the topic of breasts during the many phases of a woman's life cycle. Worry about the timing of breast development, concerns about the perceived need for augmentation or reduction, decisions regarding breastfeeding, fears about breast cancer, and adaptation to menopausal and postmenopausal breast changes are among the issues that may appear. The predominant focus of this chapter is on the psychosocial issues that can surface with a diagnosis of breast cancer and the appropriate role for the primary care physician in these circumstances. Brief comments follow on the life cycle breast changes noted above.

TEENAGE ISSUES

It is not uncommon for adolescents to struggle with issues of self-esteem. Such issues may contain a component that is engendered by a teenager's dissatisfaction and confusion with the development of her "womanly self." Teens are referred for psychotherapy less frequently when the primary care physician has picked up on a potential problem the adolescent may be experiencing with female development. Far more often there is some "acting out" behavior on the part of the adolescent that is poorly understood by the parents who bring the young woman to therapy so her problem behavior might be "fixed." These more extreme instances do not represent the norm. However, even in the more general situation, a few reassuring words from a young woman's primary care physician about normal variation in breast development can be helpful.

ADULT ISSUES

Decisions regarding breastfeeding are influenced by a woman's peer group, the current societal standard, and perhaps her obstetrician. Certainly the decision is often influenced by the women's husband or significant other, but in my experience this rarely surfaces as an issue during couples therapy except as related to the issues of power and control.

Breast size is a frequent concern. It is almost as though breasts come in only two sizes: too small or too big. Women appealing to their doctors for augmentation or reduction may have unrealistic expectations as to how these changes in breast size may affect their lives. These expectations are best brought to the surface and dealt with before surgery. At the Comprehensive Breast Center (Monmouth Medical Center, Long Branch, NJ) no woman is accepted for augmentation or reduction surgery without a psychosocial evaluation and, when indicated, psychosocial intervention.

MENOPAUSAL ISSUES

Menopause, though a normal transition, frequently calls on women to make many physical and emotional adjustments. Breast changes are only one of many physical changes a woman may experience during the menopausal and postmenopausal period. Primary care physicians should be sensitive to the emotional issues and should not hesitate to suggest support groups or individual therapy (or both) when assistance is needed during this life cycle transition.

BREAST CANCER

Women are most anxious about breast cancer. Though the perceived risk is frequently inflated, women are aware of the statistics and the implications of the family history. Women sometimes report feeling "like a walking time bomb." Many would be well served by obtaining a more realistic perspective on risk status that can be obtained by referral to programs that deal with women at high risk. However, given the limited availability of such programs, explanations from primary care physicians that put the "one woman in eight" figures in better perspective can be helpful (Table 31.1). The real impact of genetic testing on helping all women understand their risk has not yet been appreciated. There remain a great variety of issues to be resolved on this topic. Beyond refinements regarding appropriate clinical application are issues that fall into the realm of the psychological, the ethical, and the legal. The broad-based application of genetic testing awaits further study.

Emotional Impact

For the woman and her family facing a breast cancer diagnosis, our understanding of the depth and breadth of psychosocial issues that can surface has greatly

Table 31.1. Chance of developing breast cancer

By age (years)	Chance
25	1:19,608
30	1:2,525
35	1:622
40	1:217
45	1:93
50	1:50
55	1:33
60	1:24
65	1:17
70	1:14
75	1:11
80	1:10
85	1:9
Ever	1:8

Source: Marshall,[1] with permission.

expanded over the last two decades. Women contemplating the diagnosis and treatment of breast cancer face many powerful emotions. The feelings of sadness, loss, anxiety, and anger may ebb and flow along the pathway from diagnosis to treatment to rehabilitation and recovery (which may be long-lasting or yield to recurrence). These feelings do not surface in any consistent or structured fashion. There is no simple algorithm that tells the physician what a woman's emotional response will be. The only rule is that any emotion may surface at any time.

There are many ways a woman may traverse this emotional time in her life. A woman who shows virtually no emotion from the time of diagnosis through surgery and adjuvant chemotherapy may suddenly exhibit a clear and dramatic response as chemotherapy treatments come to conclusion. Alternatively, quite the opposite, another may appear almost totally consumed by an emotional reaction to the diagnosis and remain so until formal treatment is about to end. Every woman takes this journey in her own way.

Personal style plays a role as well. Some women are so intensely private that any show of emotion, even to the physician with whom she has had a long and rewarding relationship, may be anathema. Others seem to reach out to those willing to listen to a detailed emotional description of the breast cancer experience.

Many women describe the vulnerability they experience after the diagnosis of breast cancer. They may report a feeling of loss for a previous sense of balance in their lives. For some the feeling is expressed as a painful loss of control. Some women set about gaining as much control as possible, in part by gathering information. Others may choose to receive only the barest information and yearn for an earlier time when fewer options were put before them and they did not need to be involved in the decision-making. It is important that the team working with a woman through her treatment and therapy show respect for her style.

During Adjuvant Therapy

The time of diagnosis and surgical treatment may cause early emotional trauma, and adjuvant therapies may also engender such reactions. Often women report an increase in their general sadness and anxiety as they face chemotherapy and, less frequently, radiation therapy. Patients often speak of the torment of chemotherapy-induced weight gain, skin changes, loss of hair, nausea, trouble concentrating, and fatigue. Radiation therapy has a major demoralizing impact described as a consuming fatigue. Women also report distress at having been "branded" by the tattooing of the treatment boundaries. Reminders, offered in a compassionate and empathetic fashion, that many or most of these symptoms are time-limited, can be somewhat helpful. Speaking with one of the trained volunteers of ChemoCare can be helpful at this time. ChemoCare volunteers are matched for diagnosis and chemotherapeutic agent and for age/life stage whenever possible. They are available to visit in person when geographically possible or by phone (Table 31.2).

Recurrence

Fear of recurrence is ongoing. Some women speak of this fear as a constant companion that looms larger with each unexpected or unexplained symptom and around the time of repeat clinical evaluations. These women often seek counsel from their primary care physician who, one hopes, wisely does not minimize the symptoms but rather works with their oncologic colleagues to rule out recurrence or metastatic disease and then offers reassurance as soon as it is appropriate.

Many women have to face a recurrence of their breast cancer. This situation can be an even more powerful emotional blow than the original diagnosis and often prompts questions about earlier treatment decisions and guilt and remorse regarding those decisions. With a diagnosis of recurrence, vulnerability looms even larger. In an effort to recapture some hope toward their own survivorship, women often try to reach out to others who are "doing well" after a recurrence.

When Does the Fear End?

There is a myth that the psychosocial issues fade at some approximate boundary (e.g., after treatment ends or at the conclusion of a 5-year follow-up). In my experience there are longer-term survivor issues for at least a subset of women, and research has identified anxiety, fear, and anger among the ongoing emotions.[2] Unfortunately, women often stop talking about their feelings because "everyone is tired of hearing about all these 'downer' emotions." When actively queried about their ongoing emotions, women frequently own up to them and relate feelings of sadness, loneliness, and isolation. Interestingly and importantly, those feelings most often begin to resolve if women talk about them. It has been so edifying to watch women come back year after year to Reach To Recovery's (Table 31.2) annual day-long meeting and to hear conversations taking place throughout the day between women who are anywhere from newly diagnosed to approximately 25 years after diagnosis. I am convinced that the validation a woman receives from

Table 31.2. Support groups

American Cancer Society—Reach to Recovery
1599 Clifton Road NE,
Atlanta, GA 30329
Phone: 404-320-3333

ChemoCare
220 St. Paul Street,
Westfield, NJ 07090-2146
Phone: 1-800-55-CHEMO
          908-233-1103 (in New Jersey)

National Alliance of Breast Cancer Organizations
9 East 37 Street, 10th Floor
New York, NY 10016
Phone: 212-889-0606

National Breast Cancer Coalition
1707 L Street NW, Suite 1060
Washington, DC 20036
Phone: 202-296-7477

National Coalition for Cancer Survivorship
1010 Wayne Avenue, Suite 505
Silver Spring, MD 20910
Phone: 301-650-8868

Y-Me (breast cancer support program)
212 W. VanBuren Street,
Chicago, IL 60607
Phone: 800-221-2141

knowing that there are others at approximately the same stage in their recovery process who are feeling much of what she feels is as vital as the concrete information shared at the formal sessions.

Sexuality

Among the many issues to be faced short term and longer term are those of intimacy and sexuality. The sexual dynamics and difficulties are frequently complicated. A woman's existential experience of herself as a cancer patient and the impact of the cancer and treatment may collude to leave her with greatly lessened sexual feelings, at least transitionally and for some far longer. These issues must be taken seriously, as research has pointed out that problems with sexuality are among the most persistent of problems faced by women with breast cancer.[3,4]

Patients often report problems at all stages of the sexual response cycle (desire, arousal, orgasm). Part of the genesis may be physical for those women undergoing systemic therapy[5] (including hormonal therapy[6]). Nevertheless, much of the difficulty seems to be connected to a woman's perception that she is less attractive, especially to her partner. It is not unusual to hear from a breast cancer patient some variation of, "A cancer patient is not sexy." Although an open and frank discussion may have a remarkably helpful effect, most couples with whom I have spoken do not feel comfortable having these intimate and delicate conversations.

Unfortunately, problems with sexuality is an area that physicians often fail to address and one that women seldom bring up on their own. It is wise to acknowledge before treatment begins that a woman may have questions and concerns regarding sexuality and that you expect her to seek information from you. Avoidance of this topic by physicians has been connected to concerns about lack of time, discomfort with the topic, and insecurity about what actions to recommend. Yet avoidance of the topic has been offered as one of the greatest obstacles to sexual rehabilitation for cancer survivors.[7] Physicians need not feel the burden of knowing all the answers about sexual issues but may have to cause the issue to surface as a problem and refer the woman to a professional counselor as appropriate. It does not have to be a time-intensive intervention; questions that facilitate this interchange are listed Table 31.3.

Referring women and their partners to books written by breast cancer survivors that include sections on sexuality can be helpful. Such books are listed in Table 31.4.

Two U.S. organizations that certify practitioners on the topic of sexuality can make local expert referrals available. These organizations can be contacted as follows:

American Association of Sex Educators, Counselors and Therapists (AASECT)
45 N. Michigan Avenue, Suite 1717
Chicago, IL 60611
Phone: 312-644-0828

American Association of Marriage and Family Therapists
1133 15th Street, NW, Suite 300
Washington, DC 20005
Phone: 202-452-0109

Table 31.3. Questions facilitating discussion of sexual issues

1. Often women feel some change in their intimate relationship after the breast cancer diagnosis. How has this been for you?
2. People frequently feel some change sexually during this time. What have you noticed?
3. Speaking to a counselor for a few sessions is often helpful because of the impact of the cancer diagnosis and its treatment on sexuality. Would you like a list of local counselors?

Lumpectomy Versus Mastectomy

It was thought that women who underwent breast-conserving therapy (i.e., lumpectomy) would experience less emotional reaction than those with mastectomy. It was thought that women with breast-conserving surgery would avoid the negative impact on their sexuality, as they would maintain both breasts "intact." Such has not been my experience, nor has it been borne out in recent research.[8,9] It does seem true that women who have had breast-conserving surgery have greater satisfaction with their body image, but it does not appear to translate into a trouble-free sexual life. Both groups report the sense of emotional disquiet of being a breast cancer patient/survivor. Research has found no difference between these groups regarding anxiety, depression, or other measures of quality of life.[10] One recent group participant stated, "Whether I have a breast or not just isn't my major issue. What I fear is what breast cancer means to my life."

Impact on the Family

Certainly the woman diagnosed with breast cancer receives the brunt of the psychosocial blow, but her family experiences a dramatic emotional impact as well. In my psychotherapy practice, I have frequently had occasion to work with women and their family members in joint sessions. Families react to living with feelings of uncertainty stimulated by the cancer diagnosis and to confusion about what they should or should not do and say to be supportive. Husbands in

Table 31.4. Recommended reading for breast cancer patients and family

No Less A Woman: Femininity, Sexuality, and Breast Cancer, Deborah Hobler Kahane. Hunter House, 1995 (Phone: 800-266-5592)

Spinning Straw Into Gold: Your Emotional Recovery from Breast Cancer, Ronnie Raye. New York, Simon & Schuster, 1991

Upfront: Sex and The Postmastectomy Woman, Linda Dackman. New York, Viking Penguin, 1990

Man to Man: When the Woman You Love Has Breast Cancer, Andy Murcia and Bob Stewart. New York, St. Martin's Press, 1990

The Breast Cancer Companion: From Diagnosis Through Treatment to Recovery: Everything You Need to Know for Every Step Along the Way, Kathy LaTour. New York, William Morrow. 1993

When The Woman You Love Has Breast Cancer. Chicago, Y-Me, 1995 (Phone: 800-221-2141)

For Single Women With Breast Cancer. Chicago, Y-Me, 1995

particular report concern about what to tell the children and the frustration and guilt about any feelings they perceive as negative (e.g., anger at the inconveniences and struggles they personally are experiencing). Researchers have found that whole families may exhibit many of the same feelings as the person with the cancer diagnosis.[11]

The Single Woman

Cancer patients who are not in a long-term relationship (i.e., "single women") often report an added layer of concern. They feel an even greater vulnerability and worry about their financial resources. It is noteworthy and unfortunate that little of the research on the psychosocial impact of breast cancer has been conducted on single women, which leaves those of us who work with their issues to do so almost entirely based on anecdotal reports and our own clinical experience.

Support

Generally speaking, women need and respond well to receiving support during this time in their lives. Support may come from family, friends, and professionals, although the type received from each may be quite different. Support may be tangible (i.e., help with children, financial) or emotional. Many women do not find it easy to admit that they need or could benefit from some sort of emotional support. It is important that her health care team not "pathologize" this need but, rather, realize it is normal for a woman to have a broad range of emotions and that many find it helpful to talk to other women (and psychosocial counselors) at this time. Many women seem to hold to the "rugged individualist" ethic and endure this time bereft of this potentially helpful connection.

ROLE OF THE PHYSICIAN

When evaluating her treatment options, a woman often seeks the opinion of her primary care physician, particularly if there has been a satisfactory long-term relationship between them. Women often report feeling tremendously supported upon learning that their primary care provider and cancer treatment team have been in communication with each other.

Professional support may be informational. Clear, direct information unencumbered by medical jargon and delivered slowly and with time for questions is often mentioned by women as being wonderfully supportive; and they have bemoaned it when it is not available. It is clear that women need information at every step along the treatment trajectory, and that often they need to have this information repeated, as it is difficult to focus on that which is not only foreign but emotionally charged.

As I have listened to women over the years, it is clear that among the most important factors is the relationship of the woman with breast cancer and her physician. Breast cancer survivors report that they want and need their doctors' interest and understanding, and that they want their physicians to show them that they care.[12] Women speak frequently of wanting "quality relationships" with their doctors and to feel trust and confidence in them. Women need their physicians to legitimize some of what they are experiencing by letting them know which of the physical and emotional reactions are indeed within the normal range. This type of communication is immensely gratifying and reassuring.

It also appears that the primary physician is the professional from whom the advice to "speak to someone regarding this emotional time of life" is most willingly taken. Too often after a woman finally arrives at group or individual counseling do I hear that she did not come sooner because her doctor did not recommend it. In fairness, the physician is often deceived by the woman who is being a "good patient" and thus not sharing information about her emotional state. The physician who is willing to inquire about the woman's emotional adjustment in such a way that she receives "permission" to unmask her emotional needs is offering a real service indeed. All that remains then is for the physician to be prepared to offer appropriate referral. It is important to note that some women are not aware of any elevated emotional needs (often referred to as "denial"); and although it is wise to address the issue of emotions, it may also be appropriate not to press an unwilling patient but to leave the door open for later discussions.

PSYCHIATRIC/PSYCHOLOGICAL SUPPORT

At times one questions whether the depth and breadth of the emotions a woman appears to be experiencing are beyond an illness-connected grief reaction. At these times it is necessary to refer her for psychological/psychiatric evaluation to ensure that she receives the appropriate help. This intervention is important. Although the distinctions between the generally exhibited reactions of sadness, grief, and anxiety and a more full-blown depression are not always easy to distinguish, whenever there is any doubt about the patient's psychological status the physician should encourage a professional evaluation.[13] This advice, though often offered by concerned friends and family, is generally best heeded when delivered by the woman's doctor.

There are circumstances within the breast cancer experience that increase the risk for psychological morbidity. Routine psychological evaluation has been recommended for patients who are in a troubled relationship, who are poorly educated, who have undergone chemotherapy,[14] who have a psychiatric history, who have poor social support,[15,16] or who have had what appears to be a higher than usual number of stressful events within the past 5 years.[17] Referrals made in a kind but firm manner can help a woman move toward a clinical environment in which she can seek and receive support and understanding. She can then work toward resolution of the debilitating emotions with which she may be living.

SUPPORT GROUPS

Support groups, available usually with no fee at most hospitals, can be immensely validating, normalizing, and helpful for both the woman with breast cancer and her family members. Although not everyone feels comfortable in group settings, a recommendation to try a few sessions is advice well given and often well received.

It is often helpful for women to talk with others who have moved on to a normal life after breast cancer. In such cases referral to an American Cancer Society (ACS) Reach to Recovery volunteer may offer a reassuring presence (Table 31.2). These ACS "friendly visitors" have been trained in the appropriate boundaries of their helping role (i.e., never to offer "medical advice" or "medical opinion"). Telephone support of a similar variety is available through Y-Me, a Chicago-based organization that trains breast cancer survivors (and their male partners) to receive calls from women (and their male partners) across the United States who are facing a like experience (Table 31.2).

Referral from the physician to these groups is frequently cherished and seen by the patient as a direct sign of caring. A partial listing of such organizations is included in Table 31.2.

CONCLUSION

Although it is true that some women appear to move through the entire breast cancer experience seemingly untouched emotionally, I encourage physicians to inquire in kindly and empathetic fashion about the issues discussed here. Breast cancer can engender a great variety of emotional reaction at any point along the continuum. The physician who develops an awareness of these issues and makes appropriate recommendations for the patient is caring in a way that supports full recovery of her soma and her psyche.

References

1. Marshall E. SEER/NCI Surveillance Program data. Science 1993;259:618–621
2. Polinsky ML. Functional status of long-term breast cancer survivors: demonstrating chronicity. Health Soc Work 1994;19:165–173
3. Ganz P, Schag AC, Lee J, et al. Breast conservation versus mastectomy: is there a difference in psychological adjustment or quality of life in the year after surgery? Cancer 1992;69:1729–1738
4. Schag CAC, Gans PA, Polinsky ML, et al. Characteristics of women at risk for psychosocial distress in the year after breast cancer. J Clin Oncol 1993;11:783–793
5. Kaplan HS. A neglected issue: the sexual side effects of current treatments for breast cancer. J Sex Marital Ther 1992;18:3–19
6. Kaplan HS, Owett T. The female androgen deficiency syndrome. J Sex Marital Ther 1993;19:3–24
7. Auchincloss SS. Sexual dysfunction in cancer patients: brief clinical evaluation and treatment guidelines. In: Proceedings of the Workshop on Psychosexual Reproduction Issues that Affect Patients with Cancer. Atlanta, GA, American Cancer Society, 1987, pp 122–128
8. Fallowfield LJ. Psychosocial adjustment after treatment for early breast cancer. Oncology 1990;4:89–97
9. Wilmoth CM, Townsend J. A comparison of the effects of lumpectomy versus mastectomy on sexual behaviors. Cancer Pract 1995;3:279–285

10. Ganz PA, Hirji K, Sim MS, et al. Predicting psychosocial risk in patients with breast cancer. Med Care 1993;31:419–431

11. Northouse LL. The impact of cancer in women on the family. Cancer Pract 1995;3:134–142

12. Roberts CS, Cox CE, Reintgen DS, et al. Influence of physician communication on newly diagnosed breast patients' psychologic adjustment and decision-making. Cancer 1994;74:336–341

13. Andersen BL, Doyle-Mirzadeh S. Breast disorders and breast cancer. In Stewart DE, Stotland NL (eds) Psychological Aspects of Women's Health Care: The Interface Between Psychology, Obstetrics and Gynecology. American Psychiatric Press, Wash., D.C., 1993, pp 425–446

14. Shover LR, Yetman RJ, Tuason LJ. et al. Partial mastectomy and breast reconstruction: a comparison of their effects on psychosocial adjustment, body image, and sexuality. Cancer 1995;75:54–64

15. Bloom JR. Softening the psychological sequelae of mastectomy. Prim Care Cancer 1989;9:13–16

16. Glanz K, Lerman C. Psychosocial impact of breast cancer: a critical review. Ann Behav Med 1992;14:204–212

17. Maunsell E, Brisson J, Deschenes L. Psychological distress after initial treatment of breast cancer: assessment of potential risk factors. Cancer 1992;70:120–125

32 MODERN TREATMENT OF LYMPHEDEMA

Arnold Walder

Postmastectomy upper extremity lymphedema is a distressing, disabling, potentially life-threatening consequence of breast cancer treatment. The swollen hand and arm cannot be disguised or hidden by a prosthesis. Lymphedema often causes repeated episodes of cellulitis and lymphangitis, eventual disability, and the need for expensive and time-consuming antibiotic therapy. Rarely, rapidly fatal lymphangiosarcoma (Stewart-Treves syndrome) follows.

The incidence of lymphedema has been reported to be anywhere between 3% and 52% depending on several factors, such as extent of initial surgical treatment (e.g., segmental mastectomy, modified radical mastectomy, Halsted radical mastectomy) and the use of postoperative radiotherapy. Obesity has been identified as one of the leading predictors for lymphedema. Loss of contact with the operating surgeon, an attitude of "you just have to live with it," and a concern for survival from the primary disease have contributed to inadequate reporting of the incidence of the disease.

Precise identification of those most at risk for lymphedema is difficult. All patients treated for breast cancer should be instructed about activities that prevent increasing lymph production and those that restrict lymph flow. Patients are advised to avoid extreme heat (sun exposure, sauna baths), tight or restrictive garments, and high-impact exercises. They are encouraged to participate in active exercise. They are instructed in meticulous attention to skin care, the use of a skin lotion with a slightly acidic pH, and avoidance of skin puncture and blood pressure measurement using the at-risk extremity. Because of the reduction in ambient pressure at altitude, they should be cautioned to wear an appropriate compression garment for airline travel.

CONVENTIONAL THERAPY

Conventional treatment for postmastectomy lymphedema has been application of an external compression garment (sleeve), pneumatic compression, diuretics, surgical procedures, and often, unfortunately, therapeutic nihilism. The introduction of complete decongestive physiotherapy (CDP) represents a major advance and is discussed in detail.

Wearing an elastic sleeve prior to swelling reduction is of almost no value. It does nothing to reduce the swelling, delays proper treatment, and if fitted by unskilled personnel may contribute to increased discomfort and swelling.

Diuretics are useless and detrimental. They promote excretion of free water, further concentrate the remaining plasma protein, increase osmotic pressure, promote increased swelling, and because of the concentrated protein lead to fibrosis in the subcutaneous tissue.

Benzpyrones belong to a group of drugs that include the bioflavonoids and coumarin. These naturally occurring compounds increase macrophage activity, proteolysis, and the removal of excess protein from the tissue spaces, and they relieve chronic high-protein edema. Lymphedema is mildly reduced with prolonged use of these drugs. Several benzpyrones are used clinically, topically and systemically, but the U.S. Food and Drug Administration (FDA) has approved none for safety or efficacy.

Single-chamber pneumatic compression devices, and their modern incarnations using multichambered gradient pressures and sequential pumping from distal to proximal, have not been found to provide a lasting benefit. The externally applied pressure forces protein-rich fluid from the periphery to the root of the extremity into an area of the ipsilateral trunk that is already congested, without providing an alternative channel for the fluid to be restored into the general circulation. These devices are expensive, often painful, require daily use for the remainder of the patient's life, and may add to the problem. Electron microscopic studies have shown massive injury to lymphatic collectors and vessels after only minutes of exposure to pressures of 70 mm Hg.

COMPLETE DECONGESTIVE PHYSIOTHERAPY

Professor Michael Földi introduced complete (or complex) decongestive physiotherapy (CDP) based on many years of careful laboratory and clinical investigation. This treatment regimen consists of a tetrad of manual lymph drainage, compression bandaging, remedial exercises, and meticulous skin care. CDP must be performed by appropriately trained therapists. During the treatment phase (phase I) the patient undergoes one or two treatments of approximately 70 minutes daily for 2–4 weeks. During the maintenance phase (phase II) the patient maintains and may actually continue to improve the results by daily home care, including wearing an elastic sleeve during the day, wrapping the arm at night, doing a series of exercises for 10 minutes twice each day, and caring for the skin of the hand and arm. Patients are evaluated monthly to record progress and measure for a new elastic compression garment as needed.

Manual Lymphatic Drainage

Manual lymph drainage (MLD) is a gentle massage technique using four essential motions—kneading, stretching, rubbing, tapping—with a carefully designed technique to stimulate the dilatation of lymph vessels in the trunk and to channel lymph and edema fluid toward adjacent, functioning lymph basins. MLD begins with stimulation of lymph vessels in the trunk, neck, contralateral axilla, and ipsilateral groin, followed by manual decongestion of the involved trunk, shoulder, axilla, arm, forearm, wrist, and hand. Edema fluids are directed to new pathways, toward functioning lymph basins across the midline, over the shoulder, down to the groin, and around to the back. Stroking the skin should be done with no more than 30 mm Hg pressure.

Compression Bandaging

Compression bandaging is done immediately after manual lymph drainage. Three layers of material are used. The innermost lager is light nonelastic cotton gauze for absorption of sweat; the next is padding to distribute the pressure evenly; finally, an external, minimally elastic wrapping is used for compression. Foam rubber strips are inserted to ensure uniform pressure distribution and to selectively increase pressure in fibrotic areas. Bandages are applied from the fingertips to the axilla, with maximum pressure distally and minimal pressure proximally. The bandage does not constrict blood flow but increases the interstitial pressure and acts as a barrier against which the muscles can apply pressure to the dilated lymphatic vessels whose valves are not functional. External compression prevents reaccumulation of evacuated edema fluid. The edema fluid now gathering in truncal lymphatic channels then flows into the venous circulation via the thoracic duct. The kidneys filter the water, and the protein is returned for metabolic needs. Patients are encouraged to drink 1–2 liters of water daily to dilute the lymphatic fluid further and encourage more rapid flow.

Remedial Exercise

The patient performs a series of remedial (nonimpact) exercises designed to increase lymph flow in the remaining lymph vessels and the now stimulated collateral lymph channels, thereby propelling the lymph to the thoracic duct.

Skin Care

Meticulous skin care is an essential part of the program. Bacterial and fungal infections should be cleared before embarking on a course of manual lymph drainage. Patients are encouraged to use a commercially available skin cream or lotion with pH 5.5–6.0 (e.g., Euceryn, Nivea, or Stevens) to supplement the bacteriostatic effect of their bath soap.

   Patient response is evaluated by daily circumferential measurement at seven designated points on the extremity. Extremity volume determined by water displacement has been shown to bear a direct linear relation to that determined by circumferential measurement. For the purposes of one study the response to therapy was considered complete when the extremities became symmetric. Reduction of 50% or more of excess volume was considered a partial response, and anything less than 50% reduction of excess volume was entered as a nonresponse. Altogether 163 patients were treated. Because of missing values only 154 patients

Table 32.1. Comparison of lymphedema pump and manual lymph drainage

Lymphedema pump	Manual lymph drainage
Expensive	Relatively inexpensive
Lifetime use	Two daily active treatments for 3–4 weeks
Often painful	Painless
Little long-term benefit	Proved long-term benefit
Potential injury to lymphatics	Simple maintenance program
Risk of genital edema	Absolutely risk-free

were included. A total of 32 patients (20.8%) showed a complete response, 88 (57.1%) reached a partial response, and 32 (20.8%) showed considerable reduction but were considered by these criteria to show no response. Examination of the data shows that patients who have the greatest disparity in limb size (double the volume of the nonaffected limb) tend to be nonresponders, and those with 30% excess volume tend to have a complete response. The implication is that the sooner one treats the lymphedema, the more likely is a complete response.

Complete deconjestive physiotherapy (CDP) has been used by properly trained therapists in Europe, Australia, and the United States to treat thousands of patients. It is safe and effective; and if the patient is compliant, she rarely requires any further active treatment. The patient is returned to her home much improved, usually ready to assume almost all activities of daily living, with minimal maintenance required. There is no risk to the patient, no detrimental side effect, and no toxicity. The advantages/disadvantages of manual lymph drainage (MLD) are compared with those of a mechanical lymphedema pump in Table 32.1.

33 Pregnancy Before, During, and After Breast Cancer

Audrey J. Arona

ancer of the breast is the most common invasive cancer in women, now estimated to develop, during her lifetime, in one of every nine women. As many as 15% of breast cancers present during the childbearing years. The most common cancer in pregnant women is breast cancer; and although it occurs rarely, it causes significant emotional issues for all involved. Moreover, the clinical challenge is often greater than with nonpregnant women. Finally, because physicians deal with this situation so infrequently, it is easy to propagate misinformation.

Many risk factors are known to predispose women to the development of breast cancer, including early menarche, late menopause, nulliparity, no lactation, obesity, family history of breast cancer, and most of all age. Body mass and age are known to influence prognosis. Cigarette smoking is not a risk factor for breast cancer, but it is associated with axillary node involvement.

Pregnancy and lactation have not been shown to be risk factors for the development of breast cancer. In fact, women who breastfeed have a lower incidence of breast cancer. Pregnancy disrupts the cyclic ovarian function. This altered hormonal status is believed to allow proliferation of the breast epithelium, followed by differentiation and mitotic rest. Hence it is believed that lactation has a protective effect on a woman's risk for breast cancer. It is possible that lactation allows neoplastic differentiation, with removal of the noxious agents and abnormal/damaged cells associated with breast epithelium.

INCIDENCE

The incidence of breast cancer in pregnant women is low, approximately 3:10,000. Only 2–4% of all breast cancers occur during pregnancy or lactation. Whereas most patients with breast cancer are diagnosed between ages 50 and 55, the average age of pregnant patients diagnosed with breast cancer is 32–38 years. The youngest age reported for a pregnant patient with advanced/disseminated breast cancer is 18 years. Because patients are usually older, however, and because more and more women are choosing to delay their childbearing years, the incidence of breast cancer during pregnancy is expected to increase. This might be due to the loss of any protective benefit of early childbearing.

ETIOLOGY

Pregnancy and cancer have one thing in common: they are both conditions where antigenic tissue is tolerated by the immune system. However, there is no evidence to show that pregnancy is responsible for the generation or progression of breast cancer. Pregnant women do in fact have depressed cell-mediated immunity, and they are known to have hormonal changes that might be immunosuppressive, such as increased circulation of corticosteroids. These changes could allow tumor growth but probably are not responsible for its initiation. It is known that a cancer that presents during pregnancy has probably been clinically apparent for months and biologically present for years. Therefore the etiology of breast cancer during pregnancy, as in the nonpregnant patient, remains unknown.

DIAGNOSIS

Obstetricians must screen all pregnant patients for breast cancer. An appropriate history and thorough breast examination should be performed and instructions for breast self-examination given. Physicians should not hesitate to evaluate pregnant patients with breast complaints. These symptoms are often presumed to be related to the normal physiologic changes that accompany pregnancy, and biopsies are often delayed until after delivery. Serosanguineous discharge from both breasts during late pregnancy is normal. A mass with or without unilateral discharge warrants an immediate workup and diagnosis. As gestation progresses, the breast examination becomes more difficult, so it must be performed early.

Managing pregnant women with breast masses poses a dilemma. These women are at a low risk for cancer because of their age and, as with nonpregnant women of the same age, their lesions are probably benign. Nonetheless, it is impossible to be certain without histologic tissue diagnosis. Performing operations during pregnancy risks teratogenesis, low birth weight, and preterm labor; but a delay in the workup and diagnosis of a malignancy alters the stage and therefore the patient's outcome/prognosis. In pregnant patients the average delay from the initial detection of the mass to effective treatment generally exceeds 5 months. An even longer delay, often exceeding 7 months, has resulted in pregnant patients with axillary lymph node involvement.

This delay in diagnosis is probably the reason for the worsened prognosis overall for pregnant patients with breast cancer: 25% of these patients have inflammatory changes; 80% have axillary adenopathy; and 27% have evidence of metastatic disease at the time of diagnosis. Recurrences are seen in approximately 70%, and the mean survival is 18 months. One study found an average 5–15 months for the duration of symptoms before diagnosis in pregnant women. Physician and patient neglect can be responsible. It is difficult to palpate a dominant mass in the pregnant or lactating breast because of engorgement, tenderness, and breast tissue hypertrophy. The pregnant breasts become tense and multinodular. During pregnancy, masses are commonly ignored even when noticed by the patient or her physician. The plan often is to pursue evaluation after delivery if the mass persists. Screening mammography is not usually performed in pregnant or lactating women owing to the relative increase in water density and hyperplastic changes, each making the reading more difficult. Furthermore, mammography during pregnancy or lactation can be a painful experience for a woman.

Obstetricians and gynecologists can play a major role in the diagnosis of breast cancer in pregnant and lactating women. A thorough breast examination at the first prenatal visit, before breast engorgement occurs, is essential and the only means by which these patients can be diagnosed more rapidly. Physicians should perform breast examinations throughout prenatal care, paying particular attention to any changes inconsistent with pregnancy. A prenatal patient should be taught and encouraged to perform breast self-examination throughout her pregnancy and for the remainder of her life.

As with all patients with breast cancer, pregnant or lactating women with breast cancer usually present with a painless lump. To simply follow up in a few months or deal with it after delivery is inappropriate. As with all dominant masses, the clinical triad of clinical breast examination, mammography, and fine-needle aspiration (FNA) is essential and usually yields a definitive diagnosis. FNA cytology has more than 90% sensitivity and specificity. FNA is particularly applicable for obtaining a cytologic diagnosis of neoplasms during pregnancy and lactation.

A new mother may complain that her infant refuses to nurse from a breast in which a malignancy is subsequently diagnosed. This has been called the "milk-rejection sign." Occasionally, a pregnant or lactating patient presents with metastatic adenocarcinoma. In such a case, a primary breast cancer should be strongly suspected.

Mammography is not contraindicated in the pregnant/lactating patient. Modern techniques and proper abdominal and pelvic shielding prevent fetal exposure to the minimal degree of radiation present. There are no reports of damage to any fetus following mammography in pregnant patients; but because a mammogram in these cases rarely influences therapy, it seems reasonable not to obtain it. Particularly in young women, ultrasonography of the breast is an option often preferred by radiologists.

If a persistent dominant mass remains undiagnosed after FNA cytologic examination, excision biopsy is the next step. The biopsy can be performed in an outpatient operative setting by the standard technique with local anesthesia. If required, general anesthesia is considered safe to use during the second and third trimesters. Milk fistulas can be a complication following excisional biopsy in the pregnant or lactating patient, especially if the mass removed is located in a central and deep position within the breast.

PATHOLOGY

The histopathology of breast masses in pregnant patients is the same as that for nonpregnant patients. Matching age for age, the probability of a biopsy specimen demonstrating cancer is the same for pregnant and nonpregnant patients, but the axillary lymph node involvement in pregnant women is higher, ranging from 70% to 90%. It is probably due to the advanced stage of disease at diagnosis. It was previously thought that inflammatory carcinoma was more common in pregnant patients with breast cancer, but multiple studies have shown that the incidence is similar to the 1.5–4.0% reported among nonpregnant breast cancer patients.

A breast mass detected during pregnancy is usually benign, most commonly representing fibrocystic change, galactocele, abscess, or fibroadenoma. Other rare causes of a breast mass during pregnancy include leukemia, lymphoma, sarcoma, and tuberculosis.

STAGING

When a breast cancer is diagnosed, clinical staging of the disease is necessary so appropriate therapeutic decisions can be made. Except for blood work and physical examination, many of the staging procedures involve radiation exposure. There is considerable controversy over what is an appropriate staging evaluation for the patient who is pregnant. Liver tests and calcium and carcinoembryonic antigen studies may be helpful but do not provide a definitive diagnosis of metastatic disease.

Radiation risk to the fetus depends on the age of the fetus. During the preimplantation stage (days 0–10) any radiation exposure can lead to embryonic death. During organogenesis (days 11–56) radiation exposure can lead to developmental abnormalities, the most common of which is microcephaly. Doses as little as 10 rad may cause birth defects. Doses in excess of 100 rad produce abnormalities in 100% of cases (as evidenced by the atomic bomb survivors). During the growth stage (after day 57), it takes larger radiation doses to cause any significant abnormality. Beyond 25–30 weeks the fetus is more resistant to radiation injury. However, the statistics on the effects of radiation on the developing fetus were extrapolated from studies done on animals with considerably higher doses than are incurred with current human studies.

The data are insufficient to determine the long-term risk to the fetus from low-dose radiation such as that involved in most current scanning procedures. Documentation of osseous metastases might change therapeutic recommendations, so a bone scan could be important in patients who have symptoms suggestive of bone metastases. The radiation dose exposure to a fetus from a bone scan is approximately 0.1 rad. The maximum fetal exposure allowed by the Nuclear Regulatory Commission for radiation employees is 500 mrem.

The possibility of leukemia and other malignancies is of concern for children whose mothers undergo intrapartum diagnostic radiography of the abdomen.

Intrapartum radiation exposure may cause defects in development and retardation of growth, although for exposures below 5–10 rad gross congenital anomalies and intrauterine growth retardation have not been reported. Careful consideration should be given prior to performing any diagnostic radiographic procedure during pregnancy, but the more commonly used procedures expose the fetus to only a fraction of tolerable radiation levels. Therefore diagnostic procedures for staging breast cancer in pregnant women are considered reasonably safe.

The risk of carcinogenesis from radiation exposure is another concern. Even with the atomic bomb experience the association between cancer and fetal exposure to radiation has not been clearly established; therefore exposure to x-rays in utero is best avoided unless absolutely necessary. This rule does not apply to chest radiographs, as proper abdominal and pelvic shielding are protective to the fetus and ensure minimal risk. A patient with breast cancer and central nervous system (CNS) symptoms is appropriately evaluated by computed tomography (CT) scan. Suspected liver involvement can be evaluated by ultrasonography.

TREATMENT

Psychological and emotional factors overshadow the treatment of breast cancer at any time in a woman's life, but pregnancy adds to the burden for all parties involved, including the patient's physician. Many controversial questions arise about treatment options, including their effect on the developing fetus, the patient's self-image, subsequent fertility, and of course her very life. A multidisciplinary approach to the patient's treatment is best, and the team should include the patient's obstetrician, a perinatologist, a surgeon, a medical oncologist, and a radiation oncologist if radiation treatment is necessary.

During the 1940s physicians believed that breast cancer during pregnancy or lactation was so aggressive that these patients could not be "cured" by surgery and that the situation was near hopeless. It is now known that the stage of the cancer at the time of presentation/diagnosis is what determines the prognosis and overall survival. This, of course, is true for pregnant and nonpregnant patients.

Treatment of breast cancer for pregnant patients does not differ from that for nonpregnant, nonlactating patients. However, because of unanswered concerns about the well-being of the fetus, modified radical mastectomy (MRM) with or without primary reconstruction is commonly the recommended treatment for locoregional control in patients during early pregnancy with stage I or II cancers. If radiation therapy can prudently be delayed until after delivery, breast-conserving therapy (BCT) is an alternative for selected pregnant patients with early-stage breast cancer. As with any major surgery performed during pregnancy, the risk for miscarriage is estimated at less than 1%. The primary therapeutic breast surgery, including mastectomy, is usually performed as soon as possible after definitive diagnosis, although if delivery is imminent a delay of up to 2 weeks is reasonable. Breast surgery may safely be performed at the time of an obstetrically indicated cesarean section.

Termination of the pregnancy (discussed below) is not necessary and does not improve the prognosis or the survival rate. Nevertheless, the mother may elect not to continue the pregnancy.

Radiation Therapy

Fetal exposure to radiation should be avoided. Organogenesis (days 11–56) is the most radiosensitive time, with the brain, skeleton, and eyes most commonly affected. When radiation is given, the dose to the fetus (mostly from scattered radiation) is calculated depending on how far the fetus is from the center of the field of radiation, the size of the irradiated field, and the radiation energy. Radiation treatment for breast cancer involves the whole breast, generally with a boost to the area of the tumor bed. This method produces a scattered dose of radiation exposure to the fetus that is unacceptably high. Even during early gestation, if a fetus is 25 cm away from the field of radiation and if 7500 rad were to be given, the fetus would be exposed to approximately 30 rad. This dose is unacceptable and places the fetus at significant risk. When the fundus of the uterus enlarges to the xiphoid, the fetus can receive as much as 100 rad. During this later trimester, teratogenesis is markedly decreased, but radiation can still cause microcephaly and intrauterine growth retardation and can create an increased risk for childhood cancers. For these reasons, radiation therapy is usually not recommended during pregnancy. Because BCT usually requires adjuvant radiation therapy, it is not generally advisable in pregnant patients with breast cancer, unless the radiation can reasonably be withheld for a period of time. Special treatment options are made, however, for some pregnant patients who insist on BCT. It might involve primary surgical excision, followed by a small boost of radiation to the breast area, with full irradiation to the breast after delivery. Usually efforts are made to discourage patients from this approach. A more appropriate treatment plan is primary surgical excision upon diagnosis, sampling of lymph nodes, then observation until after delivery, when radiation therapy may begin.

Adjuvant Chemotherapy

For patients with breast cancer and node involvement, adjuvant chemotherapy is usually recommended. This therapy is now being offered and recommended more often to patients without axillary lymph node involvement as well. There are no current published data concerning the use of chemotherapy in pregnant patients. The cytotoxic agents are damaging to rapidly dividing tissue, and these drugs could cause major damage to a fetus, a fact that has been well established in animal studies. Chemotherapy creates an increased risk for teratogenicity during the first trimester and therefore is not usually recommended. Some chemotherapeutic agents have been used for metastatic disease during the second and third trimesters without apparent harm to the fetus. There are reports, however, that chemotherapy given during later trimesters has been associated with intrauterine growth retardation. In addition, premature labor occurs more commonly in women treated with chemotherapy. For these reasons, chemotherapy is usually delayed until after delivery even though delay may reduce the benefit of adjuvant therapy.

Adjuvant Hormonal Therapy

Tamoxifen has been used in some patients with breast cancer, but the drug has not been well studied in pregnant patients. Oophorectomy has not been shown to improve overall survival in breast cancer patients regardless of whether the woman is pregnant, nor has it been shown to delay recurrences or delay or interrupt the course of the disease, even when lymph nodes are involved.

ANESTHESIA CONSIDERATIONS

There is no evidence that breast biopsies create a significant risk to the mother or fetus, even if general anesthesia is necessary, but it is important to consider the physiologic changes of pregnancy. Blood volume increases; the heart rate increases, leading to an increased cardiac output; and the lower hemoglobin content creates difficulty maintaining oxygen saturation. Pregnancy also changes the coagulation profile by increasing the platelet count and fibrinogen levels, leading to hypercoagulation and an increased risk for thromboembolism. The enlarged uterus elevates the diaphragm, compromising lung volume by decreasing functional residual capacity, and produces a higher respiratory rate. The anesthetic build-up of vapor in the alveoli can result in more rapid induction of anesthesia. Forced hyperventilation and maternal respiratory alkalosis can cause fetal acidosis if the patient is not carefully monitored. Ventilatory balance should be maintained. Because of the hypervascularity of the respiratory tract, intubation can be hazardous. Gastric emptying during pregnancy is prolonged, approximately 60% more than normal, and the pressure on the stomach leads to increased reflux. Therefore pregnant patients require specialized intubation techniques to avoid aspiration of gastric fluids.

Studies to date have not shown any negative effects of anesthetic agents on the fetus, even during the development stages. No long-term effects on the fetus of the various narcotic and sedation agents used in conjunction with anesthesia have been confirmed. Fetal monitoring should be utilized to recognize early fetal distress. General anesthesia is considered safe for the mother and fetus so long as special care is given to the unique requirements of the pregnant condition.

CURRENT MANAGEMENT RECOMMENDATIONS

Management of breast cancer patients should be individualized, although in pregnant patients the preferred primary treatment for stage I and II (operable) breast cancers is MRM. If breast conservation is a priority, wide local tumor excision with clear surgical margins and axillary lymph node dissection (AxLND) can be performed, with plans for radiation therapy to follow after delivery. If the AxLNs are involved, chemotherapy is recommended but delayed until the second trimester or after delivery. An early cesarean section or labor induction, after fetal lung maturity is documented, is an option to shorten the delay of any necessary adjuvant therapy.

For stage III (locally advanced) or stage IV (distant metastases) breast cancers diagnosed early in pregnancy, for which both radiation and chemotherapy are strongly recommended, termination of the pregnancy should be considered. For patients later in gestation, as previously noted, adjuvant therapy following primary surgical therapy can be delayed, but the significance and ultimate risk of delaying adjuvant therapy is not known.

Clearly there are no "right" answers to the many questions concerning appropriate treatment plans for pregnant women diagnosed with breast cancer. The patient must be counseled about all known and theoretic risks and benefits inherent in any therapeutic approach. The patient's family should be participants in these difficult decisions.

PREGNANCY TERMINATION

In the past abortion was almost automatic for pregnant women diagnosed with breast cancer based on the theory that the higher levels of estrogen and progesterone might stimulate breast cancer cells. It was the basis for the previously held belief that breast cancers presenting during pregnancy were biologically more aggressive. However, no adverse affect of pregnancy per se has been documented. There are no reported prospective randomized trials demonstrating the effect of pregnancy termination on breast cancer's biologic behavior or prognosis. Aborting does not appear to affect maternal survival or the clinical course of the disease. As with nonpregnant patients, it is the stage of cancer at diagnosis that is most predictive of survival. Thus therapeutic abortions are no longer considered appropriate treatment for patients who are pregnant and have breast cancer. Similarly, pregnant patients with breast cancer are no longer encouraged to undergo prophylactic oophorectomy.

Pregnant patients fear that their breast cancer may be metastasized to the fetus. These patients should be reassured that such metastasis has not been reported with breast cancer. The cancers known to have transplacental spread to the fetus are choriocarcinoma, leukemia, lymphosarcoma, and melanoma.

It seems reasonable for patients with advanced breast cancer who are in early pregnancy to terminate their pregnancies. These patients obviously are anxious about their disease and their immediate prognosis. Pregnancy termination allows prompt adjuvant therapy and irradiation as indicated while avoiding the harmful (often disastrous) effects on the developing fetus.

PROGNOSIS

According to current data, being pregnant does not alter the prognosis of patients with breast cancer. When matched age for age and stage for stage, the 5- and 10-year survival rates for pregnant women with breast cancer are the same as those for women who are not pregnant. For pregnant or lactating women with breast cancer who do not have lymph node involvement, the 5-year survival is approximately 80%. The 10-year survival is approximately 70% with surgical therapy. If there is nodal involvement, the 10-year survival decreases to 30%.

As with nonpregnant patients, tumor size has a direct relation to the probability of axillary node involvement. When the cancer is ≤1.0 cm, the nodes are involved in 26% of cases. When the cancer is >10 cm in diameter, 80% of patients have involved AxLNs. Age is related to nodal involvement. Older women have fewer AxLNs involved. Among patients under 40 years of age, 49% have involved nodes; 42% of patients age 70 or older have metastasis to the AxLNs. No difference has been noted in the incidence of node involvement in women who have breastfed their infant(s) versus those who have not.

Age has a much greater influence on breast cancer survival than does pregnancy. Age comparisons show that the overall 5-year survival for patients under age 40 is significantly greater (75%) than for those older than 40 (55%). Pregnancy, especially if it occurs for the first time at an early age, decreases the epidemiologic relative risk for breast cancer.

Estrogen and progesterone receptor status and its prognostic value in pregnant patients with breast cancer is not well documented. It is known that the estrogen receptor/progesterone receptor ratio is decreased in pregnant patients with breast cancer, but the significance of this finding has not been determined. In cases where hormone receptor studies have been performed, approximately 70% of gestational breast cancers have been reported to be estrogen receptor-negative.

SUBSEQUENT PREGNANCY

The concern about pregnancy following breast cancer centers on the possibility that the hormonal changes of pregnancy might stimulate breast cancer cell proliferation. This is why bilateral oophorectomy used to be recommended in an attempt to improve the prognosis of premenopausal patients. Breast cancer patients were, of course, discouraged from future pregnancy. Recent studies, albeit with small numbers, have shown that pregnancy after breast cancer does not alter the prognosis. In fact, some studies have shown that survival rates are better for patients who subsequently become pregnant and deliver live children than for patients who do not. Selection bias may play a part in these results as patients who feel well opt to have children, whereas those who do not feel well probably do not.

Most breast cancer recurrences appear within 2–3 years after the initial diagnosis. Therefore breast cancer patients have been advised to avoid pregnancy during that time. This suggestion is more for the social effects of losing a mother than for any biologic effect of the pregnancy on the prognosis of the cancer. If a patient has axillary node involvement, the recommendation to defer pregnancy is usually extended to 5 years. Prior to a breast cancer survivor's attempting pregnancy, it seems prudent to have a consultation with a medical oncologist and a full evaluation for evidence of metastatic disease. The workup usually includes bone and liver scans, chest radiography, mammography, and CT scan of the brain if neurologic signs are present.

LACTATION

There is no current convincing clinical evidence that lactation or the suppression thereof improves the prognosis or survival rates of postpartum women who develop or have breast cancer. However, there are two situations in which suppression of lactation is generally recommended. First, when breast surgery is planned during the immediate postpartum period, suppressing lactation may decrease the size and vascularity of the breast, allowing the surgery to be performed with less risk. Second, if chemotherapy is planned during the postpartum period, nursing is generally not recommended, as the drugs can reach high levels in human breast milk and can cause neonatal neutropenia.

CONCLUSIONS

There are no convincing studies reporting the influence of pregnancy or lactation on the development of breast cancer. It seems that pregnancy per se does not worsen the prognosis for women with breast cancer. However, pregnancy can obscure the disease, in many cases for more than several months; and by then vascular invasion and potential metastatic process may have begun. For all women with breast cancer, it is the stage (clinical and pathologic) at the time of diagnosis and primary treatment that is predictive of survival. Many breast cancers during pregnancy and lactation are diagnosed at a late stage, accounting for the apparently adverse prognosis in these patients. Increased vigilance on the part of physicians during prenatal and postpartum care can reverse this adverse trend. Thorough breast examinations for pregnant and lactating women are essential, and complete evaluation of a palpable breast mass should not be delayed.

34 BREAST PROBLEMS SPECIFIC TO PREGNANCY AND THE PERIPARTUM PERIOD

T. Murphy Goodwin

MASTITIS

Mastitis is the most common serious breast problem related to pregnancy and usually occurs around 4 weeks postpartum. The problem is rarely seen during the first 2–3 weeks postpartum and is uncommon after 5 weeks. Fever, erythema, and tenderness are noted, with the erythema usually confined to the area of a single breast lobule. The differential diagnosis includes breast engorgement, which is almost always bilateral, and the rare inflammatory carcinoma. In the latter case the erythema and induration are usually more diffuse and skin changes are more common. The principal clue, however, is its failure to respond to antibiotic therapy.

Although it has been shown that a number of organisms can be involved in puerperal mastitis, by far the most common is *Staphylococcus aureus*. Empiric therapy directed at this organism has a high success rate unless abscess formation is present. First-line therapeutic regimens include dicloxicillin (500 mg PO q6h) or amoxicillin/clavulanate (500 mg PO q6h). For penicillin-allergic patients, erythromycin (500 mg PO q6h) may be given. Therapy should be continued for 7–10 days. The patient should be encouraged to continue nursing (or pumping) the breast during therapy, as drainage of the infected area is important to the response to therapy. The nutrition of the breast milk is unaffected by acute infection. Symptomatic support with analgesics or hot or cold packs on the breast are recommended. Patients should be seen within 48–72 hours to document an adequate response.

A number of other adjunctive measures have been recommended, including culturing milk from the affected breast and milk leukocyte counts, and from the infant a complete blood count and cultures of the nose, throat, and skin. We do not undertake any of these measures unless there is recurrent mastitis.

At the initiation of therapy it is important to confirm that there is no evidence of breast abscess formation, as the latter may not respond to antibiotic therapy alone. If an abscess is suspected on physical examination, aspiration with an 18-gauge needle can be undertaken. Ultrasound guidance (and confirmation of the abscess cavity) is useful for needle aspiration. A good response to antibiotic therapy can be expected following needle aspiration, although often aspiration drainage of an abscess must be repeated. If there is delay in the response to needle aspiration and antibiotic therapy, surgical drainage under general anesthesia should be considered. Should this be required, it is reasonable to perform a biopsy at the same time to rule out inflammatory carcinoma. When an abscess is identified, nursing the infant on the affected breast should be discouraged, as serious newborn infections may result. The principal complication of a neglected abscess is disfigurement of the breast.

Mastitis may be seen during the antepartum period. The presentation and treatment is similar to what has been described for the peripartum period. Because it is an uncommon finding, however, less common causes should be considered more prominently in the differential diagnosis. They include tuberculous mastitis, granulomatous mastitis, or the previously mentioned inflammatory breast carcinoma.

BREAST ASYMMETRY AND ENLARGEMENT

Some women notice asymmetric enlargement of the breasts during pregnancy or, even more, marked asymmetry in the involution of the breasts during the period of lactation. The cause of these changes in breast size is not known. The problem seems to be entirely cosmetic. Breast pain and tenderness, especially in the area of the nipples, are commonly noted during early pregnancy. These problems generally diminish after the first trimester, and no specific treatment is usually required.

Enlargement of the breast is normal during pregnancy beginning usually around the end of the first trimester. Occasionally massive enlargement (hypertrophy) occurs. A number of therapies for hypertrophy have been attempted, of which bromocriptine appears to be the most successful. Doses as high as 20mg/day have been reported, but a common starting dose would be 5mg in two divided doses daily. Patients may require mechanical measures to relieve pressure. When massive hypertrophy is noted, it is essential to give prophylactic antibiotics, as skin breakdown and secondary infection can be a catastrophic problem. Many patients eventually (e.g., postpartum) require reduction mammoplasty or even mastectomy in severe cases to relieve their symptoms.

Once hypertrophy has been noted in one pregnancy, it is likely to occur in all subsequent pregnancies. Unfortunately, even after reduction mammoplasty, the breast may undergo hypertrophy in a subsequent pregnancy. Breastfeeding is not recommended, as the breast may continue to enlarge during the postpartum period, and breastfeeding exacerbates this enlargement.

Mammary hypertrophy has been associated with large amounts of parathyroid hormone-related protein (PTHr-protein) in some cases. It has been shown that mammary hypertrophy can be associated with rapid bone loss due to production of PTHr-protein. The mild bone loss seen during pregnancy is not exacerbated by a 6-month period of lactation.

Ectopic Breast Tissue

Occasionally, ectopic breast tissue or supernumerary breast tissue presents for the first time during pregnancy or the puerperium. The presentation of supernumerary breasts ranges from a complete breast, the areola only, or simply a patch of hair. The true incidence is unknown, but it appears to be relatively uncommon. The axilla is the most frequent site of presentation, although any area of the milk line down the flank to the vulva can be involved and occasionally even areas outside the milk line.

Supernumerary nipples occur in 0.6–3.5% of women. Again, they are usually present along the milk line and may appear as part of a totally developed nest of ectopic breast tissue, or they may be easily confused with skin tags or nevi. Neither the supernumerary nipples, the ectopic breast tissue, nor supernumerary breasts are problematic per se. They may be associated with underlying renal and vascular disease, and they are part of a number of Mendelian syndromes. If they are identified, therefore, a careful history and physical should be undertaken. Specific treatment (e.g., surgical excision) is indicated only if they are symptomatic.

Breastfeeding During Pregnancy

Some patients may wish to continue breastfeeding a child from a previous pregnancy during the current pregnancy. In general, it presents no specific problems. After the middle of the second trimester, however, a distinct pattern of uterine contractions may be noted after suckling; and it is unknown if this poses a risk for preterm birth. It seems wise to undertake evaluation of the cervix and to observe the pattern of contractions carefully. If cervical change is noted, the breastfeeding should be discontinued.

How Pregnancy Affects the Approach to Common Breast Problems

A bloody nipple discharge, most commonly seen during the second or third trimester, can be due to proliferation of the epithelium, commonly seen during pregnancy. Cytology can be misleading owing to the rapid cellular changes taking place; as with nonpregnant women, evaluation of nipple discharge smears is not cost-effective and rarely assists in clinical management. Unless a distinct mass is noted, observation and reassurance are appropriate. The problem should be evaluated further if it persists more than 2 months after delivery.

Galactorrhea is not uncommon during pregnancy as the breast prepares for the normal postpartum period of lactation. The patient should be reassured that it represents a normal part of breast development during pregnancy.

The approach to the breast mass during pregnancy does not differ from the approach in the nonpregnant state. A persistent dominant breast mass must be definitively diagnosed. Evaluation by fine-needle aspiration, tissue core-needle biopsy, and open surgical biopsy are described in Chapter 14. The principal difference seen with a breast mass during pregnancy is that the distribution of lesions that present as a dominant breast mass during pregnancy is different. Changes specific to pregnancy and lactation that present as breast masses are cystic changes, which include the galactocele, the lactating adenoma, fibroadenomas with lactational change, and lactational changes within the breast (including lobular hyperplasia). The galactocele yields cloudy fluid on aspiration, and the mass regresses immediately after aspiration. The lactating adenoma develops during pregnancy, whereas the fibroadenoma with lactational change usually presents as a mass that was present before pregnancy that has now undergone enlargement. Above all, it is critical to avoid delaying diagnosis when a mass is discovered during pregnancy. If there is a low suspicion of malignancy, the mass may be observed for a short time (2–4 weeks), but if it persists it should be further evaluated for a definitive diagnosis.

The use of mammography during pregnancy is problematic. Contrast is reduced significantly during pregnancy owing to the increased water content and breast density. Although mammography may be performed safely during pregnancy from the point of view of radiation exposure to the fetus (<50 mrad), a negative mammography result should never be used to defer further evaluation of a dominant mass via biopsy.

Cytologic examination of specimens from fine-needle aspiration should be undertaken by a pathologist experienced with the changes characteristic of pregnancy. Proliferative nuclear changes can mimic some of the changes of the epithelial cell characteristics of malignancy in nonpregnant women.

ISSUES RELATED TO BREAST CANCER DURING PREGNANCY

When the diagnosis of carcinoma of the breast is established during pregnancy, the obstetrician is frequently the first person to talk with the patient and deal with her questions: Will the fact that I am pregnant make the cancer worse? Would terminating the pregnancy improve my prognosis? If I were to continue the pregnancy, can the disease be fully evaluated without affecting my baby? What would be the effect of treatment on the baby?

In answer to these questions, the obstetrician should be aware that the data do not support the view that termination of pregnancy improves the prognosis when breast cancer is diagnosed. The patient may elect to terminate the pregnancy for her own reasons, but this option should not be presented as medically indicated. A thorough diagnostic workup, including chest radiographs, abdominal radiographs, bone scanning, and magnetic resonance imaging, if deemed necessary, can be undertaken without known risk to the fetus.

Treatment of early (stage I and II) breast carcinoma can also be accomplished during pregnancy without significant risk to the fetus. Regimens that require adjuvant radiation therapy must be avoided, but adjuvant chemotherapy can be utilized with little apparent effect on immediate neonatal outcome, especially if use is avoided during the first trimester. Certain specific chemotherapy agents, such as aminopterin and methotrexate, must be avoided, however. Low birth weight and preterm delivery may be more common with chemotherapy, but the data available on long-term follow-up suggest that the effects are transient. The patient must be informed that long-term effects of the various chemotherapy regimens on childhood development are largely unknown.

For women who have previously been treated for breast cancer, it is usually advised that they not attempt pregnancy for 2–3 years, as this time period is when most recurrences clinically manifest. There does not appear to be any adverse effect of subsequent pregnancies on the natural history of breast cancer. Some women are able to breastfeed after certain therapies for breast cancer, such as lumpectomy and local irradiation. However, because of the variation in the radiation dose and technique and the surgical technique, it is difficult to predict the extent to which a treated breast is able to undergo lactational changes. There is no evidence that lactation in the breast previously treated for breast cancer in itself poses a risk for recurrence of breast cancer. Parents who inquire about the risk of passing the cancer cells to the fetus may be reassured that although breast cancer metastases to the placenta have been reported, there has never been a report of fetal metastasis from a primary breast cancer.

The spectrum of breast problems unique to pregnancy is limited, and the problems are usually manageable without serious consequences. Among the common breast problems that cause confusion during pregnancy, a breast mass and its definitive diagnosis is the most important. Delay in diagnosis must be avoided.

35 BREASTFEEDING AND LACTATION

Katherine Schlaerth

The idea of nursing her baby should be introduced to a prenatal patient in a casual manner on the first or second prenatal visit. The suggestion, "You'll probably be breastfeeding your baby, won't you?" elicits variations of the following responses.

"Yes, I'd like to try." In this case case you ask the multiparous patient if she has successfully breastfed before (and therefore needs a minimal level of instruction) or whether and why a prior attempt at breastfeeding had been unsuccessful.

"No, I don't want to breastfeed." Here tact is of the utmost importance. While reaffirming that bottle-fed babies grow well and are not in any sense deprived, you may wish to explore gently the reasons the patient does not desire to breastfeed. At times, incorrect information may stand between the patient and a successful nursing experience.

"I'd like to, but I'll need help." Again, an educational process, carried out throughout the pregnancy, can increase the patient's knowledge and facilitate successful breastfeeding.

EDUCATING THE PRENATAL PATIENT

First Trimester

At the initial physical examination the breasts should be examined for anatomic abnormalities that could interfere with successful lactation. Look for the following variations: inverted nipples; tubular breasts; ectopic breast tissue; ancillary nipples; any biopsies, other surgery, or injury that may have traumatized the mammary ducts; breast implants (inquire about type and placement); breast masses.

When the breasts are found to be anatomically normal, reassure the patient that her breasts will enlarge during pregnancy but that the size of the breasts has no effect on their ability to produce milk. Large breasts have greater quantities of fatty tissue, which does not contribute to milk production. However, infants can nurse quite adequately and are not smothered by large breasts. "Flat-chested" women need reassurance that the changes in their breasts during pregnancy put their ability to produce milk on a par with their more well endowed sisters.

Women appreciate knowing that breastfeeding does not disfigure their breasts or make them less pleasing to their husbands after lactation is completed. Also, the fully lactating woman who gives her baby only breast milk has considerable protection from becoming pregnant for the first 6 months. Once additional forms of nourishment are ingested by the infant, this relative infertility wanes. Women also are reassured by mention of the studies that have shown some protection against breast cancer for women who have nursed their babies. Additional benefits of breastfeeding, tailored to the interest of the patient, may be mentioned: protection for baby from enteric infectious diseases; lower rates of ear infection and other infections; protection from early development of severe allergies (especially important if the family is allergy-prone); availability and economy of breast milk; lower doctor bills for the baby; less absenteeism from work for the working mother because the baby stays healthier; and psychological benefits to both mother and baby (breastfeeding is often a calming activity for the mother).

Second Trimester

The second trimester is a good time to introduce the physiology of lactation and to clarify sources of support for the lactating mother. The breast is composed of a network of lobules in which alveoli produce milk, which then travels down ducts to a collecting system at the base of the nipples, ready for the baby to extract through suckling. Some mothers can understand the concept of breast architecture better by comparing the breast to a tree, with the alveoli being the leaves, the collecting ducts the stems and branches, and the trunk the nipple with its collecting system.

The let-down reflex, it may be explained, is often felt during the first week as "after-pains" because oxytocin causes the uterus to contract and involute more rapidly. This phenomenon is replaced by a pins-and-needles or tightening sensation in the breasts by week 2. This sensation is not painful, can occur when the baby suckles or even if the mother thinks about nursing, and is accompanied by leakage of milk from the nipples, especially during the first few months of lactation.

Mothers should be aware that if there are no complications they are generally permitted to nurse the baby right after delivery. The milk produced initially is creamy yellow colostrum, rich in factors that prevent infection. Somewhere between days 2 and 4 the mother's milk "comes in," an event heralded by engorgement of the breasts caused not just by milk but also by interstitial edema. This event may be painful and may even be associated with low-grade fever. The discomfort of engorgement is minimized significantly by frequent suckling by the infant during the first days after birth; "rooming-in" is essential for this to occur.

It is important to evaluate the pregnant patient's support system and to involve family in the breastfeeding process. Babies suckle every 2–3 hours, if not more often, during the first 6–8 weeks of life, so new mothers should not plan on keeping the house spic and span or on going immediately back to work (when it is avoidable). They need to educate their other children on breastfeeding and work out a plan to breastfeed while ensuring the safety and cooperation of their toddlers and preschoolers.

Fathers need to be involved in the decision about breastfeeding, as their support is invaluable. Often they are concerned about financially supporting their expanding family, may worry about their ability and desire to parent, and may want to be involved with the baby yet fear that the breastfeeding process will exclude them from access to both mother and child. Some men fear that their partner's breasts will belong to the baby and become jealous of surrendering their wives to the infant. Others may think that their lactating partners will no longer be sexually interested in them, or that they themselves will not be interested in a woman who is lactating. Often these fears are difficult for a man to verbalize. Men who wholeheartedly support their partner's desire to breastfeed need affirmation of their importance in the process. Those who seem reluctant need information and the assurance that their conflicted feelings are normal and shared by many new fathers. They can be told that their partner's feelings for them, while perhaps a little blunted by the fatigue of caring for their new baby (and early on by the breastfeeding process itself), will return—if not immediately, then in time. They can be complimented on their strength in making decisions to support their spouse in her effort to give their child the best start possible in life. Fathers from some cultures, where nursing a baby is the cultural norm, are often free of the anxieties that men from other backgrounds may have. The father of the baby should be offered an opportunity to join his partner on one of her visits during the second trimester, so these issues can be raised and he can obtain answers to his questions about breastfeeding.

Grandparents and others can be a help or a hindrance to the breastfeeding mother, and a clinician may wish to inquire about their attitudes and experience with lactation. The key person is the grandmother or another older woman in the circle of support. Such a woman has the benefit of prior experience, and her opinions carry weight, especially if the patient is a first-time mother. If the grandmother (or other important woman) has successfully nursed her own children, she can be a valuable resource on technique. Grandmothers who have not successfully lactated sometimes feel grief and regret that they were unable to do so. Some of these women are strong supporters of the lactation process, whereas others may react with negativism, along the lines of "If I wasn't able to do it, you probably won't be able to either." Women of the past two generations who desired to breastfeed frequently met with lack of support from physicians and nurses who had no training in breastfeeding, so this negative attitude is understandable. Educating the grandmother frequently pays dividends for the patient. This education need not take place in person but can be accomplished through the pregnant patient. She can be asked about how she thinks her mother will react to her decision to lactate. If she expresses concern, suggest that a gift be made to the grandparent-to-be of a book like Karen Prior's "The Womanly Art of Breastfeeding" or that the grandparent make contact with La Leche League

International, local chapters of which proliferate throughout the country. They can answer questions and recommend appropriate reading material.

Some myths circulate so frequently they deserve debunking.

1. MYTH: *Breast milk is thin and weak, not strong and thick like formula, and the baby does not grow nearly so well on it.* Human milk varies in composition over time attendant upon the physiologic needs of the baby. Thick, yellow colostrum is produced during the first week. This milk, though not copious in quantity (because the newborn baby needs less fluid than the older baby), is rich in antibodies that provide protection against disease in the vulnerable newborn. It is also high in protein, fat-soluble vitamins, and minerals. It facilitates establishment of the colonic flora with *Lactobacillus bifidus*, a healthy bacterium whose presence in the intestine protects against bad bacteria. Transitional milk is secreted between the colostrum and mature milk stages, approximately from the end of the first week after birth through the second week. This milk has less protein and lower levels of immunoglobins but more of the sugar, fat, and calories needed by the growing neonate. Mature milk is produced after the second postpartum week. This milk contains a lot of water and high levels of the fats needed for energy. There are more polyunsaturated fats in human milk than in bovine milk, and change in the fat composition of human milk over time may reflect the need of the infant's nervous system for different fats at different stages in its development. Cholesterol levels in human milk are 240 mg/100 g of fat, and some studies have shown fewer atherosclerotic changes in humans and rats with early exposure to cholesterol. The protein content of human milk, although lower than that in cow's milk, is of the quantity and type most needed by the human baby for growth. Iron, although also lower in quantity, is far better absorbed from human milk than from cow's milk. Immunoglobulins, which protect babies from infection, are found in mature human milk as well as in colostrum. The principal immunoglobulin of mature human milk is secretory immunoglobulin A (IgA), which coats and guards the infant's intestines from invading bacteria and viruses. Even as human milk composition and appearance varies with the age of the baby, it also varies during a single feeding. The principal carbohydrate is, of course, lactose. "Foremilk," the milk the baby ingests at the beginning of a feeding, is bluish and watery compared with formula and cow's milk. "Hindmilk" (which the mother probably does not see) comes at the end of the feeding; it is higher in fat, is creamier, and probably helps the infant feel full and drift off to sleep. Therefore human milk, despite its appearance, is richer in the nutrients a human infant needs for lifelong health, and it changes its composition in a way formulas can never do to meet the specific nutritional needs of an infant at each developmental stage.

2. MYTH: *A nervous mother may produce spoiled milk, which will harm her baby.* This myth takes the form of "susto" in women of Hispanic heritage, and variants are encountered in other cultures as well. The idea is that a frightened or nervous mother curdles or damages her milk, and the baby may sicken from it. An ancillary myth holds that if the mother drinks a cold beverage during the act of lactation, her baby may sicken or die. Mothers under stress need to be reassured that their milk is still healthy; stress may diminish their let-down reflex, not the

quality of their milk. The baby may fuss because of diminished flow. Therefore steps must be taken to support and calm the mother or lessen her responsibilities, so relaxation permits resumption of normal milk flow. The physician or other health care provider can be instrumental here by foreseeing stressful situations and using his or her authority to mitigate them. For example, visitors may be forbidden for the first 6 weeks, thereby ameliorating demands on the tired mother and diminishing the opportunity for interfamilial tensions to arise. A new mother may be instructed not to cook or clean the house for the first several postpartum weeks, freeing her from familial criticism and giving her time to rest and nurse.

3. MYTH: *Breastfeeding is disgusting and should never be witnessed by others.* This myth is present in some cultures and entirely absent in others. Queen Victoria expressed disgust at the process of lactation, comparing herself with a cow during this stage of motherhood. Other Victorian myths may have dissipated, but many people are still troubled by this one. Breastfeeding is a normal, natural act not usually associated with the sexual arousal of observers. In fact, it is helpful for children to observe the loving, nurturing relationship between a lactating mother and her infant. Little girls especially should see their mother breastfeed; it provides powerful role-modeling for the future. Many little girls want to "breastfeed" their dolls when mother nurses their sibling. The health-care provider who senses disgust for the nursing process in the prenatal patient may want to say something like, "Sometimes at first my patients are a little uncomfortable thinking about the intimacy of breastfeeding, especially as it is sometimes pleasurable for the mother; and they worry there may be something wrong in breastfeeding a child and actually enjoying it. But breastfeeding is a completely natural process, the feelings associated with it are normal and good, and it is a gift to your child. There is no guilt or shame in such a normal and natural part of being a mother." Mothers can also be reassured that if they treat lactation as a normal, necessary part of motherhood, their other children will treat it that way too. When breastfeeding in public, discrete clothing, shawls, or papooses facilitate the process, and no one else need know that a woman is breastfeeding.

4. MYTH: *Breastfeeding makes you fat.* Mothers who are breastfeeding often note a significant increase in appetite when compared with their prepregnancy appetite. The average lactating woman in fact needs more calories (about 2500–2700/day) to produce milk and often has so little time that the calories consumed may not be optimal in type. The baby, after all, ingests 500–750 or more of these calories depending on his or her weight and age (e.g., >940 kcal for the average 3-month-old). Many lactating mothers note that they shed pregnancy weight faster because they are breastfeeding. Others complain about weight gain, and for these women a dietary evaluation is in order to optimize the nutritional value of calories ingested. All nursing women should continue their prenatal vitamin pills while lactating, and fad diets are to be discouraged. Particular attention must be paid to the diets of vegens so that adequate sources of vitamins are ensured.

5. MYTH: *Breastfeeding ruins my breasts.* Some women think their breasts become larger, and some smaller, after lactation is completed. For all, a well-fitting nursing brassiere can minimize problems.

6. MYTH: *I must not eat certain foods when I am nursing.* Although an occasional infant seems to develop allergies when the mother ingests large amounts of cow's milk, and others may react to essential oils in garlic and other heavy spices, most babies tolerate their mother's diets well. Gassy foods do not cause gas in the infant. Occasionally, colic, rash, or gastrointestinal upset follows ingestion of certain fruits, melon, or allergy-inducing foods such as chocolate. A mother may have to eliminate temporarily the food she suspects is causing problems and observe the infant for cessation of symptomatology.

7. MYTH: *Babies do not grow as quickly when they are breastfed.* Actually, bottle-fed babies may be in danger of being overfed because the parents track ounces ingested rather than signs of infant satiety. The breastfed baby given free access to breast milk grows at a healthy pace, although he sometimes is not quite as fat as his formula-fed counterpart. Rapid growth and infant obesity are not always healthy.

8. MYTH: *If a woman's mother was not able to nurse her babies (because her breasts were too big, too small, or whatever), her daughter will be unsuccessful as well.* Many women were unsuccessful because the physicians and nurses of prior generations were not knowledgeable about the advantages and techniques of breastfeeding and lactation and were quick to switch to bottle feeding whenever a problem arose. Minor problems that today can be easily overcome were not even addressed a generation ago.

9. MYTH: *Breastfed babies take forever to sleep through the night.* Many breastfed babies need nocturnal feedings beyond the time when formula-fed infants awaken for them, though some do not. On the other hand, lactating mothers may welcome nocturnal feeds, which are easy if the infant is in the parental bedroom and require no preparation. Nocturnal feeds prevent morning engorgement, which can be painful for the lactating mother.

Third Trimester

The third trimester is the time when the breasts should be reexamined to be sure they are showing normal pregnancy enlargement. Test for inverted nipples by pressing the areola between your thumb and forefinger. If it retracts, a rare event, some authorities recommend the use of a glass or plastic nipple shell, although in one study the use of this device reduced the rate of breastfeeding. Other authorities point out that most babies, if put to the breast right after birth, can learn to nurse from flat or inverted nipples. Ruth Lawrence noted success with inverted nipples by using a breast pump (see Addendum 2) the first few days after birth to elongate the nipple, enabling the baby to latch onto it more easily. Mothers who have previously nursed a baby should be cautioned that babies have their own individual nursing style, and a good nurser may be followed by a sibling who is a bit sluggish at the breast.

At this point the physician should discuss parturition and the events that will take place, with special reference to lactation. The type of anesthesia may affect a neonate, with epidurals potentially prolonging labor and affecting infant behavior transiently. Immediately after delivery, healthy babies from uncomplicated deliveries can be placed on the mother's breast but may not nurse all that vigorously. Should the baby need immediate care after delivery, the mother will need reassurance in the delivery room and afterward about nursing; possible events that may interdict immediate nursing on the delivery table should be discussed and the mother reassured they will not preclude successful breastfeeding.

It is wise to discuss the fact that giving anything other than the breast, especially during those first few days when lactation is being established, is not wise: Throw out the formula gift packs and demand rooming-in.

Ask your patient what conditions will be like when she brings the baby home. Who will be there to help her? Will there be undesired visitors to attend to? Here you can help by forbidding visitors or limiting the length of their visits. How are her other children to be cared for? Who will do the shopping, cleaning, cooking? Environmental conditions must be optimized, especially as lactation is becoming established. Perhaps a home health nurse or church volunteer can be provided to assist the new mother. If you will not be providing ongoing care for the baby, this is the time to encourage a visit with a health care provider who can assist in the breastfeeding process, be that a family physician, pediatrician, nurse-practitioner, lactation consultant, or other specialist.

MANAGEMENT OF LACTATION

Skin-to-skin contact for the first hour after birth, while mother and infant are still alert, helps the infant's temperature to stabilize, normalizes blood glucose and acid-base status, helps with bonding, and gives the health care provider an opportunity to be sure the infant is latching onto the breast properly, with the aureola in his or her mouth so that tongue compression of the lactiferous ducts against the palate can take place, permitting flow of milk to the baby. The provider can demonstrate the rooting reflex where the lower cheek is brushed by the mother's breast, causing the infant to turn its head toward the breast, and the sucking reflex once the aureola is securely in the infant's mouth. The mother can compress the nipple between two fingers as she brushes the infant's cheek, making it easier for her baby to get the nipple in the mouth. The mother can be asked if she notices uterine contractions, often painful for the first few days after birth, as the release of oxytocin causes both uterine contractions and a pins-and-needles feeling in the breasts (the let-down reflex) permitting milk flow to the baby. She should be reassured that the uterine contractions she experiences with nursing help the uterus return to its normal size more quickly, that the pain soon diminishes, and that the contractions are evidence that she is releasing the hormone that facilitates breastfeeding.

Mothers appreciate a positive approach, need to know that what they are experiencing is normal, and are encouraged by praise from their physicians and nurses. Other practical pointers include how to best hold the baby for nursing with the forearm supporting the baby's back and buttocks, its head tucked in the crook of the arm (Figures 35.1 and 35.2). For twins, or after cesarean section, try the "football hold," with each baby's head in one of the mother's hands, the body

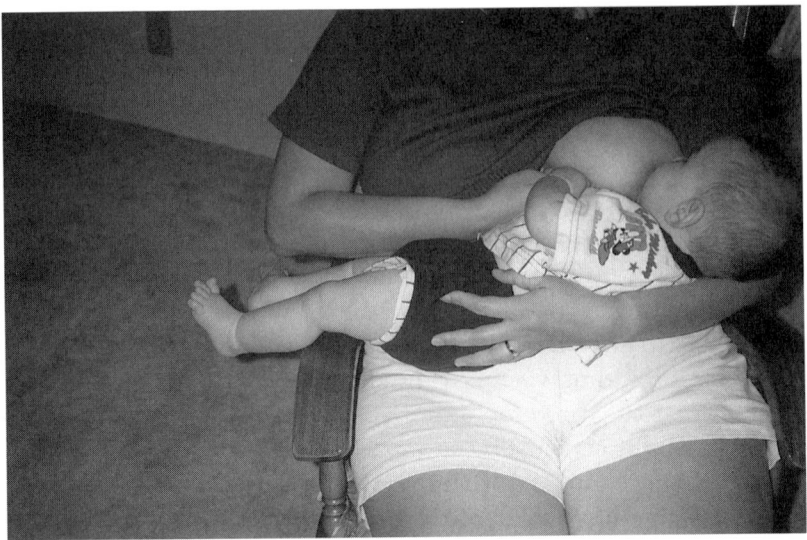

Figure 35.1. Breastfeeding positioning: baby cradled across mother's lap.

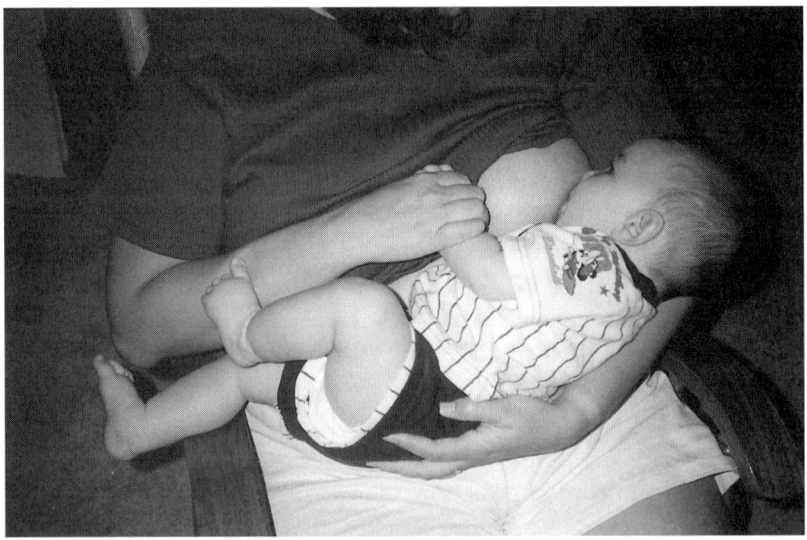

Figure 35.2. Breastfeeding positioning: baby cradled and rotated towards the mother.

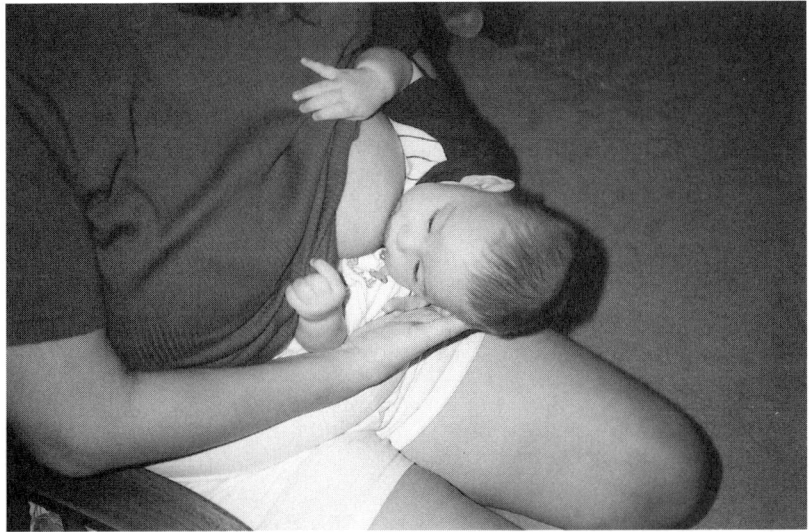

Figure 35.3. Breastfeeding positioning: "football hold" viewed from the front.

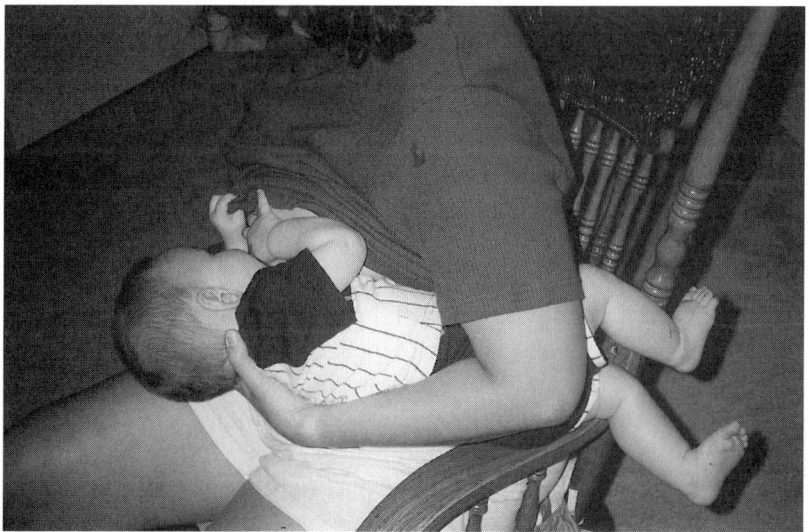

Figure 35.4. Breastfeeding positioning: "football hold" viewed from the side.

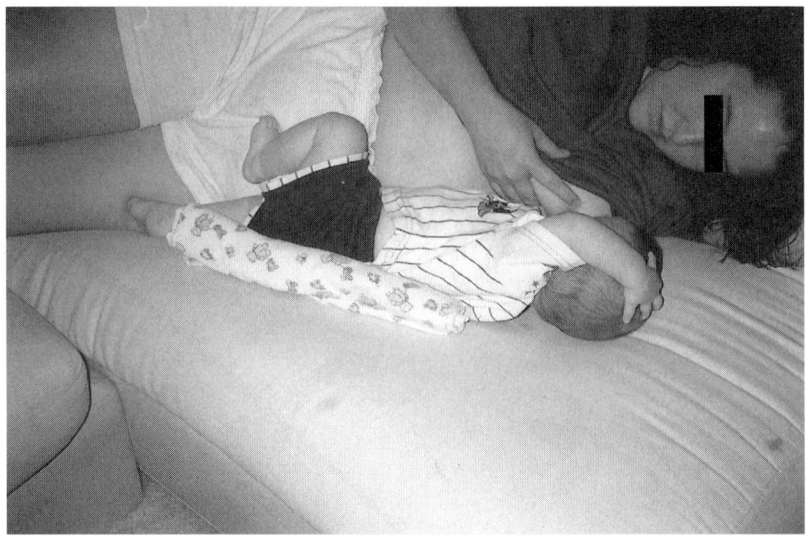

Figure 35.5. Breastfeeding positioning: mother and baby lying on their sides.

supported partially by the mother's forearm and partially by pillows (Figures 35.3 and 35.4). Two babies can then be nursed simultaneously and any abdominal incision protected from pressure. Babies can also be nursed with the mother lying on her side, baby parallel (Figure 35.5). Examine the nursing pair or have an experienced nurse or lactation consultant do so. Be sure that the infant has latched onto the breast properly, that you can hear and see the baby swallowing, and that the mother is not in too much pain after the let-down reflex has dissipated. Pain may signify that the baby has not latched on correctly but is just "chomping on the nipple" without having the lactiferous sinuses securely in a position to be suckled. Try repositioning the baby if you suspect a problem along these lines.

Engorgement occurs around the third postpartum day when the breasts become firm, swollen, warm, and variably painful. Milk is now being produced in significant quantity, and at times there is a low-grade maternal "milk fever." Much of the swelling in the breast is not milk, however, but interstitial fluid. Marked engorgement can be avoided by permitting the infant almost constant access to the breast during the 48–72 hours after birth, especially after the initial period of somnolence, which both babies and mothers experience somewhere between 6 and 18 hours after birth. Newborn babies may not be interested in the breast initially and often doze off. They can be encouraged by unwrapping their covers, jiggling them gently, or stimulating the soles of their feet. Mothers need to be told that this initial disinterest does not presage failure of breastfeeding. Lactogenesis is a critical time for breastfeeding success, when mothers need to breastfeed nearly every hour or two to secure an established milk flow. Breast pumps can be used to help this process if necessary.

Painful nipples often occur when the woman becomes overly engorged, leading to poor nipple attachment by the infant, painful lactation, fissured nipples, and even nipple bleeding and cracking. A drop of milk on the nipples after feeding may prevent inflammation, and this practice should be encouraged after each feeding. Fungal infections also frequently exacerbate painful, cracked nipples. Examine the infant's buccal mucosa for the white enanthem pathognomonic for thrush, and his or her diaper area for the red, intertrigal confluent rash of moniliasis: if either is present, consider treating the infant with nystatin oral suspension, 1 ml to each side of the mouth four times a day for a week. A topical ointment usually containing nystatin or other approved antifungal drug can be used on the affected diaper area, along with air exposure when feasible. The nystatin oral suspension can be used to coat the mother's nipples after each nursing for at least 14 days. Air exposure of painful nipples also enhances healing. Sometimes mothers have to endure a few painful feedings when they are quite engorged and suffering from irritated nipples because, always assuming the baby is properly attached, the feedings themselves reduce engorgement and assuage nipple soreness.

Routine breast care is simple with normal habits of cleanliness. No preparation is needed to sanitize the mother's nipples before feeding. A supportive nursing brassiere should be worn at all times. Encourage mothers to wash their hands before feeding their babies.

The first week is crucial for breastfeeding success, and babies should be checked around day 6 or 7 to be sure they have regained their birth weight. Most babies stool a small amount with almost every feeding and urinate 8–10 or more times a day. Breastfed babies have loose stools, with a transition from the thick, black, sticky meconium variety, through gray-brown, to the sweet-smelling yellow cottage cheese variety surrounded by a small ring of yellow water that characterizes the completely breastfed infant's normal stools at the end of the first week. Many parents interpret normal breastfed stools as diarrhea because formula-fed babies have much firmer stools. When you see the baby and mother after the first week, inspect the mother's breasts and be sure she is nursing at least 10 times in a 24-hour period. Ask her about pain, tenderness, uterine contractions, the prolactin-induced let-down reflex, whether she notices milk running out of the breast the baby is not suckling, about her own fluid intake, and about home conditions. Weigh the baby and compare it with the birth weight. If the baby is below birth weight, be sure you observe the infant at the breast, checking attachment, milk flow, and sucking efficiency. You will be able to partially see the infant's tongue compressing the aureola, hear the milk as the baby swallows, and see small amounts of milk on the baby's lips. Congratulate the mother warmly and compliment her on the richness of her milk when you find the baby growing well.

Failure to regain birth weight by a week or two mandates reexamination within 2–4 days after reinstructing the mother about feeding frequency and technique. Have her set the alarm every 2 hours at night if the baby is failing to awaken. She need not awaken the baby but just put him or her to the breast: suckling usually begins automatically. When done, the baby can be placed back in bed. Instruct the mother to call if she has difficulty. Rarely, a baby is found to be feeding infrequently and is getting dehydrated. This situation is an emergency. Primary maternal glandular insufficiency, retained placenta delaying lactogenesis, idiopathic delayed lactogenesis, maternal pain or anxiety inhibiting the let-down reflex, or parental inexperience and incorrect information about nursing frequency may mandate supplementation, consultation with a lactation specialist, or rarely hospitalization. Babies with neurologic problems may fail to nurse efficiently or be unable to synchronize the oropharyngeal movements needed to express milk efficiently, so a brief neurologic examination of the baby, focusing on his or her alertness, ability to track faces, tone, strength, presence of normal neonatal reflexes, and absence of subtle seizure equivalents such as eye deviation, lip smacking, or jerking of an extremity is in order. When a transient neurologic problem is uncovered, breastfeeding may be possible with the use of a temporary supplementing apparatus (see Addendum 2) made up of a milk reservoir with a feeding tube leading to the mother's nipple. Mother's milk can be placed in the reservoir after being expressed by a breast pump. The infant nurses, but milk flows through the feeding tube despite inefficient suckling.

The jaundiced breastfed baby often presents diagnostic problems during the first week of life. Check the total and indirect bilirubin levels in the infant's blood or do equivalent bilirubin tests. Weigh the baby. Of course eliminate causes of jaundice unrelated to breastfeeding, such as sepsis or ABO incompatibility. Babies who have lost more than 5–10% of birth weight, are not stooling and urinating often enough, or are nursing less frequently than every 2–3 hours may just need more frequent and more efficient nursing with the attendant increase in caloric and fluid intake. Evaluation of the nursing infant coupled with close outpatient follow-up is sufficient if by age 3 days the indirect bilirubin level remains below 18 mg/dl without evidence of hemolysis. Babies with so-called breast milk jaundice unrelated to inadequate calorie intake (which tends to occur during the second week) can be managed much the same way, but some authorities prefer to substantiate the diagnosis by having the mother stop breastfeeding and use a pump for 12–24 hours while the infant is supplemented with formula. Remeasure the bilirubin level at the end of this time, document the fall, and then put the baby back on the breast. The bilirubin level should not rise further, but there is a real risk of subsequent lactation failure when the baby is taken off the breast at such a critical time.

Ongoing breastfeeding routines can be discussed before hospital discharge and at well-baby visits. Once breastfeeding is initiated, mothers should be encouraged to nurse on one breast until it begins to feel lighter (roughly 10 minutes) and then switch to the other. It is important that the infant get the lipid-rich hindmilk in the first breast for caloric content and satiety. Taking only the lactose-rich foremilk and then switching to the contralateral breast for more lactose-rich foremilk can result in relative lactose overload (foremilk/hindmilk imbalance). Babies who nurse often but who consistently do not suckle one breast long enough to get the hindmilk may present with fussiness, spitting up, and large, watery, sometimes greenish stools.

The breast used first should be reversed at each feeding. Especially during the first few months of lactation, the mother should watch for bilateral milk flow soon after she experiences the let-down reflex, for rhythmic swallowing by the infant, for lightening of the breast after a feed, and for frequent stooling during the first few weeks. Urine output is usually considerably more frequent than the six to eight times a day given as a minimal frequency for the nursing neonate. Of course with the use of highly absorbent disposable diapers, frequency of urination can be difficult to assess.

Babies do best if they sleep in the parental bedroom (porta-cribs are good for the young infant) so mothers are roused when the baby starts to awaken for a feed. Parents should not be worried about lovemaking with the baby in the room. Shared sleeping quarters are as old as humanity and may even help reduce the incidence of sudden infant death syndrome (SIDS)-like episodes. For parents who prefer not to share sleeping quarters with an infant, investing in an intercom is an acceptable alternative.

Babies should be fed whenever they are hungry; but if feedings fail to spread themselves out after 3–4 weeks, when nursing is well established, a reevaluation is in order to check the growth and the adequacy of the milk supply. Many babies develop a preference for one breast over the other for reasons that are clear only to baby. To keep both breasts in full lactation, the less-liked breast should be offered first at most feedings so it is adequately stimulated. If it is not used, unilateral failure of milk production inevitably follows. Many mothers notice the effects of markedly reduced levels of estrogen a few weeks into nursing. They experience vaginal dryness, "hot flushes," and sweats. Infants too may break out in afebrile sweats from time to time. Reassurance that the mother's symptoms will resolve with the resumption of hormonal cycling when the baby is introduced to table foods is usually all that is necessary.

The premature infant without serious medical problems can usually nurse adequately if more than 34 weeks' gestational age and often when younger. However, close surveillance of intake and nutritional status is necessary. If suckling is poor, an ancillary reservoir to deliver milk through a feeding tube placed adjacent to the mother's nipple may assist in both breast stimulation and maintainance of the baby's caloric intake. Mothers of very young premature infants often can use a breast pump to provide milk to be incorporated with other nutritional sources. This practice not only helps a baby immunologically but helps the mother psychologically and can enhance bonding. The milk produced by the mother of a premature baby is uniquely constituted to meet the nutritional needs of prematurity and differs in composition from the milk produced for a full-term baby. It is higher in protein, taurine, and antioxidants and contains the perfect combination of lipids for optimal absorption.

The infant with a craniofacial anomaly is often the one who benefits most from breastfeeding. Babies with cleft lip often thrive on breast milk because the breast can conform to the shape of the labial defect and establish a seal in a way that no artificial nipple can. Vascular and cutaneous facial anomalies rarely interfere with breastfeeding. After surgical correction of a facial anomaly, nursing usually can be promptly resumed or a breast pump used transiently to obtain milk until oral feeds can be resumed.

Contraindications to breastfeeding are rare. The human immunodeficiency virus (HIV)-positive mother living in an area where safe, clean formulas are readily available should not breastfeed. A few medications given the mother, such as certain chemotherapeutic or radioactive agents, mandate temporary or complete cessation of breastfeeding. Active tuberculosis is a contraindication until treatment has been under way for 1–2 weeks, the baby having been evaluated and placed on isoniazid. Active hepatitis B in the mother may be a contraindication to breastfeeding, and the infant should be given hyperimmune globulin and vaccinated. Febrile endometritis should be treated, and when the mother is afebrile for 24 hours she can begin or resume breastfeeding. Mothers with group A streptococcal infections can resume nursing after 24 hours of effective antibiotics. In areas of the world where substitution of breast milk with a safe formula is not possible, contraindications to breastfeeding may need to be reevaluated. Some infectious diseases require temporary cessation of breastfeeding; most do not, and breastfeeding protects the baby as maternal antibodies are transferred to fight infection. Breast cancer is usually considered a contraindication to nursing a baby. Other cancers must be evaluated with respect to activity, need for chemotherapy, and viral associations. A basal cell skin cancer, for example, would hardly be a contraindication. Before interdicting maternal breastfeeding when the mother has an exotic infectious disease, it may be advisable to consult an infectious disease specialist or one of the lactation centers to obtain expert advice. The American Academy of Pediatrics may be consulted by writing to: Work Group on Breastfeeding, PO Box 927, Elk Grove Village, IL 60009-0927.

Mastitis is a common occurrence, especially during the first few weeks of lactation, and in its early presentation may be difficult to distinguish from a plugged milk duct. Plugged ducts, of course, predispose to the occurrence of mastitis, as do fissured nipples, stress, and missed feedings. Mothers with a plugged duct do not feel ill, are afebrile, and have a gradual onset of discomfort. Warm soaks and frequent nursing usually relieve symptoms. Mastitis usually presents acutely with fever, flu-like symptoms including achy bones and joints, chills, and fatigue. Often mothers complain of a pie-like wedge of erythematous, indurated, tender breast that hurts even more at the time of a let-down reflex. *Staphylococcus aureus* is the usual causative organism, but streptococcal and *Escherichia coli* infection may occur. Conversely, should a lactating woman present with flu-like symptoms and fever, always check and palpate the breasts for evidence of localized erythema, wedge-shaped tenderness, and induration.

If a breast milk sample is to be collected, the mother should clean the nipple and breast (and her hands) with water. A midstream milk collection of about 3 ml should be sent to the laboratory (using sterile technique) to be plated as quickly as possible. Treatment with an antibiotic (e.g., amoxicillin-clavulanate), a cephalosporin (e.g., cephalexin), or in the allergic patient erythromycin is usually successful but should be complemented with bed rest, a high fluid intake, frequent nursing on the affected breast, and warm soaks every 2–3 hours. Early treatment should forestall abscess formation, which though rare necessitates surgical drainage. Chronic or recurrent mastitis is often triggered by cracked nipples infected with fungi or incomplete adherence to a course of antibiotics, which must be continued for 10 days.

Food intolerance in the breastfed baby is an occasional occurrence, not associated with any one particular food. Gas-producing foods ingested by the mother cannot cause gas in an infant; but excessive intake of caffeine, 1% of which gets into breast milk, occasionally causes fussiness in neonates. Certain foods may be associated with problems, including eczema, in the breastfed baby. If a parent is suspicious of a particular food, she can exclude this food from her diet for a week, see if the symptoms resolve, and then reintroduce it and observe the infant for symptom recurrence. A mother who suspects dairy products should ingest other foods high in calcium and may need a nutritionist's advice if a dairy product is indeed causing serious symptoms in her baby. Some allergists suggest that highly allergy-prone families be selectively encouraged to breastfeed their offspring, and that milk-containing products be excluded from the mother's diet from the third trimester onward.

Mothers receiving medication need careful attention. All mothers should continue their prenatal vitamins. Over-the-counter medications are avoided wherever possible. The nursing mother should check in when she does decide to take any over-the-counter agent. If possible, delay treatment of a specific, nonurgent ailment in the mother until the baby is older. Use contraindicated medications in brief courses where possible, having mothers pump and discard the milk produced while the offending medication is in their systems. Check with texts that address the metabolism of drugs in the pregnant and lactating woman to see which needed drug is likely to be the most benign or least secreted in milk. Use a topical instead of a systemic medication when possible, as it is less likely to reach high concentrations in breast milk. See if you can manipulate the timing of the dose to avoid peak levels of nursing. Use alternative treatments or medications that are friendly to breastfeeding when possible. As a rule of thumb, if a medication can safely be given to the baby, it can safely be given to the lactating, nonallergic mother. Remember that the renal threshold for sugar is reduced in some lactating women, so glycosurea is possible with perfectly normal blood glucose levels.

Nursing twins is a logistical challenge but can be done sequentially or, better yet, using the football hold (described earlier) to nurse both simultaneously. Neuropathy has been reported when mother's arms are compressed against the firm surface of an armchair or a rocking chair. Special attention must be paid to ensure that the lactating mother of twins has sufficient in-home support to allow her to care properly for herself and her infants.

Tandem nursing is the term used for nursing an unweaned toddler and a neonate at the same time. Often the nursing desired by the toddler is nonnutritive, brief, and psychologically helpful in circumventing sibling rivalry. Tandem nursing works best if the toddler has a separate time to nurse after the baby has been fed and understands that this time is special for him or her. Most mothers find they can quickly substitute storytime or a brief walk for the nursing, but the toddler needs to know that he or she has not been displaced. Once reassured on this point, the toddler generally accepts other forms of closeness.

Nursing during pregnancy is possible with special care to the mother's nutritional needs. Should the mother not want to tandem nurse after the birth of her new child, weaning should take place before the third trimester. Otherwise, the older baby may feel he has lost his or her breast rights, which have been taken over by the new baby.

Nipple confusion refers to the difficulty some infants have when attempting to nurse from a bottle after having learned to nurse at the breast or, conversely, the problem of breastfeeding a neonate who learned the bottle first. Many infants have no problems learning the tongue and palate compression skills and the rhythmic suck and swallow movements needed to extract milk from the maternal breast and can easily switch to the nipple with its automatic milk flow. Some babies, however, become frustrated when they have learned at the breast and then are "flooded" with bottle milk from a self-flowing rubber nipple. Even the most sophisticated nipple and bottle designs do not mimic the special physiologic interactions between the suckling baby and its mother's breast. Conversely, a neonate used to the ease with which bottle milk flows may become frustrated when trying to learn the skill of extracting milk from the maternal breast, which is an active, not a passive, task. Nipple confusion is most problematic for the mother who must return to work. One solution that works for many mothers, as the difficulty a baby ultimately has is not predictable, is to use a breast pump to extract milk from one breast while nursing on the other. Someone else, ideally the father, can bottle-feed the baby this milk later on. Mothers must be cautioned not to use formula for this task. When mothers attempt to bottle-feed their own milk, some babies are smart enough to refuse because they know the mother has breast milk. Once a child has learned to take from both bottle and breast, bottle feeds do not have to be given often.

The mother who works outside the home can continue to breastfeed her infant and in fact should be vigorously encouraged to do so even more than the at-home mother. Infants in day care, especially those 3–4 months of age, experience a waning of maternal transplacental IgG and are vulnerable to infectious diseases. Breastfeeding provides antibodies to cover this immunologic gap [mostly surface IgA (sIgA)]. Breastfeeding mothers, in fact, have less absenteeism from work. Studies have shown that full-time working mothers breastfeed as long as at-home mothers, and part-time workers breastfeed longer than full-time workers.

A mother who must return to work may wish to avoid nipple confusion by introducing bottles of her own milk within the first 2 weeks of her baby's life. These bottles need be given only once or twice a week, or less, as they are for learning purposes only. If part-time or take-home work or even bringing the baby to work are options for the breastfeeding mother, she should take advantage of them. When the nursing woman does return to work, she should plan on using a manual or a mechanical pump (during breaks and at lunch) to aspirate milk and promptly refrigerate it. Sterilized bottles and nipples can be used initially; clean bottles are probably all that is necessary after about 6 months of age. If a refrigerator is not available at work, a small ice chest supplied with ice from home works as well if the ice stays frozen. Mothers should nurse immediately before leaving for work; many mothers can get two before-work sessions in. When baby is picked up from the sitter another nursing should take place immediately, at the sitter's or day-care center if things will be too chaotic when they return home. Nursings ought to be frequent after work. Some mothers even set the alarm to awaken a couple of times at night to nurse their babies if the babies do not awaken on their own. Nighttime feeding usually does not mean fully waking the baby. Many babies put to the breast suckle well and drift off to sleep without completely awakening. Catch-up nursing on the weekends can keep the breast at prime production levels. The working nursing mother probably would do well to avoid elaborate social or housekeeping tasks on weekends.

Periods of rapid growth and developmental change are vulnerable periods for both mother and infant and should be anticipated amd discussed by the health care provider. The first several weeks, of course, are critical to the establishment of breastfeeding, and infants usually gain anywhere from 0.5 to 2.0 oz of weight a day. Frequent feeding is the norm during the first two to three critical growth months, and especially during the first few weeks. The normally lactating mother should never be given a formula gift pack when she leaves the hospital: it is too much of a temptation. The use of a formula gift pack, however brief, has been shown to interfere with lactogenesis at a critical time.

Somewhere around 6–8 weeks, babies experience rapid growth and nurse more frequently. The breast, being a demand organ, complies within a day or two with increased production. Mothers may interpret this increased nursing frequency as an indication that they are not producing enough milk. They should be told that growth periods do not reflect their adequacy as lactating mothers but, rather, represent the intricate balance between baby's changing physiologic needs and the ability of the breast to meet these changing needs in a way formulas never can. They can also be told that their milk even changes somewhat in composition over time as their baby's optimal growth demands specific quantities of certain nutrients. When a baby reaches 2.0–2.5 months, eating becomes more social; and he or she frequently stops nursing to look around or smile at the mother. Mothers frequently interpret this social behavior as rejection of the breast. Sometimes a mother even weans a baby who she believes is rejecting her milk. She needs to be told that this behavior can occur and is not a personal rejection. She should be instructed to reintroduce the nipple to the baby while gently drawing his or her attention away from socialization until the feed is completed.

Women often believe their femininity is associated in some way with their ability to nourish a child at the breast. Failure of lactation, or even the fear of it, is a great blow to self-esteem for some women, whereas success breeds more success. The physician or nurse who praises a mother's ability and compliments her on her baby's progress plants the seeds for further success, as the mother's motivation is often the most important component of long-term breastfeeding.

Pacifiers and biting are capable of sabotaging successful breastfeeding if not handled with discretion. Some infants do fine with a pacifier, and pacifiers can be helpful in the premature nursery when used by babies who cannot yet take oral feeds reliably. However, there are risks: Some babies suckle less at the breast and have subsequent poor weight gain, and some develop nipple confusion; babies who have poor sucking coordination at the breast may aggravate this condition by using a pacifier.

Biting becomes a problem when teeth appear. It is a behavior quickly extinguished in most infants by a look of surprise, disapproval, or a yelp of pain from mother, coupled with a gentle smack on the cheek and a firm, "No!"

Parents commonly raise questions about the use of vitamins and the introduction of solids. Mothers are advised to continue their prenatal vitamins. Fluoride drops (0.25 mg/day) should be added at 6 months if the local water supply contains less than 0.3 ppm of fluoride. Vitamin D (200–300 IU/day) is needed only where sunlight exposure is lacking (<2 hours a week, infant clothed, without head covering).

Vitamin K, of course, is routinely given at birth (0.5–1.0 mg IM) and is especially needed by the nursling who is at risk for hemorrhagic disease of the newborn. Strict vegen mothers especially need a daily vitamin to provide B-complex vitamins, including vitamin B_{12} and pyridoxine.

Solids do not help an infant sleep through the night. In fact, breastfed babies should not sleep through the night: the baby needs nocturnal nutrition, and the mother needs her breasts emptied. Many, if not most, breastfed babies are still awakening for a nighttime feed at 1 year of age. Most motivated mothers accept these inconveniences, and all should be made aware that breast milk is much more rapidly digested (1.5 hours) than is formula milk (up to 4.0 hours) because of its optimal nutrient content, and therefore breastfed babies get hungry more quickly.

Six months of age is an optimal time for the introduction of solids; 4 months is the minimal age. The gut has matured by this time and is more impermeable to macromolecules, which could trigger an allergic problem. Oropharyngeal muscular coordination is better, and the tongue thrust has dissipated, so food has a good chance of being swallowed rather than thrust out of the mouth. The introduction of solids reduces the quantity of maternal milk produced, with the latter being the optimal food for the first 6 months of life. Cereals are usually introduced first, followed by vegetables, fruits, and meats, although this order is not absolute. Introduction of one new food every 3–7 days permits recognition of any food that may produce an untoward reaction, such as eczema, in the baby.

Diarrhea and other illnesses are treated with the continuation of breastfeedings, and mothers should be urged to offer the breast even more when a child has gastroenteritis. Never stop breast milk, not even to put the baby on clearfluids. Breast milk facilitates healing in the gut, shortens the period of illness, and transmits maternal antibodies to the infant.

Water supplementation is not needed even in hot weather. Studies have shown that frequent feeding of breast milk meets the free water needs of children in hot or tropical regions of the world. The frequency of nursing can be increased in hot weather. Hypernatremia has been reported rarely in breastfed babies but not specifically in association with warmer ambient temperatures. Rather, this problem has arisen in the context of poor maternal milk supply and insufficient lactation.

Failure to thrive (FTT) by a breastfed infant is defined as failure to gain adequate weight. A growth chart should be consulted by the clinician at each office visit of the breastfed infant. Weight gain during the first few months is usually in the range of 1.5–2.0 lb a month (0.5–2.0 oz/day), the infant needing about roughly 120 kcal/kg/day during this period for optimal growth. Breastfed babies as a group tend to grow a bit more slowly than some of their formula-fed counterparts—which is not necessarily a bad thing. Should the clinician suspect FTT in a breastfed baby, the history is of great importance. Ask about maternal breast development during pregnancy, infant stooling patterns (starvation stools are mucoid and dark green in contrast to yellow, seedy, and frequent), total number of feedings per 24-hour period and duration of each feeding, number of wet diapers per 24-hour period, onset of lactogenesis, adequacy of the let-down reflex and contralateral flow of milk, pain associated with feedings, use of hormones, and past lactation history. Inquire into the baby's ability to communicate hunger, latch on, suck vigorously and synchronously, and gulp milk, a sound recognizable to the mother. Some babies seem disinterested in nursing, sleep for long periods, do a lot of nonnutritive sucking, and do not make their needs known to the mother. Some mothers then misguidedly think nursing four or five times a day is the norm.

Look for frequent, brief feedings, which may not permit ingestion of the more calorically dense hind-milk. Ask if the baby has been ill. Examine the infant with special attention to signs of malnutrition (loss of subcutaneous tissue, wizened look), dehydration (dry mucous membranes, sunken fontanelle, excessive tachypnea, lethargy, rarely mottling and shock), and hypernatremia (doughy skin). Check the infant neurologically for alertness, Moro's reflex, grasp, rooting and suck, tone, and ability to track and respond to sound; perform a brief general physical examination.

Observing the nursing pair during the process of feeding is of utmost importance. Look for problems with latch-on, coordination of suck and swallow, milk production, even behavior of the infant, and pain in the mother. Check the mother's breasts for size and weight (heavier and somewhat boggy before, and lighter after, a successful feed) and the presence of mastitis or a plugged duct. Medical conditions in the infant are sometimes recognized through his or her feeding behavior. For example, the infant who starts to nurse vigorously and "just poops out" after an ounce or so, breaking out in a sweat and appearing fatigued, could have a congenital cardiac defect. A nursing diary is not a bad idea if the cause of FTT is still obscure, and close follow-up (1–3 days) is needed. Most FTT is uncovered by this point, the most common correctable causes being infrequent feedings, poor latch-on, poor infant suck and swallow, and a suboptimal let-down reflex. One specialist recommends the use of oxytocin nasal spray for a couple of days (never more), which sometimes helps with the latter problem. More often a stressful situation in the mother's life is interfering with her let-down reflex and must be addressed.

Should the cause or treatment of lactation-associated FTT still be a problem, consultation with a lactation specialist may be helpful. Prior breast surgery on the mother may or may not affect her ability to lactate or may affect the amount of milk she can produce. The key is whether the lactiferous ducts have been interrupted. This happens with reduction mammoplasty when the nipple is repositioned for cosmesis. Silicon or other implants generally do not damage the ducts or nerves, but concern has arisen about their ability to harm the nursing baby through silicon diffusion.

Weaning is carried out when the nursing couple is ready, but the mother must be careful not to misread the infant's clues about readiness. The 4-month-old who frequently unlatches herself from the breast to smile at the mother or look at siblings is not showing a desire to be weaned. She is merely making her meal into a more social event, and her attention must be brought back to the task of eating. A 7-month-old who bites is unaware he is causing his mother pain, and it must be made clear to him with a tap to the cheek and a firm, emphatic "No!" Physicians, nurses, and other providers should gently explore the reasons a mother may want to wean early, especially if weight gain is suboptimal because the mother may have lost confidence in her ability to produce good milk. She may not really wish to stop nursing and may be helped to continue by referral to a lactation specialist.

Breastfeeding up to and beyond a year is optimal. Two years or more is the norm encouraged by the World Health Organization. Mothers who are breastfeeding should never be ashamed of this activity, even though mothers breastfeeding a toddler may experience negativism even from health care personnel.

Generally, a child is weaned by eliminating one feeding every few days. Nighttime (not bedtime) feeds, those that occur between meals, and those at inconvenient times are the first to go, with wake-up, naptime, and bedtime feedings usually the last. As the feedings are gradually spaced out, the breast diminishes its production gradually, without the engorgement and pain associated with abrupt weaning. After a few weeks to months, nursing becomes a token activity and eventually ceases altogether. Mothers sometimes experience sadness or even depression as the weaning process proceeds, especially if they plan to have no more children. It helps at such times to remind them that they are doing what is best for the child, motherhood being a process of slowly making oneself less and less necessary to one's offspring.

The breast of a woman who has recently weaned, especially if the weaning was done rapidly, is lumpy for up to a month. Abrupt weaning should be avoided if possible, as it is emotionally and physically painful and may be accompanied, especially if done within a month or two of birth, by "milk fever," a flu-like illness lasting 3–4 days and accompanied by fever, chills, and malaise. Binders and cold packs do little to lessen the pain but can be used. Psychological support is important.

Fertility during lactation depends on the age of the baby, and whether he or she is breastfed exclusively. Suckling seems to be the most important factor in determining fertility. Babies who are exclusively breastfed and suckled on demand, which usually means during the night and in the daytime, induce a period of lactational amenorrhea and reliable infertility in the mother lasting 6 months, the age in our culture at which solids are generally introduced. Once solids or supplemental feedings are introduced, the contraceptive effect of lactation is no longer reliable. Ovulation before the end of lactational amenorrhea occurs variably in 14–75% of nursing mothers, thereby making amenorrhea in itself not a reliable marker for lactation-induced infertility.

ADDENDUM 1: RESOURCES FOR INFORMATION AND REFERRALS FOR LACTATION-RELATED PROBLEMS

Lactation Study Center (Ruth A. Lawrence, M.D., author of *Breastfeeding: A Guide for the Medical Profession*)
University of Rochester Medical Center
Rochester, NY 14627
Phone: 716-275-0088 (weekdays 8 a.m. to 5 p.m. EST)

La Leche League International
PO Box 1209
9616 Minneapolis Avenue
Franklyn Park, IL, 60131
Phone: 708-455-7730, 800-LA-LECHE

International Childbirth Education Association
PO Box 20048
Minneapolis, MN 55420
Phone: 612-854-8660

International Lactation Consultant Association
Phone: 312-541-1710

Center for Breastfeeding Information
Phone: 847-519-7730 ext. 245 or 241

ADDENDUM 2: AIDS FOR BREASTFEEDING

Nursing supplementer: Container for milk with tubing taped to the breast to augment and increase the supply of maternal milk. Indications: prematurity, Down syndrome, infant cardiac problems, poor suck for other reasons, maternal lactational difficulties. Some available products:

> *Axicare Nursing Aide*
> Colgate Medical Ltd.
> Fairacres Estate
> Edworth Road, Windsor, Berks SL4LE
> Phone: Windsor 60378

Lact-Aid
    Lact-Aid International
    PO Box 1066
    Athens, GA 37303
    Phone: 615-744-9090

Medela Supplemental Nursing System & Medela Starter SNS
    Medela, Inc.
    PO Box 660
    McHenry, IL 60051-0660
    Phone: 800-835-5968

Breast pumps: Manual, small electric, and battery-powered models; choices based on intended use. Indications: working mother who wishes to feed her milk to the baby; a baby with weak suck who is fed by eyedropper, feeding syringe, or nursing supplementer, or who is premature and in hospital. Some available products:

> *Manual breast pumps*: available in most pharmacies, various brands
> *Battery-operated breast pumps*: available in medical supply stores and pharmacies
> *Electric breast pumps*: through hospital rental and other rental supply stores
> *Lactina Breast Pump*: rental information through local hospitals; or Medela, Inc. (800-435-8316 or 800-TELL-YOU) or Ameda/Egnell/Hollister (800-435-4060) will provide lists of local rentals

Recommended Reading

Freed GL, Clark SJ. Breastfeeding and maternal illness. Contemp Pediatr 1996;13:49–61

Lawrence RA. Breastfeeding: A Guide for the Medical Profession (4th ed). St. Louis, Mosby, 1994

Layde PM, Webster LA, Baughman AL, et al. The independent associations of parity, age at first full term pregnancy, and duration of breastfeeding with the risk of breast cancer. J Clin Epidemiol 1989;42:963–973

Neifert MN. Early assessment of the breastfeeding infant. Contemp Pediatr 1996;13:142–166

Powers NG, Slusser WS. Breastfeeding update 2: clinical lactation management. Pediatr Rev 1997;18:147–161

Slusser W, Powers NG. Breastfeeding update 1: immunology, nutrition and advocacy. Pediatr Rev 1997;18:111–119

Stashwick CA. When a breastfed infant isn't gaining weight. Contemp Pediatr 1993;10:116–136

36 MEDICAL LEGAL CONSIDERATIONS FOR THE PRIMARY CARE PHYSICIAN REGARDING CARE OF THE BREAST

R. James Brenner

Intercepting cancer at a point where the natural progression of the disease can be halted for a significant number of patients is one of the primary goals in medicine. Such is the case with invasive breast cancer now that clinical screening trials have demonstrated statistically convincing evidence that case fatality rates can indeed be altered. For a disease that was estimated to affect more than 180,000 women in 1997, many of them in the premenopausal years, such an opportunity has now become a public health challenge.

Concomitant with the enthusiasm for detecting and treating breast cancer with increasingly sophisticated management approaches and procedures has been a rising number of malpractice lawsuits against physicians for delay in diagnosing breast cancer. According to the Physicians Insurers Association of America (a national consortium of physician-owned liability carriers that pool claims data) in their Breast Cancer Study of 1995, delay in diagnosis of breast cancer is the leading cause of lawsuits against physicians. The reasons are manifold and likely reflect such factors as the high expectations of a public well addressed by articles in lay publications on the subject, the high incidence of the disease, the relative lack of physician training in clinical examination of the breast, and a contingency fee basis (i.e., a percentage of the award as remuneration) for attorneys representing the patients, many of whom are young women with the prospect of attracting potentially large awards.

The clinician evaluating a woman for breast cancer need not fear the potential repercussions of the legal system. Appropriate care and attention to the signs and symptoms of cancer are generally sufficient to defeat claims of malpractice. Although a poor outcome is often the trigger for a medical malpractice lawsuit, it is the conduct of the physician, not the outcome for the patient, that determines liability. A woman whose cancer is discovered at a time that she thinks has been unnecessarily delayed may believe that her medical providers have failed her; the ensuing lawsuit, generally speaking, is an attempt to determine the facts of the case and either provide restitution to the plaintiff if negligence can be shown or exonerate the defendant.

Many forms of law relate to the practice of medicine. Usually such actions (e.g., malpractice suits) fall under the category of civil law, which governs the actions of individuals or groups of individuals. Criminal law sanctions may apply to medical practice where the aggrieved party is the state, county, or federal government. Thus the federal Justice Department may seek criminal sanctions for fraud and abuse against physicians in violation of federal statutes prohibiting certain types of conduct. Criminal law may include incarceration as a form of punishment, whereas civil law usually provides money damages to compensate an aggrieved party.

Civil law is derived from two primary sources: statutory law and common law. Statutory law is that law passed by legislative bodies at the local, state, and federal levels. The Mammography Quality Standards Act (MQSA) of 1992 is a federal law, enforced by the Food and Drug Administration (FDA), that establishes standards that must be met by every mammography facility in the United States. The Act establishes explicit standards of care that require no expert testimony. In like manner the Occupational Safety and Health Administration (OSHA) sets standards for clinical practice; the standards are established by law, and physicians (and their offices and staff) must comply.

Common law arises from decisions of appellate courts in each state that have precedent-setting value, a concept derived from eighteenth century English common law where decisions of the court would establish conduct for professions with a public calling, a process referred to as *stare decisis*. Certain principles regarding medical practice have been discussed by appellate courts in the United States, helping to guide physicians as to what is considered acceptable; virtually all of these opinions pertain to clinical care.

Medical malpractice cases are usually tried under the civil law, or *tort of negligence*. It is important to recognize that although most medical insurance liability policies cover negligence, some actions (e.g., criminal) fall outside that coverage. If a case is not settled prior to trial—and most are—a judge or jury attempts to decide the truth from disputed facts and render a judgment. Medical malpractice cases are rarely subject to appeal to higher courts because appeals deal with matters of law and not of fact.

Negligence is a term of art, notwithstanding its disparaging connotation, and is defined by four elements: duty, breach of duty, causation, and damages. The element of duty is defined in several ways during this discussion, helping the clinician understand the relation of the law to medical malpractice. In general, it is the duty of a physician, in the context of breast cancer evaluation, to obtain a complete history from the patient and to perform a reasonable and complete examination (the parameters of which are discussed in other chapters of this text). Complete documentation of such history and examination is essential. In a busy office practice, medical record entries are often cursory. The clinician is advised that entries must be complete enough to substantiate any given management plan.

Standard abbreviations and mnemonics are appropriately used when making entries to the chart, with their definition and meaning substantiated in a manual of office policy and procedure. The omission of sufficient notations may be construed as evidence—not proof—of a lack of history-taking or physical examination. Consider the case of a woman diagnosed with breast cancer whose anxiety and fear, which are normal under such circumstances for both the patient and the treating physician, prompt a review of her care. She believes that she mentioned a specific lump in her breast to her physician a year or two previously and thinks that her diagnosis was unreasonably delayed by lack of proper care. The medical record that validates a proper history and complete examination during the past 2 years and fails to identify any concern for such a lump can serve two purposes. The first is to defeat an unreasonable claim of negligence by indicating that no such sign of breast disease was either presented to or identified by the clinician. The second is to reinforce to the patient that the medical system has not necessarily failed her, an important psychosocial condition for her future care.

Medical records are an exception to the hearsay rules of evidence during a trial, which exclude indirect information or conversations from being presented to the *trier of fact* (judge or jury). Legally, a medical record is considered to be a form of "regular business records" and sufficiently reliable to help determine the truth of the situation. It is not proof, but rather evidence, of what has happened in the past, because recollections of events occurring 1 or 2 years ago may be both difficult to recall and subject to dispute. Again, the purpose of a trial is to resolve disputed facts.

It must be emphasized that the medical record should *never* be tampered with or altered. When a physician receives notice of a lawsuit, there is a natural tendency to review the medical record of the plaintiff patient. Often there is an understandable temptation to add or modify notes, if only for the sense of completion and assistance to anyone reviewing the chart. This conduct must be resisted and avoided. There is probably no more damaging evidence against a physician during trial than a medical record that has been altered after a complaint has been filed. Handwriting experts can and often do identify such alterations. The clinician faced with a lawsuit is urged to "freeze the moment in time and place," permit the defending attorney to work with the bona fide information that is available, and allow the process to unfold, as frustrating and anxiety provoking as it may be.

All conversations regarding the care of the patient must be restricted to the attorney, because anything discussed about the patient after a lawsuit has been filed is "discoverable" under oath. A clinician who seeks comfort and endorsement of his or her actions from another health care provider may subject that person to testifying under oath about the nature of such a discussion; and if such were to be unfavorable to the defendant physician, unnecessary and unintended problems in the defense of the case could result.

The clinician obtaining a proper history and completing a proper physical examination may be confronted with the common findings of a "lumpy-bumpy" breast, sometimes referred to as fibrocystic changes. Where a dominant mass is not identified by either the physician or woman, but multiple masses or lumps are appreciated, it may be appropriate to see the patient on several occasions at short intervals to establish that no particular area is of increasingly prominent concern. The parameters of this approach depend on the individual case and cannot be generalized, except to indicate that short-term follow-up approaches are used in various aspects of clinical medicine and have been advocated for mammographic abnormalities which, following sufficient evaluation, are reasonably considered probably benign.

Written (recorded) documentation is important. Consider two cases based on appellate court decisions, each where a woman developed a lump diagnosed as cancer. Previous lumps were thought to represent cysts and were successfully aspirated. However, both women contended that the original lumps were in fact the cancer, which was allowed to grow. In one case the clinician prevailed because a convincing drawing in the medical record showed the position of the original cyst to be in a distinct and separate location from that of the eventual cancer. With insufficient information in the medical chart, the second clinician's contention was subject to the opinion of the jury as to whether the original lesion was a cyst and not the cancer. Where proper care is given, documentation of such care is persuasive, if not convincing, for defeating a claim of negligent conduct.

The advisability of ordering screening mammography for asymptomatic patients and the periodicity of such examinations is an undecided issue. Different medical societies and health care organizations have proposed different guidelines. The ordering of a screening mammogram as a standard of care has not been established as a matter of law, although two appellate courts have taken "judicial notice" of such guidelines. From a risk management standpoint, screening mammography properly performed can serve two purposes. First, it permits the opportunity to detect cancer at a preclinical stage (i.e., before it is palpable). Second, it preempts the allegation that "had a screening mammogram been performed the cancer would have been detected earlier." This argument may be more persuasive if a mammogram taken at the time of cancer diagnosis shows a mass with calcifications. Although no direct correlation has been proved, some plaintiff experts may advance the proposition that an earlier (screening) mammogram would have demonstrated the calcifications, thereby prompting biopsy and earlier diagnosis, prior to the development of a palpable mass.

Appellate court decisions support the use of diagnostic mammography when areas of clinical concern have been identified. The use of mammography in such circumstances should be viewed by the clinician in two respects. The first is that the mammography study and ancillary studies such as ultrasonography may help characterize the areas of clinical concern. Clinicians should insist that the referring radiology facility specifically address any given area of clinical concern with pertinent comments, whether positive or negative, rather than the universal disclaimers often used. It remains a clinical standard of care that biopsy of a suspicious palpable area should not be deterred by a negative (i.e., with no preceived significant abnormality) mammography report. Thus the inability to characterize an area of clinical concern by imaging limits the basis of the clinical management plan to the history and the physical examination findings.

Management plans should be deliberate and reasonable. When cancer is discovered, an aggrieved plaintiff may contend that the area should have undergone excisional biopsy. This decision remains within the purview of clinical judgment, which itself is subject to expert testimony. Different reasonable approaches, especially evidence-based, may survive legal challenge.

Consider, for example, a solid mass in a woman that by imaging parameters is smooth and highly suggestive of a fibroadenoma. A fine-needle aspiration showing sufficient cellular material to indicate a probable fibroadenoma cytologically (i.e., sheets of cohesive, normal-appearing ductal epithelial cells, abundant "naked nuclei" indicating evidence of myoepithelial cells, and benign stroma) provides a rational basis for surveillance instead of excision. However, if such findings occur in a postmenopausal woman and the mass continues to grow, especially if she is not on exogenous hormonal therapy, the presumption of a fibroadenoma should be questioned. Although the initial diagnosis may have been reasonable, the continued diagnosis may not be when the clinical course is inconsistent with the initial diagnosis. Then the management needs to be altered. Thus *reasonableness*, which is the legal test of compliance with duty, depends on the given patient and the associated circumstances.

Duty, as the first element of the tort of negligence, is variable. The breach of duty, if it is the *cause in fact* and *proximate cause* of injury, such as delay in diagnosis of cancer, constitutes negligence. If the unreasonable conduct of a physician bears a substantial causative relation to an injury incurred, and if a reasonable and prudent physician in similar circumstances would not have acted in a similar manner, the defendant physician may be liable under the legal theory of negligence.

For a lawsuit to be filed and a summons and complaint issued, there must be a reasonable expectation of damages that will serve as a measure of restitution. For example, if an unreasonable and inadequate physical examination is performed so a clinically suspicious mass is not identified, but an immediate mammographic study detects malignant features associated with that mass prompting a biopsy and diagnosis, it is unlikely that "damages" secondary to delay can be shown, even though the duty of the clinician was breached. In the legal sense, there lacks a "causative" nexus (connection) to delay in diagnosis because there was no significant (actual) delay.

Another allegation that not infrequently arises in the context of delayed diagnosis of breast cancer is the infliction of mental distress (either intentionally or negligently). The issue is not trivial because the discovery of breast cancer is almost by definition "distressing" to all individuals concerned, including patients and health care providers. In the prior case example, the patient may claim distress from the inadequate examination. Lawsuits for mental distress usually require the preliminary showing of negligence, but occasionally courts award a patient damages for distress alone.

Because patient compliance with any management plan may not occur, clinicians often use tickler files or other systematic methods (e.g., computerized programs) for tracking their patients. For example, if a physician requests a patient to return in a month for reevaluation of one or more areas of her breast and she does not return, the physician may send her an additional reminder. In such a case, where a cancer diagnosis ensues, the patient may claim that the physician did not sufficiently instruct her to return or advised her to return only as needed. The court usually sees the physician as possessing superior knowledge regarding the potential seriousness of a given medical situation. When a lawsuit for delay in diagnosis of cancer is claimed, the patient may be shown to be "contributorily negligent" (the effect of which is to decrease the eventual damage award), but it does not relieve the physician of some potential liability. During legal proceedings the particular circumstances of the case are evaluated on their individual merit.

Several other medical legal aspects relating to clinical practice, all relating to the various duties the law imposes on practitioners of medicine, should be brought to the physician's attention. The *duty to refer* is imposed when medical attention or procedures are required beyond the scope of expertise of the clinician. The *tort of negligent referral* may be claimed when a clinician refers a patient to another health care provider or facility the referring clinician knows, or has reason to know, cannot provide sufficient services. Consider, for example, the referral of a patient to a mammography facility that has been denied FDA certification repeatedly. If subsequently a substandard mammographic study is performed and a cancer is undetected, both the mammographic facility and the referring physician may be subject to a lawsuit: one for negligence, the other for negligent referral.

In additon, clinicians must be aware of the tort called *abandonment*. Legally, parity does not exist in the patient–physician relationship. The patient may choose to leave a physician's care at any time, but the converse is not necessarily true. If a patient under the care of a physician requires additional care, and the physician for any reason does not wish to care for that patient anymore, the physician must provide for the proper transfer of care and should document such efforts. The more acute the medical situation, the greater must the effort be to provide reasonably prompt transfer of care. When such transfer is not undertaken, the tort of abandonment may be claimed. This situation may arise for a variety of reasons, including nonpayment for services or breakdown in the physician–patient relationship. Whatever the reason, the physician is required to provide reasonable efforts to transfer care to another qualified provider. The documentation of such efforts is important to defeat the claim of abandonment if the patient declines to participate in appropriate future care.

All states have a "statute of limitations" that requires an aggrieved patient to bring a lawsuit against the physician within a certain designated time (usually 1 or 2 years) after the patient discovers, or has reason to discover, that potential negligence has occurred. The justification for such statutes is beyond the scope of this discussion, but the intent can be understood when one considers that actions brought many years after an event are difficult to investigate because of loss of records and poor recollections. Suppose a patient with a small, misdiagnosed cancer did well for 10 years and then presented again but this time with metastatic disease. Although it is understandable that the physician might want to mitigate anxiety regarding the prior management plans, it is essential to avoid withholding or incorrectly stating any material (i.e., significant facts) even with the best of intentions. Under usual circumstances, a claim of negligence with respect to the initial diagnosis is barred; but if fraud can be shown, the lawsuit can proceed.

The *law of agency* imposes liability on the physician for errors or omissions of those personnel working under his or her control and for his or her benefit. The importance of this law, which is sometimes referred to as vicarious liability, or the *doctrine of respondeat superior*, is illustrated by the example of a significantly abnormal laboratory or imaging result being received by a clerk who does not notify the physician. Should an adverse consequence develop, the error of the clerk is attributed to the physician under whose supervision the clerk's conduct is judged.

The *law of consent*, especially *informed consent*, is frequently misunderstood. The *intentional tort of battery* (the unlawful touching of another individual), which is not usually covered by medical liability insurance policies, is defeated by obtaining consent. When an invasive procedure is performed, informed consent, which is judged under the law of negligence, is required. Informed consent requires that the physician disclose to the patient all material risks of the procedure and alternatives. For example, clinicians performing fine-needle aspirations or large needle-core biopsies of palpable lesions should obtain informed consent and include in the discussion the limitations inherent in the results of the test, including the need for compliance associated with further clinical surveillance if excisional biopsy is not performed.

The conduct of a physician is evaluated with respect to what a reasonable and prudent physician would do under similar circumstances. For example, for clinicians, who elect to perform ultrasonography of the breast in their office, the standard of care expected is determined accordingly. It is of little value to disclose to a patient that the skill and experience of the operator is limited and obtain an "informed consent" permitting the study to be done under such conditioned circumstances. This kind of consent is not valid in defending against an unreasonable examination.

The rise in medical malpractice lawsuits has prompted some clinicians to seek refuge in ordering more tests of questionable indication, a practice colloquially referred to as "defensive medicine." Such an approach is not likely to survive the restrictions of managed care and is of little legal importance. Rather, the effort of *defensible medicine* should be urged where deliberate management is based on evidence-based rationale, sound clinical judgment is well documented, and there is awareness by the patient of the intended goals and limitations of a given plan. Some of the suggested risk-management approaches discussed above may sound adversarial, though they are not so. The adversarial nature of a lawsuit is virtually antithetical to the relationship desired between a patient and a physician. The legal conditions under which physicians practice, however, must be recognized so that behavior patterns are established that serve the dual goals of sound medical practice and minimized legal exposure. There is virtually no way to insulate oneself totally from a malpractice lawsuit, the existence of which can be devastating and demoralizing to the physician. Practices that incorporate reasonable medical approaches with prudent risk management, however, are usually positioned to defeat unreasonable claims.

Recommended Reading

Brenner RJ. Breast cancer evaluation: medical legal and risk management considerations for the clinician. Cancer 1994;74:486–491

Brenner RJ. Evolving medical legal concepts for clinicians and imagers in evaluation of breast cancer. Cancer 1992;69:1950–1953

Brenner RJ. Medical legal aspects of breast cancer evaluation and treatment. In: Harris JR, Lippman ME, Morrow M, et al (eds) Diseases of the Breast. Philadelphia, Lippincott-Raven, 1996

Brenner RJ. Medical legal aspects of breast imaging. Surg Oncol Clin North Am 1994;3:67–85

Brenner RJ. Medical legal consideration in breast cancer for the primary care physician. Prim Care Cancer 1991;11:45–51

Brooks PG, Brenner RJ. The Gynecologist's Role in the Detection and Management of Breast Disease. Chicago, Year Book, 1984

37 THE BREAST DIAGNOSTIC CENTER: EXPERIENCE AND PROTOCOLS

William H. Hindle

The Breast Diagnostic Center (BDC) first began operation in July 1988 at the extensive health care facilities run jointly by Los Angeles County and the University of Southern California Medical School (LACUSCMC). The BDC was created to serve two goals: (1) provide for the breast care of women presenting to the Department of Obstetrics and Gynecology (inpatients and outpatients); and (2) fill the pressing need for education and experience in breast care for obstetrics and gynecology resident physicians.

The BDC, a mammography unit, outpatient clinics for women, operating rooms, and the Department of Obstetrics and Gynecology are all conveniently located under one roof in Women's and Children's Hospital (W&CH). Three other clinics at LACUSCMC provide breast services: two Breast Surgery Clinics, run by the Department of Surgery, and the USC/Norris Breast Center, within the Norris Cancer Hospital and Research Institute, for private patients. The LACUSCMC outpatient clinics are referral clinics; that is, the patients must be referred for consultation by a physician. The BDC is an exception to this restriction in that a woman can self-refer (i.e., can directly contact the facility and make her own appointment for a perceived breast problem). About 13% of the BDC initial encounters are self-referred patients. The BDC is not designed to do routine breast examinations.

On-site services for patients at the BDC include (1) mammography, (2) evaluation of breast concerns and symptoms, (3) evaluation of breast masses, (4) fine-needle aspiration of palpable dominant breast masses, (5) treatment of benign breast disorders, and (6) expeditious referral of patients with diagnosed breast cancer (or high suspicion thereof) to the appropriate LACUSCMC clinics for treatment.

PATIENT VISITS

From July 1988 through June 1997 there were 11,828 patient visits to the BDC, of which 10,763 (91%) were new patient encounters. By BDC policy and protocol, the clinical objective is to complete a breast evaluation during one BDC visit. Follow-up is provided at the regional Los Angeles County Community Health Centers, which are generally located closer to the patient's neighborhood than is W&CH. Thus BDC patients are returned to their primary care providers with a completed evaluation, treatment plan, and instructions for follow-up (e.g., continuing treatment or subsequent breast examinations). During 1996–1997 the weekly half-day BDC clinics have evaluated an average of 42 patients per session of whom 39 are new patients with breast problems. Because the "failed appointment" rate is currently approximately 40%, about 70 appointments are made for each BDC clinic. A woman with a perceived breast mass is given priority and scheduled for the next weekly BDC session.

PATIENT AGE AND ETHNIC BACKGROUND

The mean age of the women seen in the BDC (July 1995 through June 1997) is 39 years (range 9–91 years). About 85% of the BDC patients are Hispanic, and most of them speak limited English, if any (Table 37.1).

PRESENTING COMPLAINTS

The most common presenting complaint of patients attending the BDC (July 1995 through June 1997) is a perceived breast mass: 44% complained of a mass only and 8% complained of a mass and pain (mass only + mass and pain = 52%). Clinical breast examination (CBE) confirmed the presence of a palpable dominant breast mass in 56% of the women presenting with a perceived (by the patient or her referring physician) breast mass as the chief complaint. Breast pain (31%) was the next most common presenting complaint: 23% complained only of pain and 8% of pain and a mass.

Only 4% presented complaining of nipple discharge, among whom, when specifically questioned, fewer than 25% described spontaneous nipple discharge, thereby reducing the incidence of spontaneous nipple discharge as a presenting

Table 37.1. BDC patient demographics: July 1995 to June 1997 (n = 3311)

Self-referred	13%
Age, mean	39 years (range 9–91 years)
Self-declared race (ethnic background)	
Hispanic	85%
Black	5%
Caucasian	5%
Oriental	3%
Other	2%

complaint to less than 1%. The percentages of presenting complaints by women attending the BDC from July 1995 through June 1997 are listed in Table 37.2.

The accuracy of the clinical impression recorded by the resident physicians (after taking the breast-oriented history and doing a CBE) compared to the FNA final diagnosis was 70% for fibroadenomas, 61% for fibrocystic changes, and 58% for cysts (Table 37.3).

FINE-NEEDLE ASPIRATION

By BDC protocol, a palpable dominant breast mass is evaluated by fine-needle aspiration (FNA). From July 1988 through June 1997 FNA was performed on 3267 dominant breast masses (30% of BDC new patients underwent an FNA). The final cytology diagnoses are listed alphabetically in Table 37.4 and by frequency percentages in Table 37.5. Fibroadenoma was the most common (29%) cytologic diagnosis followed by various forms of fibrocystic changes (20%), including benign ductal epithelium (13%). Cysts accounted for 6% (hence 94% of the lesions were solid). Cancer was diagnosed by FNA in 7%. Thus slightly more than 2% of all new patients presenting to the BDC with a palpable dominant mass were diagnosed by FNA as having carcinoma. This small percentage of malignancies probably relates to the relatively young age of the patients seen in the BDC (mean age 39 years) and the low incidence of breast cancer in Hispanic women (see

Table 37.2. BDC presenting complaints at primary patient encounters: July 1995 through June 1997 ($n = 4820$)

Complaint	%
Mass	44 } 52
Mass/pain	8 }
Pain only	23 } 31
Abnormal mammogram	12
Follow-up	8
Nipple discharge	4 (spontaneous 1)
Other	1
Mastitis/abscess	<0.5

Table 37.3. BDC resident physicians' clinical impression prior to FNA of a palpable dominant breast mass: July 1996 through June 1997 ($n = 566$)

Clinical impression	% Confirmed by FNA
Fibroadenoma	70
Fibrocystic changes	61
Cyst	58

Table 37.4. BDC FNAs of palpable dominant breast masses: cytology reports: July 1988 through June 1997 ($n = 3267$)

Cytology report (listed alphabetically)	%
Abscess	<1
Acellular	2
Adenocarcinoma	7
Adipose tissue	3
Atypical ductal cells	4
Benign ductal epithelium	13
Cyst	6
Epidermal inclusion cyst	<1
Fat necrosis	<1
Fibroadenoma: consistent with, definitive, probable, suggestive of	29
Fibroadenoma/fibrocystic change	4
Fibroadenoma/phyllodes	<1
Fibroadipose tissue	1
Fibrocystic change	4
Galactocele	1
Inadequate for cytologic diagnosis	<1
Inflammation	2
Lactational adenoma	<1
Lactational change	5
Lymph node	<1
No malignant cells identified	1
Nondiagnostic	<1
Other benign conditions	3
Stroma	<1
Unsatisfactory	11

Fig. 1.4). Furthermore, within LACUSCMC there are two weekly half-day Breast Surgery Clinics staffed by the Department of Surgery to which most obvious breast cancers are directly referred (either from inside or outside LACUSCMC). The summary percentages of the final FNA cytologic diagnoses are listed in Table 37.6.

In cytology reports "acellular" means no identifiable cells are seen, a designation of no clinical value. Close follow-up is then essential. If CBE within 1–2 months reveals a persistent palpable dominant breast mass, a repeat FNA or other diagnostic procedure (or referral to a breast specialist) is required.

"No malignant cells identified (noted)" requires further reading of the written report. Benign ductal cells may be present or stroma and adipose tissue without ductal cells. If no ductal cells are seen and the clinical or mammographic impression is of a cellular neoplasm, the FNA should be repeated or other diagnostic

Table 37.5. BDC FNAs of palpable dominant breast masses: cytology reports: July 1988 through June 1997 (*n* = 3267)

Cytology report (listed by % frequency)	%
Fibroadenoma consistent with, definitive, probably, suggestive of	29
Benign ductal epithelium	13
Unsatisfactory	11
Adenocarcinoma	7
Cyst	6
Lactational change	5
Atypical ductal cells	4
Fibroadenoma/fibrocystic change	4
Fibrocystic change	4
Adipose tissue	3
Other benign conditions	3
Acellular	2
Inflammation	2
Fibroadipose tissue	1
Galactocele	1
No malignant cells identified	1
Abscess	<1
Epidermal inclusion cyst	<1
Fat necrosis	<1
Fibroadenoma/phyllodes	<1
Inadequate for cytologic diagnosis	<1
Lactational adenoma	<1
Lymph node	<1
Nondiagnostic	<1
Stroma	<1

Table 37.6. BDC FNAs of palpable dominant breast masses: cytology reports: July 1988 through June 1997 (*n* = 3267)

Cytology report	Summary %
Fibroadenoma	29
Fibrocystic changes, normal breast	20
Inadequate for cytologic diagnosis	13
Adenocarcinoma	7
Cyst	6
Other (<5% each)	25

procedures performed. However, if the clinical and mammographic impression indicate a benign lesion or normal breast tissue, and benign ductal cells are identified, it can be assumed that the lesion is benign and should be followed or treated as the clinical impression indicates.

"Inadequate for cytologic diagnosis" means that no well-preserved ductal cells are noted (or so few that the cytopathologist cannot make a judgment). Nevertheless, the report may contain clinically helpful information. For example, a cytology description of "normal stroma and adipose tissue" would be consistent with the clinical and mammographic impression of a lipoma, and the lesion could be treated or followed with confidence.

Thus correlation of all the clinical information with the entire FNA cytology report is vital. It was found that an estimated 97.5% of all the FNAs over the entire BDC experience (1988–1997) contained pertinent material (clinical information). Review of 100 consecutive cases (during 1996–1997) that traditionally would have been called "false-negative" FNAs, revealed that in 82 of the 100 cases clinically useful information was contained in the written text of the cytology report that could appropriately be used for the clinical management decision. The final cytology diagnoses that might have been classified as "false-negative" are listed in Table 37.7; they constitute 14% of all the FNA reports during the BDC experience. The written descriptions of the cellular material in these 100 reports are listed in Table 37.8. In fact, none of the "false-negative" FNAs in this review was truly false-negative; that is, none represented a missed diagnosis of a malignancy.

Open Surgical Biopsy Diagnoses

For comparison to the final cytologic diagnoses of the FNAs performed in the BDC, the final histologic diagnoses from all breast open surgical biopsies (OSBx) of a palpable dominant mass performed at the LACUSCMC during 1993–1995 ($n = 1269$) are listed alphabetically in Table 37.9 and in order of percentage frequency in Table 37.10. Of the specimens, about one-fifth (20%) were malignant; somewhat less than one-third (29%) were fibroadenomas; about one-third (33%) were various forms of fibrocystic change including benign ductal epithelium; and the remaining 18% were various other types of benign lesions (Table 37.11). These OSBx data answer the clinical question, "What is the histopathology of palpable

Table 37.7. BDC "false-negative" FNA cytology reports

Final cytologic diagnosis	No.
Unsatisfactory	14
Nondiagnostic	91
Inadequate for cytologic diagnosis	270
Acellular	82
Total	457 (14% of 3267 FNAs)

Table 37.8. Retrospective review of 100 consecutive "false-negative" FNAs, 1996–1997

Cellular material description	No.
Benign ductal epithelium	25
Fat (adipose tissue)	22
Cyst (gross fluid)	17
Normal breast tissue	10
Fibroadipose tissue	3
Stroma	3
Milk	1
Squamous cells	1
Subtotal	72
No cells identified	18 (2.5% of all FNAs 1988–1997)
Total	100

Table 37.9. LAC + USC Medical Center open surgical biopsy pathology reports of palpable dominant masses: 1993–1995 ($n = 1269$)

Pathology report (listed alphabetically)	%
Abscess	1
Adenomyoepithelioma	1
Adenosis	<1
Atypical hyperplasia	<1
Benign breast tissue	13
Ductal carcinoma in situ (DCIS)	1
DCIS with microinvasion	1
Ductal carcinoma, invasive	12
Epidermal inclusion cyst	<1
Fat necrosis	<1
Fibroadenoma	29
Fibroadipose tissue	4
Fibrocystic changes	15
Fibrosis	3
Granuloma	1
Hyperplasia, nonatypical	3
Inadequate	1
Inflammation/mastitis	3
Intraductal papilloma	2
Invasive ductal carcinoma with DCIS	3
Lobular carcinoma, invasive	1
Other carcinomas and sarcomas	3
Phyllodes tumor, benign	<1
Phyllodes tumor, malignant	0
Sclerosing adenosis	<1
Tubular adenoma	<1

Table 37.10. LAC + USC Medical Center open surgical biopsy pathology reports of palpable dominant masses: 1993–1995 ($n = 1269$)

Pathology report (listed by % frequency)	%
Fibroadenoma	29
Fibrocystic changes	15
Benign breast tissue	13
Ductal carcinoma, invasive	12
Fibroadipose tissue	4
Fibrosis	3
Hyperplasia, nonatypical	3
Inflammation/mastitis	3
Invasive ductal carcinoma with ductal carcinoma in situ (DCIS)	3
Other carcinomas and sarcomas	3
Intraductal papilloma	2
Abscess	1
Adenomyoepithelioma	1
DCIS	1
DCIS with microinvasion	1
Granuloma	1
Inadequate	1
Lobular carcinoma, invasive	1
Adenosis	<1
Atypical hyperplasia	<1
Epidermal inclusion cyst	<1
Fat necrosis	<1
Phyllodes tumor, benign	<1
Sclerosing adenosis	<1
Tubular adenoma	<1
Phyllodes tumor, malignant	0

Table 37.11. LAC + USC Medical Center open surgical biopsy pathology reports of palpable dominant masses: 1993–1995 ($n = 1269$)

Pathology report	Summary %
Fibrocystic changes/normal breast	33
Fibroadenoma	29
Carcinoma	20
Other benign lesions	18

dominant breast masses?" Furthermore, they allow correlations, for both type of lesion and percentages, with the FNA cytology diagnoses. However, the patients having FNAs at the BDC and those having OSBx at General Surgery are distinctly different populations, particularly as to age and clinical impression of cancer.

BREAST DIAGNOSTIC CENTER PROTOCOLS

Appointments

Appointments are accepted for any woman with a breast complaint from a referring physician or the patient herself (self-referred). A block of appointment "slots" are kept open for women with a breast mass, and such patients are given priority and seen usually within 1 week (2 weeks at the most).

Interviews and Physician Evaluation

All patients are initially seen by a nurse (or equivalent) who is fluent in Spanish and who fills out the BDC Patient's History Intake Form. Patients are then seen by the obstetrics and gynecology resident physicians, who review the Patient's History Intake Form, take a full breast-oriented history and whatever other history they deem clinically appropriate, perform a complete bilateral clinical breast examination, fill out the BDC Initial Evaluation form, and present the case to the staff or a staff-designated senior resident physician.

Palpable Dominant Breast Masses

All palpable dominant breast masses are definitively diagnosed. The obstetrics and gynecology resident physicians, under staff supervision, perform the initial FNA, using needle-only technique (see Chapter 8). If an adequate cell sample is not obtained, a repeat FNA is performed either by the resident physician or a cytopathologist (staff or resident). If the second FNA is acellular, a third FNA is performed by staff (usually with a pistol-type syringe holder utilizing negative pressure in the syringe and often with ultrasound guidance to ensure a successful third procedure). If the third FNA is acellular, a tissue core-needle biopsy (TCNB) is performed with ultrasound guidance.

If the TCNB histology is not diagnostic and the mass is suspicious for malignancy, the patient is sent to the Department of Surgery for OSBx. If the histology of the TCNB is not diagnostic and the clinical impression and mammogram suggest a benign lesion (including atypical cells), OSBx is performed by the Department of Obstetrics and Gynecology following the National Surgical Adjuvant Breast and Bowel Program (NSABP) lumpectomy protocol (see Chapter 12).

A logbook is kept of all the FNAs performed in the BDC with a listing of: (1) date; (2) patient's name; (3) LACUSCMC identification number; (4) patient's age and description of the mass (side and size); (5) clinical impression before the FNA; (6) preliminary impression of the cytology in the BDC; (7) final cytology diagnosis; and (8) appointments or follow-up.

Palpable Fibroadenoma

When concordance of the findings of CBE, mammography, and FNA (the diagnostic triad) confirms the diagnosis of a fibroadenoma, the patient is offered the choice of excision by OSBx (to be performed at a time convenient for the patient) or continuous follow-up with the next CBE scheduled at the BDC in 6 months.

Palpable Cyst

When a palpable cyst is identified by FNA, all the fluid is completely drained from the cyst. The area is palpated to be certain there is no residual or underlying mass. If there is a palpable mass, it is subjected to FNA for cytology. If there is doubt as to complete drainage of the cyst, ultrasonography is utilized to resolve the dilemma. FNA slides are not made of cyst fluid at the BDC, but because of an ongoing clinical research project all cyst fluids are sent to cytopathology.

Follow-up of a cyst is scheduled at the BDC in 2 months for palpation of the aspirated area to be certain that the cyst has not reformed (refilled). If the cyst has refilled, it is aspirated with ultrasound guidance and confirmation of complete removal of all the cyst fluid. BDC protocol requires that if a cyst refills a second time the lesion must be definitively diagnosed by OSBx; to date, however, this situation has not occurred.

Cyclic and Diffuse Noncyclic Mastalgia

Mastalgia is treated in a progressive stepwise fashion: That is, if the first step does not resolve the problem to the patient's satisfaction, the next step is recommended. In order, the steps followed are (1) reassurance; (2) mechanical measures; (3) premenstrual salt restriction; (4) intermittent analgesia; (5) low dose oral contraceptives; and (6) danazol. In fact, danazol is rarely prescribed.

Mastitis and Abscess

Mastitis is treated with antibiotic therapy immediately upon clinical diagnosis (or even suspicion). The patient is seen for follow-up every 3 days, and the therapy is continued if the problem is resolving. It the mastitis does not respond, the antibiotics are changed. If the second antibiotic therapy is not successful, a skin biopsy is performed and consultation obtained.

Ultrasonography is utilized to confirm a liquid center if an abscess is suspected and the clinical examination is uncertain. Abscesses are treated by 18-gauge needle aspiration. The needle aspiration is repeated every 3 days until the abscess and associated infection subsides. Ultrasound guidance is used for draining the abscess and to be certain the entire accumulation of pus has been removed. If needle drainage does not clear the abscess and achieve a complete clinical response, open surgical drainage under general anesthesia is performed. It has rarely been necessary.

Nipple Discharge

A galactogram (ductogram) is ordered for spontaneous, single duct opening nipple discharge. Clinically diagnosed non-pregnancy-related galactorrhea cases are referred to the Endocrine-Infertility Division, Department of Obstetrics and Gynecology. Other types of milky nipple discharge are evaluated, diagnosed, and treated in the BDC. Smears of nipple discharge are not utilized.

Diagnostic Mammography

Diagnostic mammography is ordered for all women over the age of 30 who present to the BDC unless they have recent films in hand (taken within 1 year). Films brought in are sent to the LACUSCMC mammography service for interpretation and a written report. If the clinical impression is breast cancer in a woman younger than 30 years, arrangements are made by staff directly with a LACUSCMC mammographer for diagnostic mammography.

Screening Mammography

Annual screening mammography is ordered for all women beginning at age 40. For a woman whose first-degree relative has been diagnosed with invasive breast cancer, annual screening mammography is begun 10 years earlier than the relative's age at diagnosis: for example, if the mother was diagnosed with invasive breast cancer at age 45, her daughter begins annual screening mammography at age 35. Screening mammography is deferred during pregnancy.

Open Surgical Biopsy by the Obstetrics and Gynecology Department

Open surgical biopsy (OSBx) is performed at the patient's request when a woman has an FNA-diagnosed fibroadenoma (see Chapter 20). Other benign (by FNA cytology) dominant breast masses are excised by OSBx if the patient requests removal. Other masses that are clinically benign, including those with FNA-diagnosed atypical cells, are excised following the NSABP lumpectomy protocol. All masses that are clinically suspicious of malignancy are referred to the Breast Surgery Clinic (Department of Surgery), as are those that the staff prefers not to excise.

Nonpalpable Lesions

By agreement with the Departments of Radiology and Surgery, all nonpalpable lesions are evaluated and followed by the Mammography Service of the Department of Radiology. Those lesions for which biopsy is recommended are presented and discussed at a weekly joint mammography–surgery conference.

Malignant Lesions

All lesions deemed malignant (including suspicious lesions) by FNA, clinical impression, or mammography are referred to the Breast Surgery Clinic, Department of Surgery, for evaluation and treatment.

Follow-up

Every attempt is made to complete the breast evaluation at a single visit to the BDC, except for suspicious lesions and aspirated cysts, which require return visits.

Appointments to other departments and for other services are made before the patient leaves the BDC.

Reports, such as for screening mammography, that do not require further studies or therapy are sent to the patients by mail. Reports that require further studies or therapy are communicated to the patient by phone by the BDC nurse supervisor (who is fluent in Spanish).

All women seen in the BDC are instructed to return to their primary care providers for periodic evaluations and an annual CBE. Annual screening mammography is advised for all women age 40 years or older. All women seen in the BDC are given breast self-examination (BSE) booklets and encouraged to perform monthly BSE. All women are instructed to return to the BDC if their breast symptoms persist or progress.

Records

A copy is made of all BDC forms after each visit and retained in a secured confidential BDC file. These copies are utilized for responses to phone calls and clinical research. All BDC original forms, reports, and notes are filed in the patient's LACUSCMC medical record.

Patient Tracking

The BDC nurse supervisor maintains a patient tracking system for all BDC abnormal reports and findings. All BDC referrals are similarly tracked. The clinical courses of all breast malignancies are followed and recorded by the BDC nurse supervisor. LACUSCMC mammography reports, FNA reports, operative reports, and pathology reports are, or soon will be, available to the BDC by computerized systems.

38 BREAST CARE AND SURGERY BY OBSTETRICIAN/ GYNECOLOGISTS IN A RURAL SETTING

James A. Hall

The Women's Health Center of Logansport (WHCL) has provided obstetric and gynecologic care, including total breast care and surgery, to rural north central Indiana since 1948. The county is served by a single 120-bed acute care hospital with a market area of approximately 120,000.

The WHCL offers a full range of obstetric and gynecologic services. There are three obstetrician-gynecologists, a certified nurse-practitioner, and a women's counselor on staff.

A large referral practice for breast disease has been developed. Patients with breast complaints are seen routinely and are not set apart in a separate breast clinic. Same-day appointments are offered to patients with breast problems. We strive to arrive at a diagnosis and therapeutic conclusion as rapidly as possible. A standardized report form (Fig. 38.1) with breast diagrams has facilitated accurate charting and proved valuable for longitudinal care (by multiple physicians) and as medicolegal documentation.

Patients of the WHCL are offered in-house mammography; the films are read by off-site radiologists. Mammography services are also offered by the hospital, but there is no local mammographic stereotactic biopsy service. Breast ultrasonography is performed by the physicians of the WHCL.

All breast surgery, including needle aspiration, open surgical biopsy (OSBx), and cancer surgery (lumpectomy, axillary node dissection, mastectomy) are performed by WHCL obstetrician/gynecologists. Breast surgery is performed at our local hospital. The privilege to perform breast surgery is approved through the hospital credentialing process. Training in breast surgery has been gained through individual effort, observation, and monitoring by other surgeons who do breast procedures. The founding physician of our group was residency trained in breast surgery and has provided leadership and training to subsequent physicians in the group.

As part of our ongoing quality assurance, we have charted our results for accurate removal of nonpalpable lesions by OSBx (Table 38.1) and compared our success rate with that of series reported in the literature (Table 38.2). Our statistics

Women's Health Center *of Logansport*
BREAST DIAGNOSTIC REPORT

NAME_____   DATE_____

Age_____   G_____ P_____ A_____   Referred by_____

Reasons for visit: Mass_____Mammo Lesion_____Pain_____Nipple Discharge_____Other_____

Right / left History:_____

_____

Past Breast History:_____

_____

Family History:_____

BREAST ULTRASOUND   YES / NO

Approximate location of abnormality

Right   Left

Findings:_____
Recommendations_____

YES / NO

NEEDLE ASPIRATION

Solid / Cyst   Fluid_____cc.   Color_____   Blood yes / no   Resolution   yes / no

Approximate location of abnormality

Right   Left

Cytology   yes / no
Cytology Result   yes/ no   _____
Recommendation_____

1201 Michigan Avenue, Suite 170
Logansport, Indiana 46947
219/722-3566
Fax 219/753-6118

Bernard R. Hall, M.D.
James A. Hall, M.D.
Duffy C. Murphy, M.D.
Jeffrey A. VanCuren, M.D.
Beth A. Ruff, R.N.C.,O.G.N.P.

American College of Obstetrics and Gynecology

Figure 38.1. Standardized medical record form for women presenting with breast symptoms or findings.

Table 38.1. Surgical misses (failures to remove target lesion) during open biopsy for nonpalpable mammographic abnormalities: Women's Health Center of Logansport 1980–1996

No. of biopsies	461
No. of failures	3
% Failure	0.6

Table 38.2. Rate of successful removal of mammographic abnormality with initial biopsy

Series	Biopsies successfully removed on first attempt (%)
Hall (WHCL)	99.4
Ostro	97.0
Leis	98.0
Norton	
General anesthesia	92.0
Local anesthesia	78.0
Powell text (multiple reports)	98.0

Adapted from: Ostro LB, Dubois JJ, Rofer RA, et al. Needle biopsy of occult breast lesions. South Med J 1987;80:29–32.
Leis HP, Cammarata A, Laraja BD, et al. Breast biopsy and guidance for occult lesions. Int Surg 1985;70:115–118.
Norton LW, Zeligman BE, Pearlman NW. Accuracy and cost of needle localization breast biopsy. Arch Surg 1988;123:947–950.

Table 38.3. Abnormal mammographic areas confirmed to be malignant by biopsy

Series	% Malignant
Hall (WHCL) 1980–1993	12
University of Kentucky 1981–1989	19
Hall (WHCL) 1993–1996	21
University of Kentucky 1990	31
Multiple series (Powell text)	25

Adapted from: Powell DE, Stelling CB The Diagnosis and Detection *of Breast Disease*. St. Louis, Mosby, 1994

for detecting malignant cancers by OSBx from mammographically abnormal areas are listed in Table 38.3, and the analysis for specific mammographic abnormalities is given in Table 38.4. Our overall experience with OSBx from 1978 through 1996 is presented in Table 38.5.

A plastic surgeon is not locally available, but the need for immediate reconstructive procedures after mastectomy has become rare with the trend toward breast-preserving procedures. WHCL physicians take a leadership role in making sure patients are appropriately referred to consulting physicians for radiation therapy, medical oncology, and plastic surgery. These consultants are available to patients within an hour's drive or at local satellite offices.

The primary care physician has the responsibility for screening, as it is only through early diagnosis that there can be a significant reduction in breast cancer mortality. We find more breast malignancies per year in our practice than all other malignancies combined (Table 38.6). Hospital-wide cancer statistics reveal that breast cancer is the most frequent female malignancy diagnosed (Table 38.7). Even if one does not provide surgical management of breast disease, it is imperative to provide diligent screening for early breast malignancy and to arrange prompt referral. It is important to be knowledgeable about breast problems and disorders, as patients look to their primary care physician for answers to their questions.

Table 38.4. Yield rate of breast cancer of specific mammographic abnormalities (published 1993)

Abnormality	%
Asymmetric density	
Hall (WHCL)	2.0
Bauer	6.6
McQuery	6.0
Abnormal calcifications	
Hall (WHCL)	22.0
Baute	31.0
Bauer	15.8
McQuery	29.0
Mass	
Hall (WHCL)	11.0
Baute	36.0
Bauer	9.7 (spiculated 63.0%)
McQuery	3.0 (spiculated 45.0%)
Mass with abnormal calcium	
Hall (WHCL)	21.0
Baute	54.0
McQuery	20.0

Adapted from: Bauer TL, Pandelidis SM, Rhoads JE, Owens EB. Mammographically detected carcinoma of the breast. Surg Gynecol Obstet 1991; 173:482–6.
McCreery BE, Frenkle G, Fzost DB. An analysis of the results of mammographically guided biopsies of the breast. Surg Gynecol Obstet 1991;172:223–6.
Baute PB, Thibodeau M, Newstead G. Improving the yield of biopsy for nonpalpable lesions of the breast. Surg Gynecol Obstet 1992;174:93–6.

Table 38.5. Indication for and results of breast biopsy: malignancies found per indication of discovery: Women's Health Center of Logansport, 1978–1996

Year	Palpable mass	Abnormal mammogram	Nipple discharge	Prophylactic mastectomy	Total
1978	2/10	0/0	0/1		2/11
1979	2/15	0/0	0/0		2/15
1980	6/17	0/1	0/0		6/18
1981	3/15	0/2	0/0		3/17
1982	4/18	0/4	0/2		4/24
1983	1/17	0/3	0/1		1/21
1984	6/25	0/18	0/1		6/44
1985	8/26	3/24	0/2		11/52
1986	5/15	1/8	0/0		6/23
1987	7/32	2/15	0/0		9/47
1988	6/24	3/16	0/0		9/40
1989	6/25	4/13	0/3		10/41
1990	7/55	6/69	0/0		13/124
1991	17/54	9/87	0/0	1/1	27/142
1992	3/26	5/37	0/0		8/63
1993	9/35	7/30	0/0		16/65
1994	6/22	8/33	0/0		14/55
1995	5/28	7/40	0/0		12/68
1996	4/40	12/61	1/1		17/102
Total	107/499 (21%)	67/461 (14%) (21% 1993–1996)	1/10 (10%)	1/1	176/971 (18%)

Table 38.6. Malignancies diagnosed at Women's Health Center of Logansport, 1992–1993

Site	No. of patients
Breast	24
Uterine	7
Ovary	3
Colon	3
Pancreas	2
Lung	2
Vulva	1
Cervix	1
Vagina	1
Oral	1
Total	45

Table 38.7. Female cancer distribution 1991: Logansport, Indiana (total hospital statistics)

Site	Percent of all cancers
Breast	50
Colon/rectal	12
Uterus	9
Lungs	8
Leukemia/lymphoma	6
Pancreas	3
Ovary	1
Melanoma	1
Urinary	1
Other	9

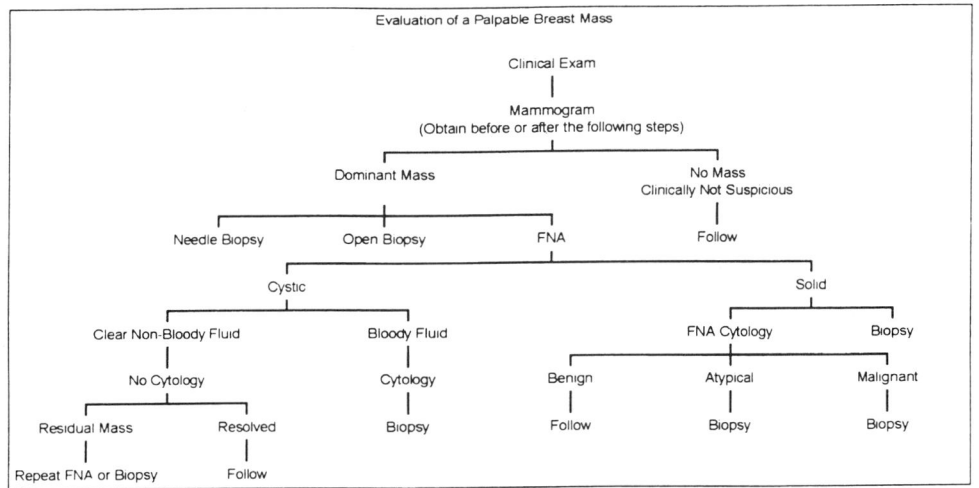

Figure 38.2. Evaluation of a palpable breast mass.

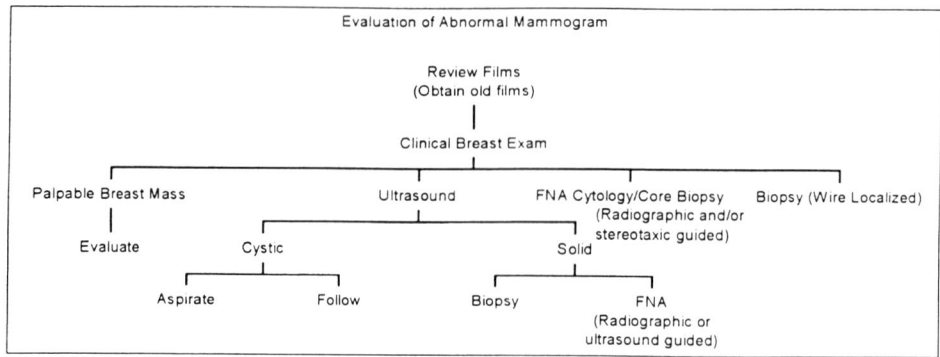

Figure 38.3. Evaluation of an abnormal mammogram.

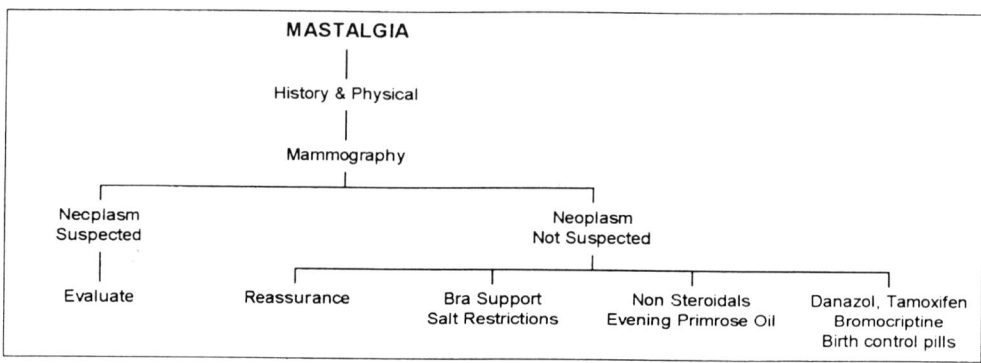

Figure 38.4. Evaluation of mastalgia.

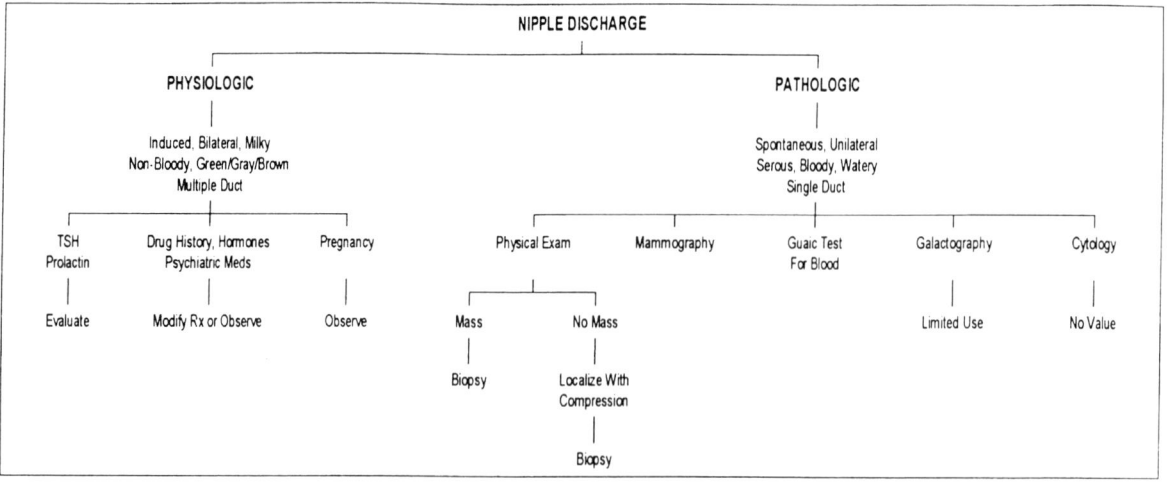

Figure 38.5. Evaluation of nipple discharge.

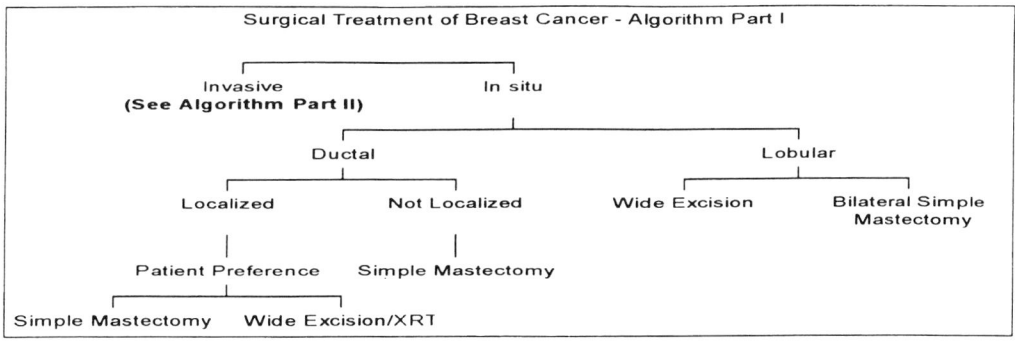

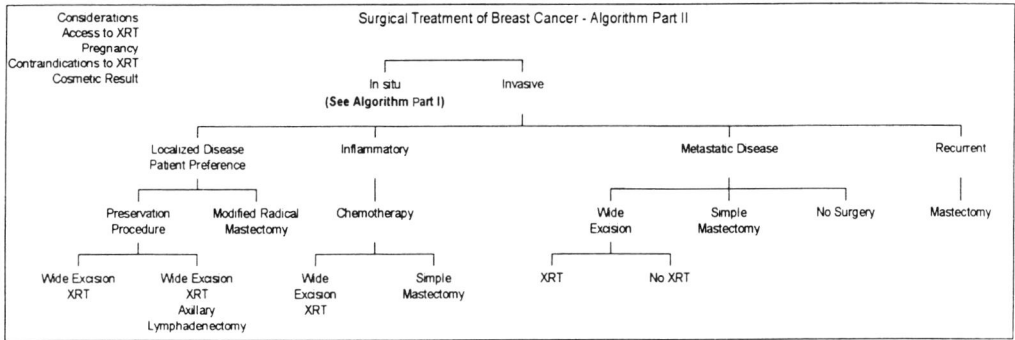

Figure 38.6. Surgical treatment of breast cancer. XRT = x-ray therapy.

Primary care physicians must be available to patients for long-term follow-up. Most patients look to their primary care physician for integration of their breast cancer treatment with other ongoing health concerns. The specialist is rarely involved in other health issues, and most patients feel more comfortable with their primary physician. Management of breast cancer requires teamwork between all health care providers, and it is our belief that the primary care physician must be involved.

The WHCL algorithms for the evaluation of the common clinical breast problems are shown in Figures 38.2–38.5: for a palpable breast mass (Fig. 38.2), an abnormal mammogram (Fig. 38.3), mastalgia (Fig. 38.4), and nipple discharge (Fig. 38.5). An algorithm for the surgical treatment of breast cancer is offered in Figure 38.6.

39   BREAST CARE BY PRIMARY CARE PROVIDERS IN RURAL AREAS

Suzanne M. Taylor

Much has been written about breast care delivery in breast care centers and multidisciplinary settings, but often the options they provide are not available in a rural setting. Certainly these services can be had by a patient who is willing and able to travel several hours and several hundred miles. For many patients, however, such travel is not an option. In the area where I currently practice it is not uncommon for a woman to choose mastectomy simply because she cannot travel to a center for the radiation therapy that accompanies breast-saving lumpectomy.

To a board-certified family physician who practiced breast care exclusively for 5 years and is now in a rural family practice, this dilemma is a real concern. Here there is no mammography or ultrasonography, and there is no hospital. A mobile mammography unit comes to town twice a month to provide screening mammography services. If a problem is found on the screening mammogram, the patient must travel 60 miles for a diagnostic workup or surgical consultation.

Because of my experience in breast care, it is not uncommon for my primary care colleagues in the area to ask me the question, "How does one provide good breast care in a rural area?" I have learned that approaches to breast care in the rural area can range from "I don't do breast care," to sticking with what worked last time, to keeping up with the literature and adapting it as best you can to your particular setting.

Regardless of the level of involvement in breast care you choose, you as the primary care physician have certain "musts": (1) taking a careful breast history; (2) doing a thorough clinical breast examination; (3) knowing what to order for a breast workup; (4) understanding the surgical procedures; (5) being able to interpret breast pathology reports; (6) having a clear understanding of the various treatment options; (7) knowing how to follow up on any treatment and what to look for in the future. These "musts" are important because the role of the primary care physician is especially critical when the patient must travel any distance for treatment not available at home. It is not uncommon for a patient to see the specialist in the city and come into my office the next day to "check out" what the specialist said. The rural primary care physician is "The Doctor." The specialist is important but has yet to develop the relationship and trust the primary care physician has cultivated over time with the patient and her family. This is true, of course, whenever a primary care physician makes referrals, but it is complicated in the rural setting because of the distance between the patient and the specialist. The primary care physician is accessible—the specialist is far away.

Thus you must be at least conversant with the total process of breast care. It requires close communication with the mammographer, surgeon, pathologist, medical oncologist, radiation oncologist, and plastic surgeon to whom you may refer your patients. It is important to be able to interact with these people, to know how they interact with each other, and most significantly how they interact with your patient and her family.

REFERRING THE PATIENT

Breast History

It is essential to communicate pertinent material in the medical record when you refer your patient, including the chief breast complaint, the history of the current problem, any applicable risk factors, previous breast surgeries, and a review of previous pathology reports. All information in the history should be up-to-date.

Clinical Breast Examination

The breast history and a careful clinical breast examination (CBE) determine whether to refer the patient for screening or diagnostic mammography. It is imperative to communicate any abnormalities found on CBE or in the history to the mammographer. The exact location of any areas of concern must be identified so the mammographer can give a specific answer to any question.

If an abnormality is noted on a screening mammogram, the mammographer notifies the primary care physician and recommends a diagnostic workup. When you send your patient for a diagnostic workup, you should have a clear understanding of the radiographic evaluation, which may include special mammographic views, ultrasonography, fine-needle aspiration (FNA), or stereotactic breast biopsy. The mammographer consults with you regarding any perceived radiographic abnormalities.

Surgical Consultation

It is essential to understand the surgical options available for the patient. In some instances, primary care physicians in rural areas perform incisional or excisional breast biopsies or may assist a surgeon who travels to the rural hospital. Often the primary care physician provides the postsurgical care for the patient who has surgery in another city. Thus it is critical for the primary care physician to have a working knowledge of postoperative care.

Pathology Reports

It is a medicolegal requirement that the primary care physician receive a copy of the complete pathology report if a breast biopsy is undertaken. It is not enough to receive a note from the surgeon simply stating that the finding was "benign," just as it is no longer appropriate for a surgeon to receive such a report from the pathologist. It is necessary to understand the meaning of the entire pathology report and, for example, such terms as nonproliferative, proliferative, atypia, ductal carcinoma in situ (DCIS), and invasive carcinoma. Each of these pathology findings has a determining risk factor for the patient and thus has a role in the follow-up evaluations.

Other Therapy

It is important for the primary care physician to know and have a clear understanding of the options offered the patient by other medical specialists. You may need to confer with the medical oncologist about chemotherapy or the radiation oncologist about radiation treatments; or you may need to discuss reconstruction with the plastic surgeon. You should insist that these specialists communicate with you in writing so you may document any visits, tests, treatment, or surgery.

ONGOING ROLE DURING TREATMENT

It is critical to maintain your role as the primary care physician to be certain that nothing "falls through the cracks." Even though the patient may not feel the need to see you while the workup or treatment for a breast problem is under way, it is important to remind her that other primary health issues must not be ignored (i.e., Papanicolaou smear, blood pressure, diabetes) and that it is your responsibility to be sure she has followed through with any treatment, tests, or surgeries recommended by the specialists. It is still your responsibility to care for the patient and to be certain that she has not "dropped out" of the treatment protocol or delayed or refused a recommended surgical procedure.

FOLLOW-UP

Finally, it is imperative for the primary care physician to have a clear understanding of the follow-up recommendations for patients with and without breast problems. Follow-up for women without breast problems, previous breast surgery, or a strong family history of breast cancer is usually easily accomplished by following the recommendations or breast screening guidelines established by the American Cancer Society (i.e., monthly breast self-examination, annual CBE, and annual screening mammography).

Breast problems to be followed up include such breast biopsy diagnoses as nonproliferative, proliferative, atypia, DCIS, or invasive carcinoma and any other previous breast surgery (breast augmentation, breast reduction, or breast reconstruction). Follow-up must often be individualized for patients with breast problems, previous breast surgery, previous breast cancer, or those in high risk categories for developing invasive breast cancer.

MEDICOLEGAL CONSIDERATIONS

In this litigious society, primary care physicians are included in the litigation regardless of the level of involvement, especially if the patient did not follow the recommendations for surgery, chemotherapy, or radiation therapy. It is essential to remember that documentation can be the health care professional's best friend or worst enemy. The legal standard of care is applicable in rural areas as well as the city and is defined as the degree of care and skill utilized by a reasonable professional practicing in the same or similar circumstances. Delivery of breast services in rural areas should address the patient's total well-being as well as the accepted and expected standard of care. Even in rural areas, consumers are educated and expect health care providers to act as educators and gatekeepers. To meet the demands of these professional roles, all personnel in the rural physician's office should be aware of policies and procedures that affect the delivery of breast care, new technologic advances that enable more accurate diagnosis and treatment, and the ever-changing needs of the patients. Understanding these responsibilities creates a stronger doctor–patient relationship and subsequently a more efficient and effective health care delivery system.

CONCLUSIONS

The patient in a rural area must rely on the primary care physician for guidance over the long course. The primary care physician may continue to treat the whole patient, even one with breast cancer, for the rest of her life. The breast specialist's milestones of 6, 12, and 24 months or 5 years are but a fraction of the time in the rural area where care is provided for multiple generations of families. We may not have treated "grandmother" when she had her breast cancer, but we need to know how to follow her; and we need to know how to care for her daughter, her granddaughter, and her great granddaughter.

Primary care physicians in the rural area have frequent special opportunities to care for patients with breast problems and even breast cancer. We can observe the natural course of breast cancer develop over time. Although we often must defer to our specialist colleagues in cities miles away, it is important to know the process of evaluation and to stay involved with our patient, her treatment, and her lifelong follow-up.

Recommended Reading

American Cancer Society. American Cancer Society national conference on breast cancer. Cancer (suppl) 1994;74:219–536

American Cancer Society. Cancer Facts and Figures 1997. Atlanta, American Cancer Society, 1997

American Cancer Society. International conference on breast cancer research: current issues—future direction. Cancer (Suppl) 1994;74:991–1192

Barker LR, Burton Jr, Zieve PD (eds). Principles of Ambulatory Care Medicine (4th ed). Baltimore, Williams & Wilkins, 1995

Bassett LW (ed). Breast imaging current status and future directions. Radiol Clin North Am 1992;30:1–290

Blank KI, Copeland EM (eds). The Breast: Comprehensive Management of Benign and Malignant Diseases. Philadelphia, Saunders, 1991

Breast Cancer. Vol 1: Reprints from The New England Journal of Medicine Books. Waltham, MA, New England Journal of Medicine Books, 1990

Davis PL (ed). Breast imaging. Magn Reson Imag Clin North Am 1994;2:505–723

DeGowin RL, Brown DD, Christense J. DeGowin & DeGowin's Diagnostic Examination (6th ed). New York, McGraw-Hill, 1994

Donegan WL, Spratt JS (eds). Cancer of the Breast (4th ed). Philadelphia, Saunders, 1995

Hayes DF (ed). Atlas of Breast Cancer. London, Mosby Europe, 1993

Hindle WH (ed). Breast Disease for Gynecologists. Norwalk, CT, Appleton & Lange, 1990

Hughes LE, Mansel RE, Webster DJT (eds). Benign Disorders and Diseases of the Breast. London, Baillière Tindall, 1989

Jackson VP (ed). Breast imaging. Radiol Clin North Am 1995;33:1027–1290

Leucht W (ed). Teaching Atlas of Breast Ultrasound, Stuttgart, Theime, 1992

Marchant DJ (ed). Contemporary management of breast disease. I. Benign disease, Obstet Gynecol Clin North Am 1994;21:421–554

Marchant DJ (ed). Contemporary management of breast disease. II. Breast cancer. Obstet Gynecol Clin North Am 1994;21:555–804

Obergfell AM. Law and Ethics in Diagnostic Imaging and Therapeutic Radiology with Risk Management and Safety Applications. Philadelphia, Saunders, 1995

Seidel HM, Ball JW, Dains JE, et al. Mosby's Physical Examination Handbook. St. Louis, Mosby-Year Book, 1995

Tabar L, Dean PB (eds). Teaching Atlas of Mammography (2nd ed). New York, Thieme-Stratton, 1985

Tohno E, Cosgrove DO, Sloane JP (eds). Ultrasound Diagnosis of Breast Diseases. London, Churchill Livingstone, 1994

Trojani M (ed). A Color Atlas of Breast Histopathology. Philadelphia, Lippincott, 1991

Tucker AK (ed). Textbook of Mammography. London, Churchill Livingstone, 1993

40 ALTERNATIVE AND COMPLEMENTARY THERAPIES FOR BREAST PROBLEMS

Maida Taylor

Almost every culture recommends some sort of herbal, botanical, or plant medicine to initiate lactation, improve breast milk quantity and quality, and assist in weaning. Additionally, there is an array of botanicals supposed to decrease breast pain, lessen premenstrual mastalgia, and improve symptomatic "fibrocystic disease."

Plant materials recommended for breast health often are also purported to lower the risk of breast cancer. A wide variety of nutritional, vitamin, and dietary supplements and interventions are promoted by practitioners of alternative and complementary medicine, but our ability to evaluate and assess the efficacy of these traditional remedies is limited by several factors.

1. Few controlled studies have been done on herbal and botanical interventions in disease processes.

2. Most of the trials that do exist have been done in Europe and Asia, and the literature is not accessible in English.

3. A good deal of the literature about botanicals is anecdotal, limited to reporting sporadic cases.

4. Experimental work on the effects of herbs and plants on animal metabolism and physiology is often freely interpreted and applied to humans. Plant practitioners presume that identical or similar effects occur when a plant preparation is given to people, despite the fact that humans and animals differ drastically in their responses to dietary and pharmacologic interventions. Data derived from animal studies must be carefully interpreted, critically reviewed, and cautiously applied.

5. Long-term interventional studies on dietary modification to lower the incidence of breast cancer and other diseases do not exist as yet. However, population-based studies clearly demonstrate over and over the important role that fruits and vegetables play in disease prevention. A high-fiber diet lowers the risk of colon cancer. High fruit and vegetable intake is associated with a major reduction in the risk of stroke. Vitamin E supplements help to maintain the patency of cardiac bypass grafts and angioplasties. New reports surface every week about the benefits of vegetarianism and of low intake of animal protein and fat, but most studies are done on populations with lifelong histories of "correct"

dietary practice. Can one's diet be modified at age 20, 30, 40, or 70 and still provide significant health benefits? Will that diet be palatable to someone who has grown up eating our "deadly" Western diet?

This chapter seeks to review any and all objective documentation of the claims made for dietary interventions and plant medicines in the treatment and prevention of benign breast diseases. The most commonly touted alternative therapies for breast problems are (1) high-phytoestrogen diet; (2) high-fiber diet; (3) herbal/botanical remedies; (4) vitamin therapies; and (5) limiting methylxanthine intake.

Phytoestrogens

Phytoestrogens are defined as naturally occurring plant sterols that appear to exert effects similar to those of estrogen. Phytoestrogens fall into three groups.

1. *Isoflavones*, particularly genistein and daidzein, are plant sterol molecules found in soy and garbanzo beans and other legumes; they are most often consumed in products such as tempeh, soy, miso, and tofu.
2. *Lignans* are a constituent of the cell walls of plants and are bioavailable through the activity of intestinal bacteria on grains. The highest amounts are found in seed oils, especially flaxseed.
3. *Coumestans* have steroid-like activity but are not important as a source of phytoestrogens for humans. High concentrations are found in red clover, sunflower seeds, and bean sprouts. They are known to have estrogenic effects when ingested by animals, the best known example being subterranean clover, which causes sterility in Australian sheep.

Soy-derived phytoestrogens are abundant in traditional Asian diets. In population-based research studies in countries such as China and Japan, where the local diet is high in soy foods, women offer few menopausal complaints; and, coincidentally, the incidence of breast cancer is low. A similar trend is seen for prostate cancer in Asian men.

A commonly held opinion is that our diet plays a significant role in the high rates of breast cancer in the Western world. Likely mechanisms for this increased risk have been postulated. American and European diets elevate plasma levels of sex hormones and decrease sex hormone-binding globulin concentrations, thus increasing the exposure of peripheral tissues to the effects of circulating estrogens. Diet also lowers the activity of intestinal bacteria on lignans and lowers the isoflavonoid phytoestrogens. Diphenols are produced from phytoestrogens and are thought to be likely candidates for cancer protective substances. Diphenols modify hormone metabolism and production and also appear to limit cancer cell growth.

Given our high levels of sex hormones, low levels of binding globulins, and low levels of lignans and isoflavonoids, the Western diet produces a complex interaction of factors that increase the risk of malignancy. Postmenopausal breast cancer patients have been found to have lower rates of excretion of lignans and isoflavones, and the rates of cancer vary with isoflavonoid excretion patterns. Diet alone, however, may not be the sole operative cause for these trends.[1] Persky and Van Horn[2] indicated that there is sufficient "epidemiologic evidence supporting the hypothesis that phytoestrogens inhibit cancer formation and growth in humans."

Asian women typically ingest 40–80 mg of isoflavones per day, whereas Americans average less than 3 mg/day. High isoflavone intake depresses luteinizing hormone (LH) levels and thereby may exert an antiestrogenic effect. Ipriflavone, a type of isoflavone, slows bone reabsorption and stimulates bone collagen synthesis. A pharmaceutical quality ipriflavone supplement of 600 mg/day is approved in Europe and Japan for treatment of osteoporosis in postmenopausal women.[3]

High isoflavone intake also favorably affects the lipid profile and cardiac disease risk. Work in Finland has found an inverse relation between isoflavone intake and coronary heart disease in both women and men.[4] A meta-analysis of U.S. population-based studies of diet found that high soy intake is associated with significant improvement of lipid profiles. An intake of 37 mg/day yielded both a decline in total cholesterol and a rise in high density lipoprotein (HDL).[5]

As yet no interventional studies have been reported on the impact of isoflavones on menopausal symptoms, such as hot flashes, dyspareunia, and vaginal dryness. Several trials are currently in process,[6] and some oral abstracts were reported recently at the Second International Symposium on the Role of Soy in Preventing and Treating Chronic Disease (September 1996, Brussels, Belgium). One paper reported that a nutritional bar containing 40 mg of isoflavones did not ameliorate hot flashes, and another report stated that an isoflavone intake of 160 mg/day produced a 50% reduction in the frequency and intensity of mild to moderate vasomotor symptoms. At the same meeting, Lamartiniere and associates reported that the isoflavone genistein, a component of soy, prevented the induction of mammary tumors in rats. Using the dimethybenzanthracene mammary cancer model, they found that prepubertal genistein treatment resulted in a decreased incidence and the number of tumors in the treated rat. Treated rats also displayed mammary glands with fewer terminal end buds and more differentiated lobules. They stated that "more differentiated [lobules are] less susceptible to carcinogenesis."

The flavonoids genistein and daidzein suppress carcinogen-induced DNA replication errors and may be partly responsible for the protective effect of soya products.[7] Lignans and isoflavonoids affect uptake and metabolism of sex hormones by participating in the regulation of plasma sex hormone-binding globulin (SHBG) levels and help modulate excretion of estrogens, thus lessening the exposure of tissues to high levels of endogenous steroids. Phytoestrogens interact with the estrogen receptors of human breast cancer cells in culture and therefore may modify estrogen-mediated events in these cells.[8]

The interactions of phytoestrogens with estrogen receptors have also been studied in the human breast cancer cell line MCF-7. A study using coumestrol, genistein, and formononetin, and the mycotoxins (zearalenone and its reduced derivative) found that all of these substances, except formononetin, compete for estradiol-binding sites on both cytoplasmic and nuclear receptors.[9]

In addition to direct effects on the breast, soy products may lower risk by lowering effective circulating levels of potent estrogens. In a study by Lu et al.[10] women were fed 36 oz of soy milk a day for one menstrual cycle. The calculated intake of isoflavone in this amount of soy milk is approximately 100 mg of daidzein (mostly as daidzin) and 100 mg of genistein (mostly as genistin). Serum 17β-estradiol levels dropped by as much as 31–81% at various times in the menstrual cycle during the feeding cycles. The effects of soy feeding persisted for two or three menstrual cycles after they were stopped. Luteal-phase progesterone levels fell by 35% and dehydroepiandrosterone sulfate levels by 14–30%. Menstrual cycle length increased from 28.3 days to 31.8 (±5.1) days during the month of soymilk and did not return to prestudy length until five to six cycles later. Thus phytoestrogens appear to lower ovarian steroids and adrenal androgens. Short-term use also alters menstrual function profoundly for long periods. A study from the National Cancer Institute confirmed that changes in the endogenous endocrine milieu take place rapidly after a high isoflavone diet is initiated. These findings suggest mechanisms by which phytoestrogens modulate the risk of breast and other cancers.

Prepubertal effects of isoflavones in rats and in vitro effects in tissue culture cannot be extrapolated to postmenopausal women, the group most motivated and most likely to implement dietary changes in an effort to lower breast cancer risks. It does seem clear that foods rich in isoflavone offer profound benefits for middle-aged persons. Soy products are an excellent source of plant proteins, and using them as substitutes for animal sources of dietary protein lowers the risk of malignancy and vascular disease. Whether dietary supplementation with isoflavones proves to be a successful therapeutic intervention to lower the risk of breast cancer in premenopausal or postmenopausal American women remains to be seen. Clinical trials studying dietary modification are currently under way.

FIBER

Diphenols, as noted earlier, may lower cancer risk and are abundant in fiber-rich unrefined grain products, various seeds, beans, peas, and berries. Fiber also modifies the level of sex hormones by increasing gastrointestinal motility and by altering bile acid metabolism, causing partial interruption of the enterohepatic circulation.[11] These changes serve to increase the amount of estrogen excreted by limiting reuptake of estrogen in the enterohepatic system. High fiber intake and increased gastrointestinal motility are associated with decreased rates of breast, colon, and endometrial cancers.

BOTANICALS USED FOR BREAST DISORDERS

Most of the herbals and botanicals used in the United States for breast problems come from old-English, European, and colonial American folk medicine practice. Many of these plants and botanicals, in addition to containing large amounts of vitamins A and C, β-carotene, and other B vitamins, are rich sources of phytoestrogens and antioxidants. As noted earlier, botanicals containing phytoestrogens also mitigate the impact of estrogen by competitively binding to estrogen receptors. When the whole plant is ingested, the fiber in botanical and herbal preparations may promote estrogen excretion through the enterohepatic route, reducing circulating steroids. The high concentrations of antioxidants found in plants may also lower the risk of cancer.

Herbs and botanicals commonly recommended for breast problems include the following.

Breast pain and fibrocystic changes

Arnica flowers	*Arnica montana*
Chasteberry (vitex)	*Agnus castus* L *verbenaceae*
Dandelion	*Taraxacum officinale*
Echinacea	*Echinacea* spp.
Evening primrose oil	*Oenothera biennis* L family Onagraceae
Goldenseal	*Hydrastis canadensis*
Green tea	
Herbal squaw vine	
Mullein	*Verbascum thapsus*
Parsley	*Petroselinum crispum*
Pau d'arco	*Tabevuia avellanedae*
Pokeroot	*Phytolacca decandra*

Cancer prevention

Burdock	*Arctium lappa*
Chaparral	*Larrea divaricata*
Chickweed	*Stelleria media*
Dandelion	*Taraxacum officinale*
Kelp and other iodine sources	
Red clover	*Trifolium pratense* L Fabaceae
Sassafras	*Sassafras albidum*

Galactogogues to bring in milk

Aniseed	*Pimpinella anisum*
Blessed thistle	*Cnicus benedictus*
Borage	*Borago officinalis*
Caraway	*Carum carvi*
Dill	*Anethum graveolens*
Fennel	*Foeniculum vulgare*
Goat's rue	*Galega officinalis*
Milk thistle	*Silybum marianum*
Vervain	*Verbena officinalis*

Mastitis

Balmony compress (bitter herb)	*Chelone glabra*
Black cohosh	*Cimicifuga racemosa*

Calendula compress	*Calendula officinalis*
Pokeroot	*Phytolacca decandra*
St. John's wort for "caking"	*Hypericum perforatum*

Other vitamins and minerals recommended for breast health
β-Carotene
Choline
Iodine
Methionine
Vitamin B complex

Herbs to aid in weaning

| Garden sage | *Salvia officinalis* var. *rubia labiateae* |

Botanicals commonly recommended for menopause

Black cohosh	*Cimicifuga racemosa*
Blue cohosh	*Caulophyllum*
Chamomile	*Matricaria recutita, Anthemis nobilis*
Chasteberry	*Agnus castus* L Verbenaceae
Cramp bark	*Viburnum opulus*
Life root, squaw weed	*Senecio aureus*
Motherwort	*Leonurus cardiaca*
Saw palmetto	*Serenoa serrulata*
St. Johns wort	*Hypericum perforatum*
Uva ursi	

Herbs with estrogenic activity—possibly contraindicated in women with breast cancer

Dong quai	
Fenugreek	
Ginseng	
Gotu kola	
Licorice	*Glycyrrhiza glabra*
Sarsaparilla	*Smilax* spp.
Wild Mexican yam	*Dioscorea mexicana*

Evening Primrose (Evening Primrose, Evening Star, Oenothera biennis L Family Onagraceae)

Evening primrose is the most commonly recommended herbal remedy for mastalgia, and it is heavily promoted for the treatment of premenstrual syndrome (PMS) and menopausal symptoms. Evening primrose produces seeds rich in oils containing γ-linolenic acid (GLA). It also contains unknown anticoagulant substances. The whole plant is eaten in pickles, soups, and sautés; and the seeds are pressed to extract the oils. An extensive literature exists in nutrition journals about the use of GLA for lipid disorders. Commercial preparations available contain both the gamma and *cis* forms of linolenic acid. Typical preparations contain GLA 45 mg + *cis*-linolenic acid (LA) 365 mg per capsule. The recommended amounts for PMS, mastalgia, and menopausal syndrome range from 1 to 12 capsules a day. At a cost of 25¢ per capsule, the therapeutic use of evening primrose oil can prove to be expensive.

One should be wary of a product praised too loudly. GLA is touted as a "miracle" fatty acid, its appeal reinforced by nonsense presented as profound physiology. GLA is produced by the placenta, and high concentrations are found in breast milk. Promoters imply that GLA is a perfect fatty acid, just as proponents of natural progesterone claim it is the one and only ideal progestin. GLA is touted as a cure or preventive for a wide range of disorders, including atopic dermatitis, bladder function, cyclic mastalgia or fibrocystic changes, diabetic neuropathy, eczema, hepatitis B, migraine headache, multiple sclerosis, PMS, sensitive skin (acne, dry skin, slow aging of skin, hair, and nails) visual acuity, and wound healing.

One study in the current literature reported an uncontrolled trial[12] wherein GLA administration lowered the rate of migraine. GLA has been disappointing in the treatment of dermatologic problems in well constructed controlled studies.[13,14] Another report said that GLA lessened signs and symptoms of rheumatoid arthritis by 25% compared to corn oil given to controls.[15] GLA has not proved effective against hepatitis B.[16] A meta-analysis was published in the United Kingdom reviewing the "clinical trials" of evening primrose oil for premenstrual syndrome. Seven placebo trials were found, and only five of the seven were randomized. Well controlled trials failed to establish any impact of GLA supplements on the symptoms of PMS.[17] The most that can be said is that GLA does offer some interesting possibilities as an essential fatty acid and that its clinical utility has not been fully elucidated. Most of the folk remedy claims made for GLA, however, appear to be poorly substantiated.

Chasteberry Vitex (Agnus castus L Verbenaceae)

Also known as chaste tree, monk's pepper, agnus castus, Indian spice, sage tree hemp, and treewild pepper, vitex contains hormone-like substances that competitively bind receptor sites and thus exert antiandrogenic effects. Promoted as a means of reducing libido in men, chasteberry is also recommended for women at menopause suffering from vaginal dryness, low libido, and depression. Its antiandrogenic effects seem antithetical to its use for symptoms of androgen deficiency in older women.

Vitex's anti-hormonal activity presumably explains its purported ability to decrease mastalgia. No studies could be found to document its effects.

Green Tea

The antioxidants found in green tea, particularly the potent polyphenols, have been proposed as agents that offer protection from malignancy. Epidemiologists have begun to speculate that the high consumption of green tea in Japan may account for the fact that although Japanese men smoke more than Americans they have only half the rate of lung cancer. Antioxidants such as those in green tea have sparked a great deal of interest and speculation by researchers and epidemiologists. Other antioxidants similar to those in green tea include proanthocyanidin, a type of bioflavinoid found in grapes, tree barks, and berries. Other bioflavinoids with high antioxidant activity are also found in pine and lemon tree bark, hazel nut tree leaves, cherries, blueberries, and cranberries. The highest amounts are found in purple grapes. The major role of this class of antioxidants appears to be to protect fruit from damage by fungus and mold. Studies have suggested that these substances also may be the active compounds in red wines and grape juices that lower cancer risk.

Other Plants

Red clover is a forage plant containing phenols and tannins. Although it remained in the U.S. Pharmacopeia formulary until 1946, it was cited as having no therapeutic utility 30 years earlier. A woman would be hard-pressed to eat enough red clover for it to have a clinically important impact on endocrine function.

Arnica flowers are used in a tincture for breast pain. Arnica does contain flavonoids and so may offer some competitive inhibition of estrogen-induced symptoms. Burdock, dandelion, chickweed, and parsley, though good sources of dietary vitamins, provide no medicinal or therapeutic effects.

Echinacea and goldenseal are used together most commonly to treat symptoms of colds and flus. They are reputed to enhance immunity and resistance to infection, and they are most often used as supportive treatments for urinary or respiratory infections. How they affect breast health is not clear from the herbal literature available for review. Mullein is offered as a "cure-all" but has, according to experts, no therapeutic utility.

Pokeroot is also reputed to be a panacea for a great number of ailments, but all parts of the mature plant, except the ripe red berries, are highly toxic. Severe illnesses and deaths have been reported after ingesting even small amounts.

Chaparral is also known as the creosote bush. The chemical creosote is toxic and carcinogenic, and it is used to treat wooden pilings to protect them from damage by marine worms. Chaparral ingestion has led to a number of cases of nonviral hepatitis, including some fatalities. It should be regarded as unsafe; more importantly, it has no clinical utility.

Pau d'arco is a Latin American herb used in Inca medicine. During the 1960s one constituent of pau d'arco, lapachol, was found to have limited success in the treatment of a variety of animal sarcomas. In human trials the side effects were so profound the studies were stopped.

Sassafras was used as a flavoring for beverages, and the roots and bark were brewed as teas until the discovery that the volatile oils in sassafras contain a substance called safrole, which is carcinogenic in small research animals (e.g., rats and mice). The U.S. Food and Drug Administration (FDA) has banned the use of sassafras in food flavorings, although it continues to be cited and recommended in herbal texts.

Herbs reputed to promote lactation and increase breast milk flow include a number of plants from the dill family, including dill, aniseed, caraway, and fennel. No studies could be found documenting any impact on milk production or let-down using these culinary herbs. Perhaps stimulating the nursing mother's gustatory senses improves her nutrition and thus augments milk production.

Plant Medicines to Avoid During Lactation

Common garden sage supposedly causes uterine contractions, and herbalists recommend that it not be used during pregnancy. These two ideas seem contradictory, as substances with pitocin and oxytocin-like activity simultaneously stimulate uterine contractility and induce the milk let-down reflex. Proof of either of these claims for sage could not be found. Sage also is said to assist in drying up lactation. The notion that it is drying and astringent no doubt comes from its high tannin content.

Sage has some estrogenic effect when injected into mice, but sage oil has a toxic effect similar to that of wormwood, the notorious plant used to produce absinthe. Both sage and wormwood produce a substance called thujone, which is toxic, causing seizures when taken in large amounts.

Pediatricians sometimes advise nursing mothers to avoid onion, garlic, and other members of the allium family. Supposedly they cause gas in the infant. The aromatics in these plants can cross into breast milk and may impart a taste that newborns find unpleasant and unpalatable. Poor sucking may then lead to air swallowing, gas, and distention.

Plant Medicines to Avoid After Breast Cancer

Botanicals reputed to have estrogenic activity include ginseng, fenugreek, licorice, sarsaparilla, gotu kola, wild Mexican yam, and dong quai. Herbal texts often recommend that women who have had breast cancer avoid estrogenic herbs and botanicals based on the assumption that estrogens induce and promote breast cancer. The role of exogenous estrogens in breast cancer causation is being hotly debated, contested, and argued; and it remains unclear. Even if these plants provided substantial amounts of estrogen, their use might not be contraindicated. On the contrary, many of the plants considered estrogenic compete for estrogen-binding sites and exert antiestrogenic effects through competitive inhibition of more potent estrogenic compounds. It thus seems that the proscription about taking these herbs in the face of breast cancer is unfounded.

The only literature available about these herbs and breast cancer comprises sporadic, anecdotal case reports. Typically, a woman with previously diagnosed breast cancer uses some sort of estrogenic herbal substance and suffers a recurrence of her breast disease. Such reports offer no evidence of causation but do intimidate both conventional and alternative practitioners.

Mexican wild yams contain dioscorea, which is used as a precursor in the production of such steroids as progesterone and dihydroepi and rosterone (DHEA). There is no biopathway for the conversion of dioscorea to other active steroids in humans. Dioscorea does not have any appreciable estrogenic activity, as the yams have to be eaten raw and in huge quantities to provide enough diogenin to affect biologic processes.

VITAMIN E AND OTHER ANTIOXIDANTS

Several controlled trials have been done to see if high doses of vitamin E can alter symptoms and findings in mastalgia and palpable "fibrocystic disease." The University of California, San Francisco did a double-blind, randomized trial of the effect of vitamin E on palpable clinically benign breast findings. Seventy-three women were assigned to either a daily regimen of 600 IU vitamin E ($n = 37$) or a placebo ($n = 36$). Breast findings were determined at the outset and rated. Of these women, 32 and 30 in each group, respectively, finished the full 2 months of the trial. No differences were found between the vitamin E and placebo groups in terms of breast findings, scores of the findings, or premenstrual breast pain. Vitamin E appeared to have no beneficial effect.[18] In another study, 105 women with mammographic evidence of benign disease were randomly assigned in a double-blind, placebo-controlled crossover trial. The use of vitamin E 600 IU offered no improvement in subjective or objective findings. Breast examination and mammograms in the two groups were unchanged.[19] Another study was done of women with confirmed dysplastic disease of the breast. Patients were given a placebo or 150, 300, or 600 IU of D-1α-tocopherol per day for 2 months. Before and at the end of the study period breast examinations, sonography, and thermography were performed during the mid-luteal phase. No significant objective effects were noted in any of the outcomes. Measures of estradiol, progesterone, DHEA sulfate, and testosterone were also unaffected.[20].

Although these well constructed trials seem to prove that vitamin E offers no alleviation of breast pain or improved findings, some decrease in symptoms was reported in one study, although the decrease was not statistically significant. Other smaller and uncontrolled trials have found that vitamin E lessens breast pain. Vitamin E has been reported to slow the progression of Alzheimer's disease and has been found to have a role in primary and secondary coronary disease prevention. Therefore although it cannot be recommended for breast disease, vitamin E offers other important clinical health benefits.

CAFFEINE AND OTHER METHYLXANTHINES

Decreasing methylxanthine intake (caffeine, theophylline, and theobromine: the substances found in coffee, tea, colas, and chocolate) is reputed to decrease mastalgia and to reduce palpable nodularity on breast examination. Women and their doctors speculate about how much caffeine is found in common beverages such as cocoa, expresso, black tea, and orange tea, all the while believing that the elimination of methylxanthines can somehow improve breast health.

The University of California, San Francisco conducted a study of 158 women who presented with breast symptoms or problems. Women were assigned to two groups: One was told to limit methylxanthine intake; the other was given no instructions. Methylxanthine consumption was estimated by intake interview. Breast findings were rated on a scale of 0–4 (no nodularity to confluent hard "dysplasia"). Examinations done 4 months later yielded a statistically significant reduction in clinically palpable breast nodularity, but the changes were minor. The predictive and preventive importance of these minor reductions was thought to be insignificant. A subset of women also underwent mammography, and again no real demonstrable differences were seen.[21]

A smaller study was done with 56 women thought to have proliferative breast disease. They were divided into three groups and then randomized to control, cholesterol-free, and caffeine-free dietary interventions. Symptoms were recorded at the outset, and breast findings were rated on a scale of 0–3 (0 = normal, fatty tissue; 1 = little seedy bumps or fine nodularity; 2 = discrete nodules or ropy tissue; 3 = confluent areas, hard or soft masses). After undertaking the advised dietary changes, they were examined at visits 2 and 4 months later. There were no changes found in the occurrence of breast nodules, pain, or tenderness with either of the "therapeutic" diets compared to controls.[22]

As is the case with vitamin E, restriction of methylxanthine intake appears to offer no objective improvement in breast findings or symptoms. The recommendation to limit caffeine intake is so ingrained in medical mythology, however, it may be difficult to contradict this fanciful notion.

CONCLUSIONS

Breast pain and nodularity are not predictors of breast cancer, but they do complicate our ability to diagnosis serious disease and may obscure other coincidental findings. Mastalgia also creates marked degrees of anxiety in midlife women.

Herbal, botanical, and vitamin therapies may provide some subjective decrease in symptoms. If we agree that reducing patient anxiety and fear is a worthwhile outcome, these interventions have some utility. The mitigation of symptoms and lessening of fears may limit the development of other types of somatization and may help reduce inappropriate utilization of health services. Lessening patient worry and anxiety may also reduce the likelihood of developing additional stress-related complaints and disorders. Many botanicals, herbals and nutritional interventions provide benefits beyond simply reducing symptoms, as many alter the effects of circulating endogenous estrogen by competitive binding, increasing estrogen excretion, and modulating levels of sex hormone-binding globulin.

Nonpharmacologic interventions, including decreasing methylxanthine and increasing vitamin E intake, appear to provide a subjective, though barely significant, reduction in mastalgia. Neither of these interventions is expensive. For the aging female, limiting caffeine holds other potential benefits, such as reducing the incidence of palpitations and transient benign tachyarrhythmias, often harmless but annoying and anxiety-provoking medical problems. Vitamin E appears to provide no "measurable" effect on benign breast disease but has many other health benefits.

Current research clearly shows that the use of soy and other isoflavone-containing legumes induces a vast array of physiologic changes that are beneficial. In addition to replacing dietary animal proteins and fat with plant-based proteins and improving lipid profiles, isoflavones and related substances lower the risk of malignancy. A diet rich in fruits and vegetables provides protection from breast, colon, endometrial, and prostate cancer. Some new data suggest that a diet high in phytoestrogens may also lower the risk of lung, esophageal, laryngeal, stomach, pancreatic, and bladder cancer.

Eating whole vegetables and fruits probably provides more protection against disease than taking isolated vitamins, supplements, or concentrates of plant phytochemicals. Consuming the "whole" food ensures the intake of all constituents in the plant that limit and control abnormal cell proliferation, thereby protecting the body from malignant degenerative changes. Interventional trials using nutritional and botanical substances are currently under way. In the near future, we may have a good deal more knowledge and certainty about how to utilize vitamins, minerals, botanicals, and phytoestrogens as preventive and therapeutic agents.

References

1. Adlercreutz H, Mousavi Y, Hockerstedt K. Diet and breast cancer. Acta Oncol 1992;31:175–181

2. Persky V, Van Horn L. Epidemiology of soy and cancer: perspectives and directions. J Nutr 1995;125(suppl 3):709S–712S

3. Valente M, Bufalino, L Castiglione GN, et al. Effects of 1-year treatment with ipriflavone on bone in postmenopausal women with low bone mass. Calcif Tissue Int 1994;54:377–380

4. Knekt P, Jarvinen R, Reunanen A, Maatela J. Flavonoid intake and coronary mortality in Finland: a cohort study. BMJ 1996;312:478–481

5. Anderson JW, Johnstone BM, Cook-Newell ME. Meta-analysis of the effects of soy protein intake on serum lipids. N Engl J Med 1995;333:276–282

6. Knight DC, Eden JA. A review of the clinical effects of phytoestrogens. Obstet Gynecol 1996;87:897–904

7. Giri AK, Lu LJ. Genetic damage and the inhibition of 7,12-dimethylbenz[a]anthracene-induced genetic damage by the phytoestrogens, genistein and daidzein, in female ICR mice. Cancer Lett 1995;95:125–133

8. Zava DT, Duwe G. Estrogenic and antiproliferative properties of genistein and other flavonoids in human breast cancer cells in vitro. Nutr Cancer 1997;27:31–40

9. Martin PM, Horwitz KB, Ryan DS, McGuire WL. Phytoestrogen interaction with estrogen receptors in human breast cancer cells. Endocrinology 1978;103:1860–1867

10. Lu LJ, Anderson KE, Grady JJ, Nagamani M. Effects of soya consumption for one month on steroid hormones in premenopausal women: implications for breast cancer risk reduction. Cancer Epidemiol Biomarkers Prev 1996;5:63–70

11. Adlercreutz H. Western diet and Western diseases: some hormonal and biochemical mechanisms and associations. Scand J Clin Lab Invest Suppl 1990;201:3–23

12. Wagner W, Nootbaar-Wagner U. Prophylactic treatment of migraine with gamma-linolenic and alpha-linolenic acids Cephalalgia 1997;17:127–130; discussion 102

13. Borrek S, Hildebrandt A, Forster J. Gamma-linolenic-acid-rich borage seed oil capsules in children with atopic dermatitis: a placebo-controlled double-blind study. Klin Padiatr 1997;209:100–104

14. Whitaker DK, Cilliers J, de Beer C. Evening primrose oil (Epogam) in the treatment of chronic hand dermatitis: disappointing therapeutic results. Dermatology 1996;193:115–120

15. Zurier RB, Rossetti RG, Jacobson EW, et al. Gamma-linolenic acid treatment of rheumatoid arthritis: a randomized, placebo-controlled trial. Arthritis Rheum 1996;39:1808–1817

16. Jenkins AP, Green AT, Thompson RP. Essential fatty acid supplementation in chronic hepatitis B. Aliment Pharmacol Ther 1996;10:665–668

17. Budeiri D, Li Wan Po A, Dornan JC. Is evening primrose oil of value in the treatment of premenstrual syndrome? Control Clin Trials 1996;17:60–68

18. Ernster VL, Goodson WH III, Hunt TK, et al. Vitamin E and benign breast "disease": a double-blind, randomized clinical trial. Surgery 1985;97:490–494

19. Meyer EC, Sommers DK, Reitz CJ, Mentis H. Vitamin E and benign breast disease. Surgery 1990;107:549–551

20. London RS, Sundaram GS, Murphy L, et al. The effect of vitamin E on mammary dysplasia: a double-blind study. Obstet Gynecol 1985;65:104–106

21. Ernster VL, Mason L, Goodson WH III, et al. Effects of caffeine-free diet on benign breast disease: a randomized trial. Surgery 1982;91:263–267

22. Allen SS, Froberg DG. The effect of decreased caffeine consumption on benign proliferative breast disease: a randomized clinical trial. Surgery 1987;101:720–730

Recommended Reading

Boik J. Cancer and Natural Medicine: A Textbook of Basic Science and Clinical Research. Princeton, MN: Oregon Medical Press, 1996

British Herbal Pharmacopoeia. British Herbal Medicine Association, 1996

Castleman M. The Healing Herbs: the Ultimate Guide to the Curative Powers of Natures Medicines. Emmaus, PA, Rodale Press, 1991

Culpeper N. Culpeper's Complete Herbal and English Physician. Glenwood, UK, Meyerbooks, 1987

Dossey L (ed). Alternative Therapies in Health and Medicine. Aliso Viejo, CA, Innovision Communications/American Association of Critical Care Nurses, 1995

Herbs for Health. Interweave Press, Loveland, CO

Huang O, Ho R. Food Phytochemicals for Cancer Prevention (vols 1 and 2). 1994

Micozzi MS (ed). Journal of Alternative and Complementary Medicine: Research on Paradigm, Practice and Policy. New York, Mary Ann Liebert, 1995

Murray M. 1995 The Healing Power of Herbs. The Enlightened Person's Guide to the Wonders of Medicinal Plants (2nd ed). Toronto, Random House of Canada, 1995 (paperback)

Murrill WB, Brown NM, Zhang JX, Manzolillo PA, Bames S, Lamartiniere CA. Prepubertal genistein exposure suppresses mammary cancer and enhances gland differentiation in rats. Carcinogenesis 1996;17:1451–1457

Newall C, Anderson L, Phillipson J. Herbal Medicines: A Guide for Health-Care Professionals. Wallingford, Oxon, England, Pharmaceutical Press, 1996

Nutrition Research Newsletter. Technical Insights. New York, John Wiley & Sons

Prevention Magazine. Emmaus, PA, Rodale Press

Reynolds J (ed). Martindale: The Extra Pharmacopoeia (30th ed). Wallingford, Oxon, England, Pharmaceutical Press, 1996

Tufts Health and Nutrition Newsletter, P.O. Box 57857, Boulder, CO 80322-7857

Tyler V. The Honest Herbal: A Sensible Guide to the Use of Herbs and Related Remedies. Binghamton, NY, Pharmaceutical Products Press/Haworth Press, 1993

Tyler VE. Herbs of choice; the therapeutic use of phytomedicinals. 1994

Willoughby M, Mills S. The British Herbal Pharmacopoeia 1996. Bournemouth, England, British Herbal Medicine Association, 1996

Online Information on Medicinal Plants and Alternative Medicine

Alternative Medicine Courses Taught at U.S. Medical Schools (sponsored by the Rosenthal Center)
http://cpmcnet.columbia.edu/dept/rosenthal/guide.html

Center for Complementary and Alternative Medicine Research in Women's Health
http://cpmcnet.columbia.edu/dept/rosenthal/Women.html

Ethnobiology and Conservation Team
http://www.ethnobotany.org

Food and Drug Administration
http://www.fda.gov/fdahomepage

Medicinal Plants of Native America (sponsored by the USDA)
http://nalusda.gov:8300/cgi-bin/browse/mpnadb

Richard and Hinda Rosenthal Center for Complementary/Alternative Medicine (sponsored by Columbia's College of Physicians and Surgeons)
http://cpmcnet.columbia.edu/dept/rosenthal

Other Sources

American Botanical Council, PO Box 201660, Austin, Texas 78720

41 NATURAL HISTORY OF BREAST CANCER: CLINICAL AND BIOLOGIC FEATURES DICTATING MANAGEMENT; AN OPINION BASED ON PERSONAL EXPERIENCE

David Plotkin

As the twentieth century draws to a close, everyone interested in breast cancer, lay and professional, can agree on one point: The management of this disease and its clinicopathologic precursor lesions has been, and remains, highly controversial. The level of interest, funding of research, campaigns for earlier diagnosis, and volume of published literature on the subject have risen to a height never before seen in oncology.

Understandably, breast cancer has been an increasing source of dread to American women over the last half century. About 20 years ago the disease began to receive more serious attention from the medical profession, probably because of the highly publicized presence of the disease in the wives of some prominent political figures. Despite its current high profile and conspicuous politicization, breast cancer is not well understood by many practitioners who encounter it. Medical school curricula do not deal with breast cancer as a single focus. Instead, several disciplines—pathology, physical diagnosis, epidemiology, radiology, general surgery, radiation therapy, endocrinology, medical oncology—are all expected to contribute a part of the puzzle. Perhaps because of this diffusion of critical insight into breast cancer, clinical competence is at risk of falling short in comparison to other equally complicated medical issues, such as acute myocardial infarction, hypertension, or the use of antibiotics. Further confusion comes from the high level of controversy that has surrounded breast cancer since it became "important."

The goal of this chapter is to describe a clinical approach to breast cancer that is as minimally intrusive to patients as possible without sacrificing their survivability. To provide the rationale for these management guidelines, it is necessary briefly to review the history of breast cancer, the real and perceived accomplishments of the last century, and the problems associated with these accomplishments. Some review of the epidemiology of the disease is required. The commonly applied statistical yardsticks require scrutiny as well.

History

Just 100 years ago when breast cancer was still relatively uncommon, death from the disease was due to progression of the primary tumor. Virtually all such breast cancer would today be classified as locally far advanced (or at least stage 3). Tumors were regularly large enough to perforate the overlying skin and produce foul-smelling ulcerations that bled dangerously or provided a portal of entry for bacterial that caused fatal sepsis. Halsted's radical mastectomy largely eliminated primary breast cancer as a direct cause of death.[1] His surgical approach, which resembled a scorched earth policy, managed to postpone death by breast cancer in women who, although no longer succumbing to the progression of the primary lesion, began regularly to suffer the problems of uncontrolled metastatic disease. Halsted's conception of breast cancer treatment, which focused entirely on the breast and immediately contiguous tissues, dominated surgical thought for about 50 years. His teachings were so entrenched in American medical schools that any skepticism of the appropriateness of radical mastectomy was greeted with disdain.

Through the influence of several European doctors interested in radiation therapy came the notion that less aggressive surgery, supplemented by irradiation, might adequately substitute for radical surgery in the management of some patients with breast cancer. Little known are the observations of Hirsch during the late 1920s in this regard, long antedating the published works of Keynes, Mustakallio, and Baclesse.[2–5]

At mid-century, George Crile Jr.[6] of the United States was scorned for his suggestion that breast cancer could be treated surgically with less than the classic Halsted operation. Haagensen[1] then took the radical mastectomy baton from Halsted and improved 5-year survival of operable breast cancer during the 1950s and 1960s by doing internal mammary and highest apical lymph node biopsies. If these nodes harbored metastases he referred the patients for radiation therapy. This might be the first example of the Will Rogers phenomenon (stage shifting) of producing meaningless "better" results in both surgical and radiation-treated groups.[7]

It was not until Fisher et al. and the National Surgical Adjuvant Breast and Bowel Project (NSABP) produced the first American clinical trial (NSABP B-01) that the issue of whether less surgery for breast cancer was as good as radical mastectomy was addressed.[8] Radical mastectomy was compared to simple (or total) mastectomy with radiation therapy to regional lymph nodes for clinical stage 2 breast cancer. For clinical stage 1 disease, radical mastectomy was compared to simple mastectomy with radiation therapy versus simple mastectomy alone. This study demonstrated that the type of surgery, radiation therapy, or both directed at the primary lesion made no difference to survival. Fisher et al., remarkably late in the process of our improved understanding of breast cancer, formally enunciated the systemic nature of the disease in 1980.[9] There is now a plethora of evidence documenting the survival equivalence of lumpectomy versus modified radical mastectomy. The essentially comparable mortality rates of clinically pathologically matched cohorts of breast cancer patients managed over a wide range of surgical aggressiveness provides further confirmation of the systemic nature of breast cancer.

The first insight into the hormone dependence of some breast cancers was seen in the published work of Beatson, more or less contemporaneously with the observations of Halsted.[10] Bilateral oophorectomy was not a simple procedure then, and its use was limited. This type of "medical" thinking about breast cancer eventually led to the expanded use of surgical endocrine ablation, that is, to adrenalectomy and hypophysectomy—formidable surgical procedures even by modern standards.

In 1936 Huggins formalized the concept of endocrine ablation for hormone-dependent cancer by reporting the efficacy, albeit transient, of adrenalectomy for metastatic prostate cancer.[11] This observation provided impetus to the use of adrenalectomy and hypophysectomy for metastatic breast cancer during the years immediately after World War II. Testosterone, or a number of analogs, began to be used as "estrogen antagonists."[12] Curiously, pharmacologic doses of diethylstilbestrol (DES) were found to be generally as efficacious as the androgen but without the brutal side effects produced in women already suffering the cosmetically severe impact of classic radical mastectomy.[13]

It was not until the early 1970s in Europe and late 1970s in the United States that tamoxifen began to be used in the treatment of largely postmenopausal advanced breast cancer with an effectiveness that rivaled or exceeded adrenalectomy or pharmacologic doses of male or female sex steroids and with much less morbidity.[14] It is now clear that tamoxifen has been used far more widely than other treatments for breast cancer, medical or surgical, in both the metastatic as well as the adjuvant setting.

Chemotherapy (single agents such as Cyclophosphamide, thiotepa, and 5-fluorouracil) were used during the 1960s with occasional effectiveness in advanced breast cancer. Complete remissions were rare and partial remissions occasional. The duration of remission was typically measured in a few to several months, and side effects of the treatment were usually serious. Combination chemotherapy began to be used as the specialty of medical oncology emerged during the early 1970s. Reponses to treatment became common, and the duration of benefit was significantly extended. Measures to combat side effects were developed with some success, leading to the use of a variety of combinations in the adjuvant setting. Conversion of some incurable patients to curable, as had been the case during the preceding decade with Hodgkin's disease, was never demonstrated, however. This remains essentially true to this day.

DEFINITIONS

To manage breast disease and breast cancer rationally as we round the corner on a century of activistic treatment, we must place certain terms in context and carefully define them. Historically, nonmalignant breast disease has had multiple diverse labels (e.g., "fibrocystic disease," fibrocystic changes, mastopathy, and mammary dysplasia). By benign breast disease we refer to a range of proliferative processes from almost riskless to potentially malignant. By frank cancer we mean the entire range of neoplasia from anatomic carcinoma in situ (CIS) to invasive. Within the category of unconfined or infiltrating breast cancer are functional measurements that permit division of the disease into four categories ranging from aggressive to moderate to indolent to very indolent forms of the disease.

We are further obligated to clarify the panoply of terms used to measure outcome: for example, 3-, 5-, 10-, and 15-year survival, crude survival, relative or disease-specific survival, mortality rate per unit population unadjusted and adjusted to a previous year's population, and relative risk for relapse or death (or both).

Timed survival is recorded in the literature either as the time interval from diagnosis to first recurrence (i.e., disease-free survival, or DFS) or to death (i.e., total survival), the latter including DFS plus non-DFS. The percentage of the original cohort alive (in the case of DFS, alive and well) is reported at periodic intervals.

Usually 5 years after the diagnosis is selected as a point when the survivors in a group under examination are compared to another group that was either treated differently or not treated. Survival percentages of different stages of the disease also are often compared by 5-year survival.

When possible, survival measurements are extended to 10, 15, 20, and 25 years and occasionally even longer. If death regardless of cause is the endpoint, the term crude survival is used. When deaths due to disease other than the specific one under consideration are taken into account, a percentage of survivors appears that is almost always higher then the crude survival rate. For example, if 60% of an original cohort is alive in 10 years, the crude survival is simply 60%. If one-fourth of the 40% (i.e., 10% of the original group) died of "other illness," the corrected survival figure, using a denominator of 90 instead of 100, with the same numerator of 60, produces a 67% survival rate. Disease-specific survival, called relative survival rate in the early literature, is a more accurate measure of the thrust of mortality of the disease under study. An important but not often mentioned fact is that if there is a high proportion of deaths due to competing illness the disease-specific survival curve generated from 3-, 5-, 10-, and 15-year survival data is made to look better.

Another measure of survival is determination of the absolute number of deaths per year due to the disease being studied. Typically this figure is modified to the number of deaths per 100,000 population (or female population, in the case of breast cancer).

Sizable variations in the age groups of the population can occur. The baby boom generation originating in the several years after the conclusion of World War II, for example, is making its statistical presence felt during the last decade and a half, as reflected by the increase in the absolute number of women diagnosed with breast cancer over the last 15 years. Only by adjusting the population back to a standard reference year, 1970, is the mortality rate per 100,000 female population seen in accurate perspective.

Other measures of survival (or mortality, its reciprocal) are used. The rate (or hazard) for recurrence or death per year is compared to the same measure in a control group, and a ratio is computed assigning the control group rate as unity. Greater risk for death in the test group as compared to the control produces a number >1.0; less risk for death is seen as a number <1.0.

When trying to determine a possible significant trend over the first few years of a study, the 3- and 5-year (usually crude) survival rates and relative risk ratios are useful. For longer-term assessment of treatment of a disease, the disease-specific survival curves at 15–20 years and the number of deaths per 100,000, age-adjusted, are more reliable.

Among the more inappropriate terms used for measurement of treatment impact in breast cancer is the word "cure." More attributable to lack of understanding than disingenuousness, cure is regularly substituted for 5-year disease-free survival. If a patient is alive and well 5 years after diagnosis but during the ensuing few years develops a recurrence and dies of the disease, the recording of the 5-year survival rate that included such a patient is valid. Terming the patient cured at 5 years, however, becomes a bitter irony when 10-year survival data cannot include this patient.

In the United Kingdom, when a patient dies of a competing illness a number of years after a diagnosis of breast cancer, the literature refers to her as a "personal" cure. If the disease-specific survival curve becomes flat in 5, 10, or 15 years, the cohort below the curve is considered actuarially cured. There is a rational use of the term personal cure when some disease of truly old age overtakes a long-term survivor of breast cancer even if in a few years she would have developed a fatal recurrence. On the other hand, a combination of prevalent fatal "other" illness, if encountered within a few years of diagnosis of breast cancer, can leave the impression of a high percentage of personal cures, somewhat of a Pyrrhic victory.

ACCOMPLISHMENTS

The accomplishments of the last half-century are worthy of respectful acknowledgment but are not legion and deserve an occasional caveat. Earlier clinical discovery, a hallmark of this era, produces down-staging that has obvious practical benefit. Many women with breast cancer have undergone lumpectomy instead of modified radical mastectomy for lesions diagnosed at a size small enough (generally <4.0 cm in diameter) to permit the lesser surgical intervention.

A lesser degree of lymph node involvement with earlier clinical intervention, another example of down-staging, is also regularly cited as a noteworthy advance in the management of breast cancer. It has become clear that radical removal of large numbers of nodes from the axilla, 15–20 or even more, is not necessary. Acknowledgment of axillary lymph node involvement as having only prognostic value has led to lymph node sampling, a procedure with much less surgical morbidity than the classic dissection. Moreover, there is no difference in surgical

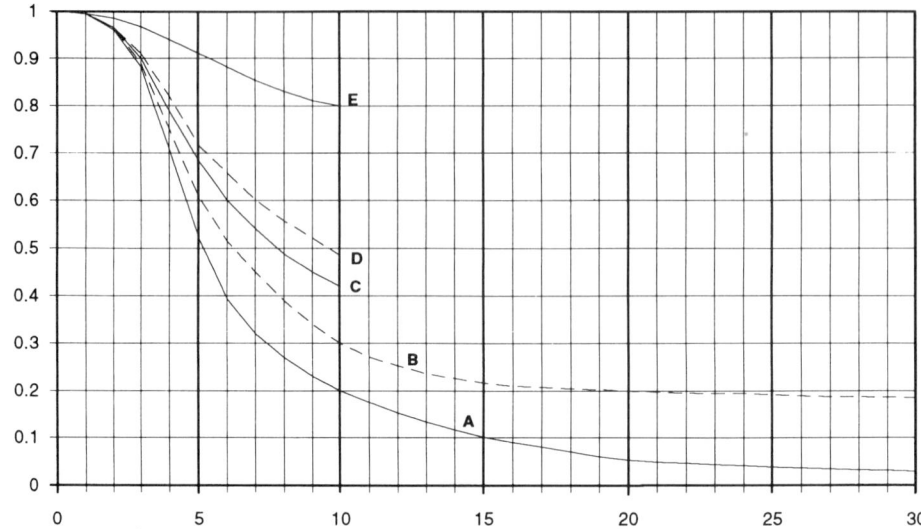

Figure 41.1. Breast cancer survival curves. A = Premammography breast cancer crude survival; B = Premammography breast cancer disease-specific survival; C = National Surgical Adjuvant Breast Project (NSABP)/Breast Cancer Trialists Organization (BCTO) crude survival; D = NSABP/BCTO disease-specific survival; E = Breast Cancer Detection Demonstration Project (BCDDP) survival: breast cancer mammography trial with selection, lead time, length biases, 30–35% diagnosed by mammography only.

morbidity after axillary node dissection following lumpectomy or following total mastectomy. There may be, on average, a few more nodes removed with modified radical mastectomy than lumpectomy, but no diagnostic advantage is attributed to this increase.

Improvement in timed survival over the last 50 years, especially 5- and 10-year survivals, are oft-repeated observations that are not to be challenged. The relation of small tumor size and less degree of lymph node involvement with better timed survival is firmly established.

There is no basis for questioning the validity of steady improvement in disease-specific survival curves extending to 10–15 years as recorded by numerous registries (Fig. 41.1). This is seen graphically as a less negative slope to the curve. Usually it is attributed to more effective treatment and better diagnosis. That a change in the biologic malevolence of what is termed breast cancer by pathologists is possibly the basis for this "improvement" has only recently been considered.[15]

One of the striking accomplishments (or consequences) of the last nearly three decades is the absolute increase in the diagnosis of breast CIS from about 1000/year to more than 30,000/year. The percentage of breast CIS diagnosed by palpation was 1–2% of the approximately 76,000 women found to have breast cancer in 1970. In 1995 the percentage of breast cancers that were in situ ranged from 10% to 20% (depending on the study) and in absolute terms was probably 30,000–35,000/year. With age adjustment of the 1995 figures to account for the baby boomer population bulge, the relative increase is still 30-fold (Table 41.1).

Table 41.1. Incidence and mortality of breast cancer, 1970 to 1995

Parameter	1970	1995
U.S. female population (FP)	104,300,000	134,000,000
No. 100,000 units of U.S. FP	1,043	1,340
Incidence		
Absolute total	76,500	212,000
Absolute total/100,000	73.3	158
Age-adjusted to 1970/100,000[a]	—	123
Noninvasive total	1,000	32,000
Noninvasive total/100,000	0.96	24
Age-adjusted to 1970/100,000[a]	—	18.5
Invasive total	75,500	180,000
Invasive total/100,000	72.3	134
Age-adjusted to 1970/100,000[a]	—	104.0
Mortality		
Absolute no. of deaths	27,000	46,000
Not age-adjusted deaths/100,000	25.8	34.3
Age-adjusted deaths/100,000[a]	25.8	26.7

[a] Age adjustment based on $1043 \div 1340 = 0.778$.

It is maintained that breast cancer, on its way to becoming invasive and metastatic, is curable if intercepted at the in situ stage. This claim is legitimate if CIS does indeed regularly progress to a life-threatening (i.e., invasive) form of the disease.

Lastly, between 1991 and 1995 a 6.3% relative decrease in the number of breast cancer deaths occurring annually has been documented. It has been attributed to earlier diagnosis and more effective treatment.

PROBLEMS WITH ACCOMPLISHMENTS

The marked increase in use of lumpectomy with a reciprocal decline in modified radical mastectomy has not been without consequence. The knee-jerk reflex addition of radiation therapy to the remaining breast poses some problems that have received scant attention. Among them are the long-term effects of radiation therapy to the involved breast, the underlying thoracic wall structures, and the ipsilateral lung. We are accumulating previously unheard of numbers of patients who have received radiation therapy for less dangerous lesions who are young enough that the full impact of radiation therapy 15–25 years down the line has yet to be encountered by many oncologists. So far, radiation heart disease is still almost anecdotal, and the approximate doubling of risk for lung cancer is not yet a major problem. Bear in mind that the cancer patients receiving radiation therapy in the past were often "spared" the long-term consequences of radiation therapy by dying of the cancer despite the radiation therapy. With data documenting only the relatively few 15-year survivors treated with lumpectomy and radiation therapy, the recognition of extra risk for ischemic heart disease and lung cancer is more worrisome by portent than by manifestation.

A seldom-made more important point is that the addition of radiation therapy to lumpectomy serves only to decrease local recurrence from the previous 30–35% to 5–10% over the 10–15 years of observation. This difference is narrowed by the adjuvant use of tamoxifen for hormone-dependent cancers. The survival of patients with local recurrence requiring a second lumpectomy and radiation therapy, or modified radical mastectomy, is not adversely affected.[16] It seems that telling a patient that she has two chances out of three of never requiring a second intervention involving the affected breast is politically incorrect. Given the clamor for health cost containment, the almost obligatory use of radiation therapy, which is not an inexpensive therapeutic modality, is an element to consider further.

To draw reliable inferences about the higher percentage of smaller cancers seen during the 1990s compared to 1970 (the reference year used for age-adjusting incidence and mortality data for breast cancer), the impact of two entirely unrelated phenomena should be examined. The incidence of breast cancer from the time of first dependable published data beginning in the mid-1930s rose by nearly 1% per year, annually compounded (Fig. 41.2). Beginning in 1980 there was a marked acceleration in the incidence to 4% per year. This increased incidence seems to have plateaued during the 1990s.

The quite steady 1% increase per year is, in my view, attributable to a change in the reproductive biology of modern Western women during this century, particularly in the last half. Earlier menarche and postponing the age at first full-term

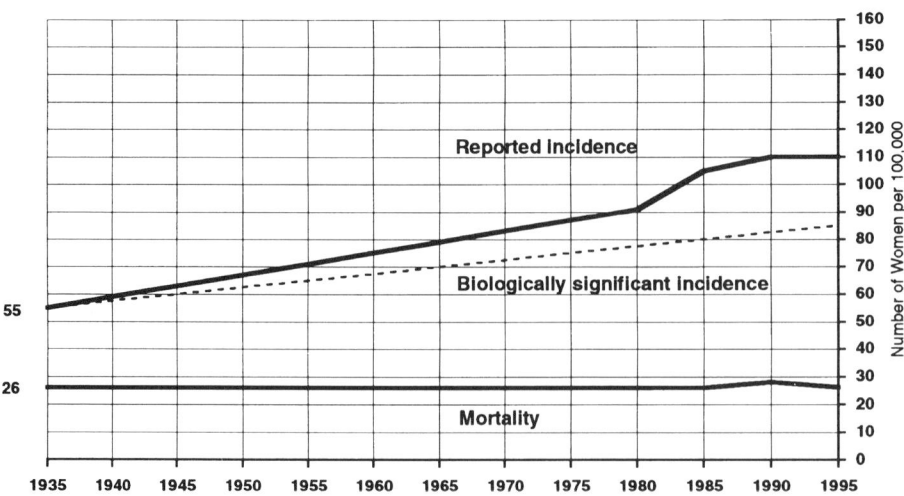

Figure 41.2. Mortality rate of breast cancer. Incidence of breast cancer reported versus biologically significant; 1935–1995.

pregnancy produces about 200 unrequited ovulations in the typical woman of North America and western Europe. This "failure" to use the organs of reproduction in the manner for which they were designed and used for countless generations produced more prevalence of three diseases: "fibrocystic disease" of the breast, cancer of the breast, and uterine leiomyomas. The endometrium of the uterus is spared hyperplasia and neoplasia somewhat by this lack of fecundity because of its monthly sloughing. It seems possible that the accumulation of a number, perhaps a 100- to 1,000,000-fold increase, of hyperplastic mammary duct and lobule cells exposed to cycle after cycle of mutagenic estrogen and progesterone is the basis for the prevalence of fibrocystic changes and breast cancer (including CIS) during the late twentieth century.

The other phenomenon superimposed on the above that accounts for the abrupt increase in incidence of breast cancer diagnoses between 1980 and 1990 has been the widespread use of mammography. The flattening of the incidence curve over the last 5 years at about 110 cases/100,000 women may well be due to saturation of the "health-oriented" part of the public. This widely used figure of 110 is between the age-adjusted rate for all breast cancers annually (i.e., 123) and the age-adjusted figure for invasive breast cancer only.

Therefore probably as a function of changed female reproductive biology plus extra case-finding, an entirely new category of breast cancer has emerged. It is a form of the disease that practically all pathologists agree is histologically confirmed breast cancer. There is a disproportionate percentage of well and moderately differentiated cancers in this new group. These malignancies are heavily sex steroid hormone-dependent. Perhaps of greatest importance, when subjected to functional analysis they are diploid tumors with slow proliferative rates. It is tempting to draw a parallel between this indolent form of breast cancer and "old man's" prostate cancer recorded as an incidental autopsy finding.

The lack of axillary lymph node involvement that parallels the size of the breast cancer at diagnosis (e.g., 1.5 cm) is of much less certain value than the patient's opportunity for breast-conserving surgery (lumpectomy). This feature of modern-day breast cancer treatment is likely a function of lead time and selection bias owing to mammographic diagnosis of nonpalpable cancers, which produces a major change in the spectrum of biologic aggressiveness of breast cancer. Moreover, the decrease in axillary lymph node involvement by routine surgical pathology is more apparent than real. When "negative nodes" are subjected to more sectioning or to immunohistochemical assay aided by monoclonal antibody assays, many more metastatic foci are uncovered.

The improvement in timed survival, usually at 5 years, is commonly cited as evidence of medical progress. The susceptibility of such a measure to lead time, length, and selection bias is scientifically documented but not adequately acknowledged. Lead bias occurs when the threshold for diagnosis is lowered. The earlier biopsy proof of a cancer's presence starts the calendar sooner. Two clinically and pathologically identical groups of cancer patients, one with the diagnosis made a year before the other, have a difference of a few percentage points in their 5-year survival but no difference in their ultimate survival. Similarly, "free interval," the time between diagnosis and first recurrence, is lengthened without having an impact on the time of death (Fig. 41.3).

Length bias is seen in mammography trials in which cancers diagnosed between screenings, the so-called interval cancers, have faster growth rates, more biologic malevolence, and shorter courses. Patients with mammographically detected cancers, compared to these more aggressive cancers, live longer (Fig. 41.4).

Selection bias is the most difficult of the biases to detect. Unbeknownst to the investigator, patients are assigned to test and control groups that are not comparable. The age of the patient, size of the tumor, and degree of lymph node involvement might all be comparable; but if the proliferative rate (e.g., high S-phase fraction in a DNA histogram) is faster on average in the control group, the test group's survival is seen as better.

The problem with the shallower slope of survival curves of breast cancer patients diagnosed during the last nearly two decades versus the analytic curves supplied by earlier investigations is that of comparing apples and oranges. As the number of women being diagnosed with breast cancer has risen (to epidemic

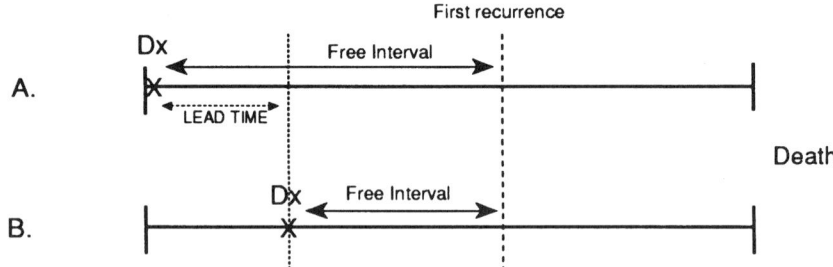

Figure 41.3. Lead time bias. The disease-free interval in A is longer than in B.

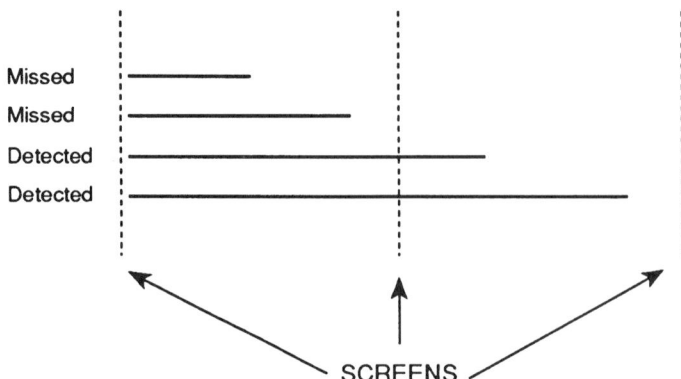

Figure 41.4. Length bias. Lines indicate the clinical life of a breast cancer.

proportions in the eyes of some), the distribution of fast-, moderate-, and slow-growing cancers has not remained the same. Indeed, it seems likely that an entirely new category of breast cancer (i.e., very slow-growing), characteristically nonpalpable and therefore detected only by mammography, is so indolent in its behavior as to be irrelevant to the patient's life expectancy. Clearly, the inclusion of such cancers, as well as an expansion of the ordinary slow-growing type into our data mix, will guarantee "better" results. If the same number of biologic aggressive cancers per 100,000 women (age-adjusted to 1970) are present, the same number of deaths per 100,000 will also persist. This is actually the case, with one minor exception to be dealt with shortly.

Many view the diagnosis of thousands more breast CISs as an unequivocal plus based on the assumption that all CIS progresses to invasive cancer and premature death. Substantially to the contrary are certain nonreputable facts. Over the course of 15 years of follow-up, only about 25% of all CIS patients develop invasive cancer. The mortality of this group has never exceeded 25% and is often reported as less; therefore the risk for death due to breast cancer within 15 years of a diagnosis of CIS probably cannot be higher than 5–6%. When this figure is further adjusted downward by death due to causes other than breast cancer, not infrequent in the half of the breast cancer population that is older than 60–65, which is the range of the mean age reported for breast cancer diagnosis, the less ominous public health significance of breast CIS is seen more clearly. It may be pondered that if occult invasive cancer is present in 1 of 16 women with CIS, and the treatment options (i.e., surgery, radiation therapy, tamoxifen) are no more effective than in the circumstance of known invasive cancer, the consequences of such treatment in the 15 of 16 women so affected who do not need it should give us pause. Only on the assumption that CIS is always on its way to becoming invasive does sure eradication of the process by bilateral mastectomy become logical. If less drastic treatments seem to produce equivalent survival of those with CIS, the premise of uniform malignant potential of this disease is challengeable.

The relative decrease in breast cancer mortality, expressed as the number of women dying of the disease per 100,000, must be viewed in perspective (Fig. 41.2). Since the mid-1930s the rate has probably crept up slightly from 26% to 27+% by the late 1980s. Mammography use rose strikingly during the 1980s, and so did the use of tamoxifen. The latter agent, producing substantial cytoreduction in hormonally dependent metastases, has unquestionably postponed the time to death for many breast cancer patients. In my view it is far more likely to be the basis for the relative 6.3% drop (consistent with a 1.7% absolute drop) than earlier diagnosis due to mammography.

Although mammography is generally accepted as a means of reducing breast cancer mortality, the data supporting this point is, in my view, open to serious question. Only two prospective randomized trials have shown statistically significant benefit. Selection bias may be a critical flaw in the Health Insurance Project (HIP) trial, and the use of death-postponing tamoxifen might have made an "occult" contribution to the better results in the Swedish two-county trial.

"How I Do It" Management Guidelines

The preceding material is obviously a lengthy preamble to the part of this treatise that now deals specifically with management guidelines that I prefer whenever possible. Only with an attempt at providing a panoramic understanding of breast cancer, its history, and the basis for claims and questioning of these claims can my approach to this disease be fairly viewed.

Having a fairly accurate understanding of the threat a breast treatment is to a patient cosmetically or, more importantly, to her life expectancy, is not enough. The influence of family and friends, as wanted or unwanted consultants, must be taken into account, as does the patient's perception of the dozens of brochures, books, and advertisements she may read, view, or hear about. How much the patient wants to know about risk for recurrence and death and her level of anxiety or composure must be acknowledged. Lastly, the specter of malpractice litigation against the practitioner must be integrated into a final recommendation.

The complexity of this mix of clinical and pathologic data and psychosocial factors provides a challenge for physicians and surgeons obligated or intrigued enough to stand up and be counted on for advice in this field. Algorithms must be created that withstand intense scrutiny.

In my view the key goal is to place the patient's malignancy in one of four categories of risk for death from breast cancer. To do this a variety of factors of varying weight should be considered.

Within the three major areas of determination—clinical, pathologic, functional—individual components are discussed. The composite effect of these determinants leads to the fairly easy exclusion of two of the four categories. Placing a patient's cancer into one of the two remaining divisions is usually possible. The prognostic category is then further weighted by the patient's age and the presence or absence of "competing illness," the latter defined as illness serious enough to shorten her life significantly independent of the coexisting breast cancer.

Usually, the least reliable parameter is the clinical history of the breast abnormality as a palpable mass. The lack of regard of such history in the evaluation is due to the unreliability of palpability. There are exceptions. Occasionally a patient or her attending physician can chronicle a growing lesion accurately enough to permit doubling time computation. Not uncommonly, serial mammograms describe an enlarging density that permits even more reliable growth rate calculation. In this circumstance the weight given clinical cancer (Tables 41.2, 41.3, columns Wt. 2) becomes dominant rather than minor.

Pathology has traditionally been relied on to provide crucial prognostic information, especially when the breast cancer is diagnosed as a palpable mass. There is no question that the larger the primary the worse are the 5- and 10-year survivals. Similarly, the degree of lymph node involvement by metastatic disease provides equivalent prognostic data. On the other hand, about 25% of women with breast cancers diagnosed by palpation that are large or have extensive axillary node metastases (or both) are alive and clinically well in 10 years. About 25% of patients with breast cancers that pathologically measure <2.0 cm and have no demonstrable axillary metastases by routine pathologic examination are dead by 10 years. These not infrequent lapses in prognostic reliability require additional scrutiny of the clinical and pathological data.

The observation of lymph node metastases by the surgical pathologist is usually confined to the number of nodes involved (reported as the numerator) over the number of nodes examined (the denominator). More weight should be given to the size of the largest metastatic deposit. If a primary is 30 mm in diameter and the largest metastatic deposit is 0.4 mm in diameter, is it as ominous as a 20-mm deposit? The 100,000-fold (or 5 log) difference in tumor cell number represented by these sizes projects to a difference in disease-free survival of 50 months with a 90-day cancer cell doubling time (Fig. 41.5).

Other prognostic information is available from the resected malignant tissue. During the last decade or so a new, important resource has emerged from what may be termed functional analysis of material still in the hands of surgical pathology laboratories. Through flow cytometry, fresh or frozen tissue or, more conveniently, tissue salvaged from archival paraffin tissue blocks is analyzable. The procedure is fairly complicated but akin to the black boxes that crank out complete blood counts CBCs and platelet counts in a few minutes. The product of this relatively rapid microscopic examination of thousands of stained tumor nuclei is electronically translated in an unusually objective form reported as the DNA index. Bizarre, usually irregularly shaped, large nuclei seen with flow cytometry translate to "aneuploidy" with a DNA index of 1.2–1.8. In many cancers fairly respectable looking nuclei (seen microscopically as round) resemble normal diploid (euploid) nuclei and have a DNA index of 1.0 + 0.1. Tetraploidy occasionally produces doubling of the DNA index (i.e., 2.0). Bear in mind that even "normal looking" cancer nuclei still harbor the malevolent capacity to replicate autonomously and to metastasize but probably not with the same virulence as aneuploid cells.

In general, the nondiploid or aneuploid cancers demonstrate clinical behavior that corresponds to what pathologists have traditionally termed "poorly differentiated" but with only fair reliability. It may be that aneuploid correlates with degree of invasiveness (i.e., how early in the life of the cancer the metastatic process begins and into which distant organs successful colonization occurs). Diploid (euploid) cancers clearly have invasive and metastatic potential, but it seems likely that the process in this circumstance of less biologic malevolence occurs later and only to organ structures where survival is less immediately threatened. The correlation between the functionally indolent and well differentiated cancers is quite strong.

The more powerful prognosticator derived from the same nuclear morphometry of flow cytometry is determination of the S-phase fraction (S = DNA synthesis). Simply put, when cancer cells are "caught in the act" of synthesizing DNA in preparation for dividing, the usual volume of DNA for the specific cancer being analyzed, whether euploid or aneuploid, shows twice the amount of DNA seen in the bulk of the cell population. This measure of the population of cells involved in DNA synthesis is reported as the percentage of cells of the total seen by flow cytometry. The higher the percentage of cells seen replicating (reasonably

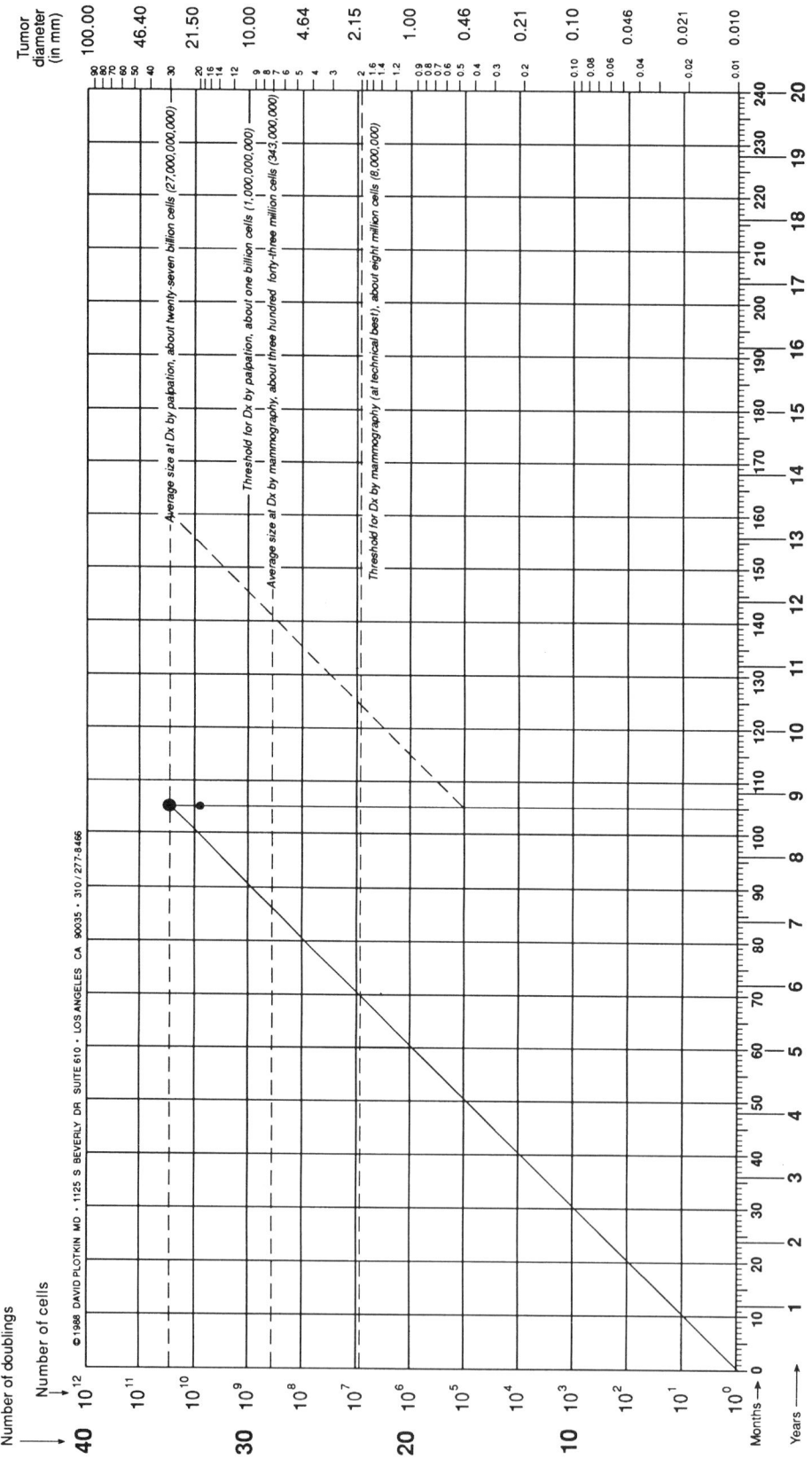

Figure 41.5. Disease-free survival in relation to size of lymph node metastases; 90-day doubling time.

Table 41.2. Cancer suspected by palpation of lump[a]

Parameter	Cancer				Wt. 1 (%)	Wt. 2 (%)
	Aggressive	Moderate	Indolent	Very indolent		
Clinical						
History (months)	<1	1–6	>6 to <18	>18	5	5
Mammographic DT[b]						35
Pathology						
Primary tumor size (cm)	≥5.0	2.1–5.0	1.1–2.0	≤1.0	10	5
LN positive	≥10	4–9	1–3	0	10	5
Size of largest LN met (cm)	>1.0cm	0.3–0.9	0.1–0.2	<0.1	15	15
Differentiation	P	P–M	M	W	10	5
Functional						
Ploidy	Aneuploid	Aneuploid-diploid	Diploid	Diploid	5	5
% of avg. SPF	≥180	70–170	20–80	≤10	25	10
ER/PR	0/0	+/+	2+/2+	≥3+/≥3+	10	10
Oncogenes	3+	2+	0 to 1+	0	10	5

Prognosis

DT average (days)	45	90	180	360
DT range (days)	30–60	61–150	151–300	301–1000
(Est) MDS (attributable to breast cancer) (years)	4.6	9.2	18.4	36.8
W/O Comp. illness				
(Est) risk of death[c] 2° to breast cancer				
W/O comp. illness (%)				
<50 years	100	95	60	15
51–70 years	95	90	50	10
>70 years	90	85	40	0
W/ Comp. illness (%)				
<50 years	80	75	50	5
51–70 years	70	60	30	0
>70 years	60	45	10	0

Wt. 1 = absence of serial mammograms permitting doubling time calculations; Wt. 2 = presence of serial mammograms permitting doubling time calculations; DT = doubling time; LN = lymph node; P = poor; M = moderate; W = well; SPF = S-phase fraction; ER/PR = estrogen/progesterone receptor ratio; MDS = Median duration of survival; W/O = without; 2° = secondary; (Est) = estimated; W/ = with; comp. = significant competing.

[a] Assumptions: biopsy positive for invasive cancer; operable breast cancer.
[b] Is actually functional.
[c] Can be refined by actuarial data.

Table 41.3. Cancers suspected by mammography[a]

Parameter	Cancer				Wt. 1 (%)	Wt. 2 (%)
	Aggressive	Moderate	Indolent	Very indolent		
Clinical						
History (months)	<1	1–6	>6 to <18	>18	5	5
Mammographic DT[b]	<60	61–150	151–300	>300		35
Pathology						
Primary tumor size	—	—	1.0–2.0	<1.0		5
LN positive (no.)	—	—	1–3	0		5
Size of largest LN met (cm)	≥1.0	0.3–0.9	0.1–0.2	<0.1	10	15
Differentiation	P	P–M	M	W	15	5
Functional						
Ploidy	Aneuploid	Aneuploid-diploid	Diploid	Diploid	10	5
% of avg. SPF	≥180	100–170	20–90	≤10	30	10
ER/PR	0/0	+/+	2+/2+	≥3+/≥3+	10	10
Oncogenes	3+	2+	0 to 1+	0	5	5

Prognosis				
DT average (days)	45	90	180	360
DT range (days)	30–60	61–150	151–300	301–1000
(Est) MDS (attributable to breast cancer) (years) W/O comp. illness	4.6	9.2	18.4	36.8
(Est) risk of death[c] 2° to breast ca				
W/O comp. illness (%)				
<50 years	100	95	60	15
51–70 years	95	90	50	5
>70 years	90	85	40	0
W/ comp. illness (%)				
<50 years	80	75	50	5
51–70 years	70	60	30	0
>70 years	60	45	10	0

See Table 41.2 for explanation of abbreviations.

[a] Assumptions: needle localization biopsy for invasive cancer.

[b] Is actually functional.

[c] Can be refined by actuarial data.

construed to be the doubling of nuclear DNA content prior to cell division), the more rapid is the proliferative rate of the cancer. The converse is also true but obviously less useful as the proliferative rate approaches 0%.

A fairly good correlation exists between aneuploidy and a high proliferative rate and, conversely, between the diploid state and a slow proliferative rate. The less than perfect symmetry one might hope for is probably largely due to pitfalls in analysis, such as inadequate sampling (e.g., material insufficient to do a statistically valid flow cytometric determination) and inadvertent sampling of large amounts of noncancer tissue or necrotic (essentially acellular) tissue. Indeed, the contribution of tumor destruction by the host, frank necrosis being the most vivid manifestation, in partially negating the proliferative capacity of a clone of cancer cells is now computable only by noting the difference in theoretic doubling time from the S-phase fraction and clinically observed doubling time. As the phenomenon of apoptosis (programmed cell death) is better understood and becomes more precisely quantifiable, the missing part of the cell kinetic equation becomes available as a reference point.

The tests for oncogenes/tumor proteins (i.e., *p53*, HER-2 *neu*, cathepsin D, epidermal growth factor receptor, among others) has thus far correlated inversely with the better established prognostic significance of estrogen and progesterone receptors. In general, the receptor-negative tumors are more likely to show the tumor-amplifying oncogenes/proteins. The frequently mixed bag of positive receptor status along with one or two oncogenes probably fits the moderate growth rate category of breast cancer better than any of the other three.

Tables 41.2 and 41.3 show how the clinical, pathologic, and functional means of assessment are weighted depending on whether the diagnosis of breast cancer is made from biopsy of a palpable mass or a mammographic abnormality. This distinction is based on the significantly different ranges of lethality posed by breast cancer that presents as a clinically palpable mass versus cancer that is not palpable at diagnosis. Note that the infrequent opportunity to calculate doubling time by serial mammographic measurements in either a palpable or nonpalpable mass is accorded extraordinary weight when placing the cancer in one of four possible groups. These examples demonstrate how the weighting of data in any individual case leads to placing the cancer's biology into the most appropriate category.

Tables 41.2 and 41.3 demonstrate the general clinical, pathologic, and functional characteristics of each of the four categories with corresponding approximations of the mean duration of survival and the range and average of doubling times. The likelihood of death due to breast cancer is then influenced by the patient's age and the presence or absence of serious competing illness. The percentages provided are simply an estimate, as the issue of "significant competing illness" adds to the complexity of any calculation. Obviously, "significant competing illness" requires listing the varying mortal thrusts over time associated with cardiovascular, pulmonary, chronic liver disease, and so on or other invasive cancers. Further definition of the risks intrinsic to each category of breast cancer but influenced variably by the absence of health in other respects is currently a subject of computer-based research.

Tables 41.4–41.7 provide an approximation of breast cancer incidence and mortality during the mid-1990s. Table 41.8 categorizes all breast cancers by their presenting stage and outlines my approach to management versus standard management. Table 41.9 shows four examples of how Tables 41.2, 41.3, and 41.8 can be used to manage breast cancer with my approach.

Table 41.4. Mid-1990s incidence/mortality

Condition	Absolute incidence		Absolute mortality	
	No./year	Percent of total	No./year	Percent of total
All breast cancer/year	212,000	100	46,000	100
CIS/year	32,000	15	2,000	4
Invasive/year	180,000	85	44,000	96

Table 41.5. Method of diagnosis

Diagnostic method	Invasive cancer		Cancer in situ	
	Absolute incidence/ year	Percent of total	Absolute incidence/ year	Percent of total
All breast cancer/year	180,000	100	32,000	100
Diagnosed by palpation with or without mammography (estimated)	120,000	67	1,000	3
Diagnosed by mammography only (estimated)	60,000	33	31,000	97

Table 41.6. Spectrum of biology of breast cancer

	Absolute incidence		Absolute mortality	
	No./year	Percent of total	No./year	Percent of total
Invasive cancer				
Aggressive	23,000	13	22,500	49
Moderate	54,000	30	21,500	47
Indolent	54,000	30	2,000	4
Very indolent	49,000	27	0	0
Total	180	100	46,000	100
Cancer in situ				
Aggressive	0	0		
Moderate	0	0		
Indolent	8,000	25		
Very indolent	24,000	75		
Total	32,000	100		

No death from breast CIS is possible without invasive component missed in diagnosis or a subsequent independent invasive breast cancer, in which case the mortality is recorded in Table 41.4.

Table 41.7. Breakdown of all breast cancer by stage at diagnosis

Stage	Absolute incidence/year	Percent of total
Cancer in situ	32,000	15
1	85,000	40
2	64,000	30
3	21,000	10
4	10,000	5
Total	212,000	100

CONCLUSIONS AND PERSPECTIVES

We do not actuarially ever cure invasive breast cancer. We can expect "personal cures" in about 50% of patients being treated today. These patients, who do not die of breast cancer, may often be treated with less surgery, radiation therapy, and chemotherapy with no risk to their longevity. We can expect a marked improvement, perhaps in excess of 50%, in personal cure rate today over the approximately 20% observed before the advent of the change in the reproductive biology of Western women and the huge surge in extra case-finding attributable to mammography. This is probably largely due to diagnosing many more breast cancers of lesser malevolence than was the situation 50 years ago. Improvements in diagnosis have made little if any impact on overall survival. Improvements in systemic treatment, notably tamoxifen, have finally dented the mortality stemming from biologically indolent, moderate, and aggressive breast cancers. The persistence of the same number of absolute deaths due to aggressive cancers despite the best surgery, radiation therapy, and chemotherapy is testimony to the lack of effectiveness of such treatments in the worst form of breast cancer.

The huge increase in the diagnosis of CIS is at best a two-edged sword. We might very well be needlessly putting tens of thousands of women through the psychological trauma of breast cancer diagnosis and the physical impact of treatments that often are the same as for invasive breast cancer.

In my view, invasive breast cancer cannot be diagnosed before the metastatic process has begun. The diagnosis and treatment of CIS may well avoid progression to invasion and metastases in some patients, but it is accomplished by overtreating many. It seems likely that a tumor marker for breast cancer, a breast-specific antigen (BSA), or perhaps a series of markers for the in situ versus invasive lesions will be found. With such molecular biologic tools, we ought to be able to compute doubling times from serial BSA assays. Hopefully our therapeutic armamentarium will also improve so we can bring to bear treatments that rationally fit specific patients. We could then abandon the widely used approach of "one size fits all" treatment that creates the current frightening level of morbidity.

Table 41.8. Breast cancer management guidelines: personal approach vs. standard approach

Stage	Aggressive (13%)			Moderate (30%)			Indolent (30%)			Very indolent (27%)		
	Standard	%	Personal approach	Standard	%	Personal approach	Standard	%	Personal approach	Standard	%	Personal approach
In situ **stage 0 (15%)**												
Local Rx	—	0	—	Lx + AND + RT	1	—	Lx + AND + RT	3	Lx	Lx	6	Lx
Syst. Rx	—		—	± tamoxifen			± tamoxifen		± tamoxifen	± tamoxifen		± tamoxifen
Stage 1 (40%)												
Local Rx	MRMx or Lx + AND + RT	1	MRMx or Lx + AND	MRMx or Lx + AND + RT	10	MRMx or Lx + AND	Lx + AND + RT	15	Lx + AND	Lx + AND + RT	18	Lx
Syst. Rx	CMF × 6		M → F × 6	CMF × 6 ± tamoxifen		M → F × 6	CMF × 6 + tamox		M → F × 6 ± Ovx/tamox	CMF × 6 + tamox		
Portacath	Yes		Yes	Yes		Yes	Yes		No	Yes		No
Stage 2 (30%)												
Local Rx	MRMX or Lx + AND + RT	8	MRMx or Lx + AND + RT	MRMx or Lx + AND + RT	13	MRMx or Lx + AND + RT	MRMx or Lx + AND + RT	9	Lx + AND	Lx + AND + RT	1	Lx
Syst. Rx	CAF × 6		CM → F × 6	CAF × 6 ± tamox		CM → F × 6 ± tamox	CMF × 6		± Ovx/tamox	CMF × 6 ± tamox		± Ovx/tamox
Portacath	Yes		Yes	Yes		Yes	Yes		No	Yes		No
Stage 3 (10%)												
Local Rx	Incis Bx + RT	4	Incis Bx	Incis Bx + RT	4	Incis Bx	Incis Bx + RT	2	Incis Bx	—	0	—
Syst. Rx	CAF × 6		CM → F × 6	CAF × 6		CM → F × 6	CAF × 6		± Ovx/tamox	—		—
Portacath	Yes		Yes	Yes		Yes	Yes		No	—		—
Stage 4 (5%)												
Local Rx	Incis Bx + RT	2	Incis Bx	Incis Bx + RT	2	Incis Bx	Incis Bx + RT	1	± Ovx/tamox	—	0	—
Syst. Rx	CAF × 6		CM → F × 6	CAF × 6		CM → F × 6	CM → F × 6 ± tamox		± Ovx/tamox	—		—
Portacath	Yes		Yes	Yes		Yes	Yes		No	—		—

Lx = lumpectomy; AND = axillary node dissection; RT = radiation therapy; MRMx = modified radical mastectomy; CMF = Cytoxan/methotrexate/5-FU; Ovx = oophorectomy; A = Adriamycin; Incis Bx = incisional biopsy; Rx = treatment; Syst. = systemic; tamox = tamoxifen.

Table 41.9. Patient examples

Patient types	Patients (%)			
	Aggressive	Moderate	Indolent	Very indolent
Patient 1				
Two-week history of palpable mass	5			
No DT				
Tumor size 4.0 cm		10		
Lymph nodes positive: 6		10		
Size of largest LN deposit: 1.0 cm	15			
Poorly differentiated	10			
Aneuploid	5			
% ave. SPF 180	25			
SR$^-$/PR$^-$	10			
HER-2/*neu* and Cath D present	5	5		
p53 EGFR absent				
Total	75	25		
Diagnosis: aggressive				
Treatment: MRMx in small breast; Lx + RT in large breast; CM → F × 6 cycles				
Patient 2				
Three-month history of lump		5		
No DT				
Tumor size 3.0 cm		10		
Lymph nodes positive: 2			10	
Size of largest LN deposit: 0.5 cm		15		
Moderately to poorly differentiated		10		
Aneuploid to diploid		5		
% avg. SPF 100		25		
ER 2$^+$/PR 2$^+$			10	
Oncogenes: no			10	
Total		70	30	
Diagnosis: moderate				
Treatment: Lx + AND followed by CM → F followed by tamoxifen × 5 years				
Patient 3				
One-year history of lump			5	
No DT				
Primary tumor size 2.0 cm			10	
Lymph nodes positive: 0/10[a]			5	5
Size of largest LN met. N/A[a]			7.5	7.5
Moderately differentiated			10	
Diploid			5	
SPF 4%/6 (ave.)			25	
ER 2$^+$/PR 2$^+$			10	
Oncogenes: absent			10	
Total			92.5	7.5

Table 41.9. *Continued*

Patient types	Patients (%)			
	Aggressive	*Moderate*	*Indolent*	*Very indolent*
Diagnosis: indolent				

Treatment: Lx + AND followed by oophorectomy in premenopausal or tamoxifen in
postmenopausal women

Patient 4				
No lump[a]			2.5	2.5
Mammographic DT				35
Tumor size 1.0			5	0
Lymph nodes positive: 0/10[a]			2.5	2.5
Size of LN met N/A[a]			7.5	7.5
Moderately differentiated			5	
Diploid[a]			2.5	2.5
SPF 2%/6			10	
ER 3[+]/PR 3[+]				10
Oncogenes: 0				5
Total			35	65
Diagnosis: Very indolent				

Treatment: Lx; no F/U treatment

DT = doubling time; F/U = follow-up; ER/PR = estrogen receptors/progesterone receptors; SPF = S-Phase Faction;
EGFR = epidermal growth factor receptor. See Table 41.8 for farther explanations.
[a]Divided between indolent and very indolent because of absence of lymph node involvement.

References

1. Haagensen CD. Diseases of the Breast (2nd ed). Philadelphia, Saunders, 1971

2. Hirsch J. Radiumchirurgie des Brustkrebses. Dtsch Med Wochenschr 1927;34:1419–1421

3. Keynes G. Conservative treatment of cancer of the breast. BMJ 1937;2:643–647

4. Mustakallio S. Treatment of breast cancer by tumour extirpation and roentgen therapy. J Faculty Radiol 1954;6:23

5. Baclesse F. Five year results in 431 breast cancers treated solely by roentgen rays. Ann Surg 1965;161:103–104

6. Crile G Jr. Treatment of cancer of the breast: past, present, and future. Cleve Clin Q 1971;38:47–54

7. Feinstein AR, Sosin DM, Wells CK. Will Rogers phenomenon: stage migration and new diagnostic techniques as a source of misleading statistics for survival in cancer. N Engl J Med 1985;312:1604–1608

8. Fisher B, Ravdin RG, Ausman RK, et al. Surgical adjuvant chemotherapy in cancer of the breast: results of a decade of cooperative investigation. Ann Surg 1968;168:337–356

9. Fisher B, Redmond C, Fisher ER, et al. The contribution of recent NSABP clinical trials of primary breast cancer therapy to an understanding of tumor biology and overview of findings. Cancer 1980;46:1009–1025

10. Beatson GT. On the treatment of inoperable cases of carcinoma of the mamma: suggestions for a new method of treatment, with illustrative cases. Lancet 1896;2:104–107, 162–165

11. Bordley J III, Harvey AM. Two Centuries of American Medicine 1776–1976. Philadelphia, Saunders, 1976, p 679

12. Nathanson IT. Clinical investigative experience with steroid hormones in breast cancer. Cancer 1952;5:754

13. Stoll BA. Hormonal management in Breast Cancer. London, Pitman Philadelphia, and Lippincott, 1969

14. Mouridsen H, Palshof T, Patterson J, Battersby L. Tamoxifen in advanced breast cancer. Cancer Treat Rev 1978;5:131–141

15. Plotkin D. The medico-legal implications of breast cancer screening. In: Jatoi I (ed) Breast Cancer Screening. Austin, Landes Bioscience, 1997

16. Fisher B, Bauer M, Margolese R, et al. Five year results of a randomized clinical trial comparing total mastectomy and segmental mastectomy with or without radiation in the treatment of breast cancer. N Engl J Med 1985;312:665–673

Appendix A: Organization of the Breast Diagnostic Center Department of Obstetrics and Gynecology

William H. Hindle

As an institutional service funded and operated by a local county government (in this case Los Angeles County, State of California) the organization, personnel, and type and location of the health care services offered have continuously changed since the Breast Diagnostic Center (BDC) was established in July 1988. However, the dual goals of providing breast care services to the patients (inpatient and outpatient) of Women's and Children's Hospital (W&CH) and breast care education and hands-on clinical experience for the obstetrics and gynecology resident physicians in training have steadfastly remained paramount. Only the format, personnel, and logistics have changed.

To avoid confusion, the descriptions that follow are given in the present tense, although changes have been made from what was orginally envisioned and implemented because of recent budget requirements and restrictions imposed by the county. We hope to reinstate any personnel or programs thus eliminated or downsized as soon as funding allows. Thus the model described represents an ideal that has worked well when fully operational. Readers should feel free to adapt our model, with restriction, to their particular situation.

Educational Presentations

During the first year resident physician (intern) orientation, an hour-long presentation, including a three-part video on breast self-examination and clinical breast evaluation (BSE/CBE), mammography, and breast mass evaluation, is given by Staff (University of Southern California Medical School Faculty). An introduction and orientation to the breast care services available through the BDC and Los Angeles County + University of Southern California Medical Center (LACUSCMC) and an illustrated CBE booklet are included in this initial presentation. Thereafter a regularly scheduled monthly breast lecture is given for the resident physicians. A typical schedule of topics for the year is as follows

July	Breast disease—an overview
August	Breast examination: clinical and self-examination: technique, frequency, documentation

September	Mastalgia: diagnosis and treatment
October	Benign breast disease
November	Mammography: case studies and film reading (resident physician participation), by the Director of Mammography Services, LACUSCMC
December	Office evaluation of breast masses and follow-up
January	Evaluation and treatment of breast cysts and nipple discharge
February	Fine-needle aspiration of the breast
March	Mammography: screening and diagnostic, diagnoses and reports
April	Pathology of the breast, gross and microscopic, by the Director of Pathology, W&CH
May	Surgery of the breast: biopsy, surgical therapy, reconstruction
June	Treatment of breast cancer: surgery, hormone therapy, chemotherapy

BREAST SERVICES ROTATION

The resident physicians participate in a month-long rotation through the various breast care support services at LACUSCMC. The weekly rotation includes attendance at and participation in:

1. Combined mammography/surgery conference, LACUSCMC
2. Breast Surgery Clinic (twice a week), Department of General Surgery
3. H. Claude Hudson LAC Comprehensive Health Center, Breast Clinic (supervised by BDC Staff)
4. Breast surgery, excisional biopsies, Department of Surgery, General Hospital, LACUSCMC
5. Breast surgery, mastectomies, Department of Surgery, General Hospital, LACUSCMC
6. Mammography reading, Department of Radiology, LACUSCMC
7. USC/Norris Breast Center, Interdisciplinary Treatment Planning Conference, Norris Cancer Center
8. Assist on breast biopsies performed by the resident physicians (usually senior residents) under Staff supervision, W&CH
9. Postoperative and other BDC follow-ups, W&CH
10. BDC repeat follow-up fine-needle aspirations (FNAs), W&CH
11. Cytology and histology review, Department of Pathology, W&CH
12. Breast cytology slide reviews by the cytopathology section of the Department of Pathology, LACUSCMC
13. Attend the BDC clinic session, W&CH

PERSONNEL

The following personnel are present at BDC clinic sessions: (1) two faculty staff, (2) four resident physicians (often additional resident physicians who are rotating from other training programs or visiting the BDC), (3) a cytopathologist, (4) a cytopathology technician, (5) the BDC nurse supervisor/specialist, (5) four nursing personnel. A computer input clerk and a mammography appointments clerk are available as needed. Not infrequently outside physicians, midwives, and nurse-practitioners visit along with interested medical students and students studying to be physician assistants, midwives, and nurses. Breast care education and the opportunity to assist (under supervision) in the BDC patient evaluations is freely offered to all those who attend the BDC sessions.

Breast Diagnostic Center Forms

New patients are first seen by a multilingual nurse who interviews the patient and fills out the BDC Patient's History Intake Form (Figs. A.1, A.2). This form is then available to the resident physician who takes a breast-oriented history, performs a CBE, and completes the BDC Initial Evaluation form (Figs. A.3, A.4). The physical findings are drawn in on the Initial Evaluation form breast diagram, and a description is added. Staff physicians are available in the BDC to review the case and suggest management. The resident physician then instructs the patient and orders appropriate tests and consultations. The bilingual nurse reviews the diagnosis and instructions with the patient. The BDC forms are designed to minimize writing and paperwork, educate the physicians as to what is required in the fundamental breast record, and allow computer input for clinical research. Ideally, the form is in a format that allows scanning, so the data can be taken directly off the form and entered into a computer program for storage and analysis. A BDC Mammography Requisition/Report form (Fig. A.5) is designed to give the mammographer the basic clinical information and permit a rapid check-off of clinically meaningful mammographic findings and recommendations. The Mammography Requisition/Report form will be revised to include the BI-RADS breast imaging assessment categories (coding) as additional check-offs. A distinctive colored (blue) border on the BDC forms allows them to be easily recognized in a large medical record.

Copies are made of all the BDC records and maintained in a chronologic file so the forms are immediately available when needed to respond appropriately to patient and physician phone calls and patient return visits. The original BDC forms are inserted into the individual patient's medical record at the end of the day. Copies are stapled to consultation requests or referral forms (e.g., when the patient or her specimens are sent for surgery, oncology, cytology, pathology, or mammography).

Physical Layout and Nurse Supervisor

The floor plan of the BDC in W&CH is depicted in Figure A.6. All the essential breast services of the diagnostic triad are available within the BDC and are performed on the patient's initial visit. Mammography and cytology reports are

County of Los Angeles   LAC/USC Medical Center   Department of Health Services
                                         Womens Hospital
                                     Breast Diagnostic Center

PATIENT'S HISTORY INTAKE FORM

Date:_____ Age:_____ Birth date:_____/_____/_____ File: _____
                                                 month   day   year

Telephone: Work (_____) _____   Home: (_____) _____

Referred by: _____

1. Reason for coming to The Breast Diagnostic Center:

   Lump   RIGHT / LEFT   How long_____   Pain   RIGHT / LEFT   How long_____

   Nipple Discharge   RIGHT / LEFT   How Long_____   Color_____

   Nipple changes _____   Skin changes _____

   Other (Explain)_____

2. Does anyone in your family have breast cancer?   YES / NO   List the age of individual at time of cancer discovery.

   Self_____   Mother _____   Sister_____

   Other _____   Relationship _____

3. Have you had breast cancer surgery?   YES / NO   Please check one:

   _____ Mastectomy   _____ Lumpectomy   _____ Other (Explain)_____

4. Have you had other breast surgery?   YES / NO   What kind _____

5. Have you had breast radiation treatment?   YES / NO   When _____

6. Have you had a biopsy?   YES / NO   Age_____   Results:_____

   When (date) _____   Which breast   RIGHT / LEFT

7. Do you know how to do Breast Self Examination?   YES / NO

8. Do you do Breast Self Examination?   YES / NO   How often _____ Occasionally _____ Monthly _____ More often

9. Do you have breast implants?   YES / NO

10. Do you have silicone injections?   YES / NO

11. Do you have skin moles on your breast?   YES / NO   Where _____

12. Do you have breast pain?   YES / NO   RIGHT / LEFT   Both sides _____

                                         [OVER]

BREAST DIAGNOSTIC CENTER
   LAC/USC Medical Center   OUTPATIENT   Name _____
      Womens Hospital   RECORD   PF# _____

Figure A.1. Patient History Intake Form, page 1.

available (by phone) on the next working day. In addition, the nurse supervisor of the BDC is available throughout the BDC clinic session if it becomes necessary to counsel a patient with a presumptive diagnosis of breast cancer. At this same time, the nurse supervisor makes the appropriate consultation appointments and instructs the patient. A "significant other" or relative/friend who accompanied the patient to W&CH are included in these counseling discussions unless the patient prefers otherwise.

[Breast Pain] If yes:

_____ Monthly: How long _____ How severe _____

_____ Burning: How long _____ When _____

_____ Premenstrual _____ Anytime _____ All the time

_____ Tenderness: How long _____ Swelling Premenstrual _____

13. Have you had an injury to your breasts?   YES / NO   When _____

     Where _____ Results: _____

14. Have you had mammograms before (breast x-rays)?   YES / NO   When _____

     Where _____ Results: _____

15. Have you ever had any kind of cancer (except breast)   YES / NO   If yes, what kind _____

16. Parity: Age of first menstruation _____   Number of pregnancies _____

                 Number of births _____   Age at first full term pregnancy _____

                 Number of children nursed over one month _____

                 Are you now pregnant? YES / NO   Are your breasts now producing milk?   YES / NO

                 Are you nursing (breast feeding)?   YES / NO

17. Date of last menstruation: _____/_____/_____
                                        month   day   year

18. Menopause: Have your periods stopped?   YES / NO   If yes, when_____

     Are you on hormones?   YES / NO   What kind _____ How long _____

19. Have you ever taken birth control pills?   YES / NO   If yes, when _____ How long _____

     Are you taking birth control pills now?   YES / NO

20. Have you had your ovaries removed?   YES / NO   When _____

21. Have you had your uterus (womb) removed?   YES / NO   When _____

22. Ethnic background: (for statistical and research purposes)

     _____ Hispanic   _____ Caucasian   _____ Oriental

     _____ Black   _____ Indian   _____ Other

23. Height _____ Weight _____   Number of pounds overweight _____

24. How many cups of coffee or tea do you drink a day? _____ How much chocolate do you eat a week? _____

25. Are you on any medication now?   YES / NO   What _____

26. Do you have any allergies?   YES / NO   To what _____

Breast Diagnostic Center
LAC/USC Medical Center
County of Los Angeles   Womens Hospital   Department of Health Services

Figure A.2. Patient History Intake Form, page 2.

PATIENT TRACKING

A patient tracking system utilizes log books, report files, chart files, and computers (for the mammography reports and follow-up). The BDC future goal is to create a comprehensive patient tracking system for all women seen in the BDC or who have mammography in W&CH with integration of all pertinent reports and follow-up in a completely computerized system. All BDC forms (the retained copies), mammography reports, cytology reports, surgical notes, pathology reports, consultations, and any other essential medical records of BDC patients

County of Los Angeles   Department of Health Services

LAC/USC Medical Center
Womens Hospital
Breast Diagnostic Center

INITIAL EVALUATION
(Circle Choice)

Date:_____ Age:_____ Referred by:_____

Hispanic   Black   Caucasian   Oriental   Other

Reason for visit: PAIN   MASS   NIPPLE DISCHARGE   MAMMO LESION

RIGHT/ LEFT   DURATION_____

_____

_____

Family history breast cancer: YES/ NO _____

Past medical Hx:_____

Past surgical Hx:_____

Previous breast Sx: Prior Br Bx YES/ NO   When_____Where_____

    Pathology_____

    Other breast Sx_____

Hormone therapy: YES/ NO   Oral Contraception YES/ NO   PAST/ PRESENT_____

    Estrogen replacement YES/ NO   PASTPRESENT_____

Medications: YES/ NO   Allergies: YES/ NO

_____   _____

_____   _____

LMP_____ Menarche_____ Menopause_____

Gravida_____ Para_____ Spontaneous AB_____Elective AB_____

Prior Mammography YES/ NO When_____ Where_____

    Report:_____

Breast self exam: YES/ NO   Monthly   Occasionally

Current Mammogram: Date_____ WH LAC Elsewhere_____

    Report: NORMAL/ ABNORMAL_____

    Advise: Annual Mammo   6 Months   Recheck   U/S_____

BREAST DIAGNOSTIC CENTER
LAC/USC Medical Center   **OUTPATIENT**   Name_____
Womens Hospital   **RECORD**   PF#_____

Figure A.3.   Initial Evaluation, page 1.

returned to W&CH are reviewed by Staff, and educational/informational feedback is given to the resident physician who originally saw the patient.

Telephone communication has proved to be the most effective way to contact the population served by the BDC. When the patient cannot be reached, letters and telegrams are used. Postcards are used for reporting normal screening mammograms. The BDC nurse supervisor/specialist coordinates patient tracking and follow-up. She also conducts patient education and patient and family counseling;

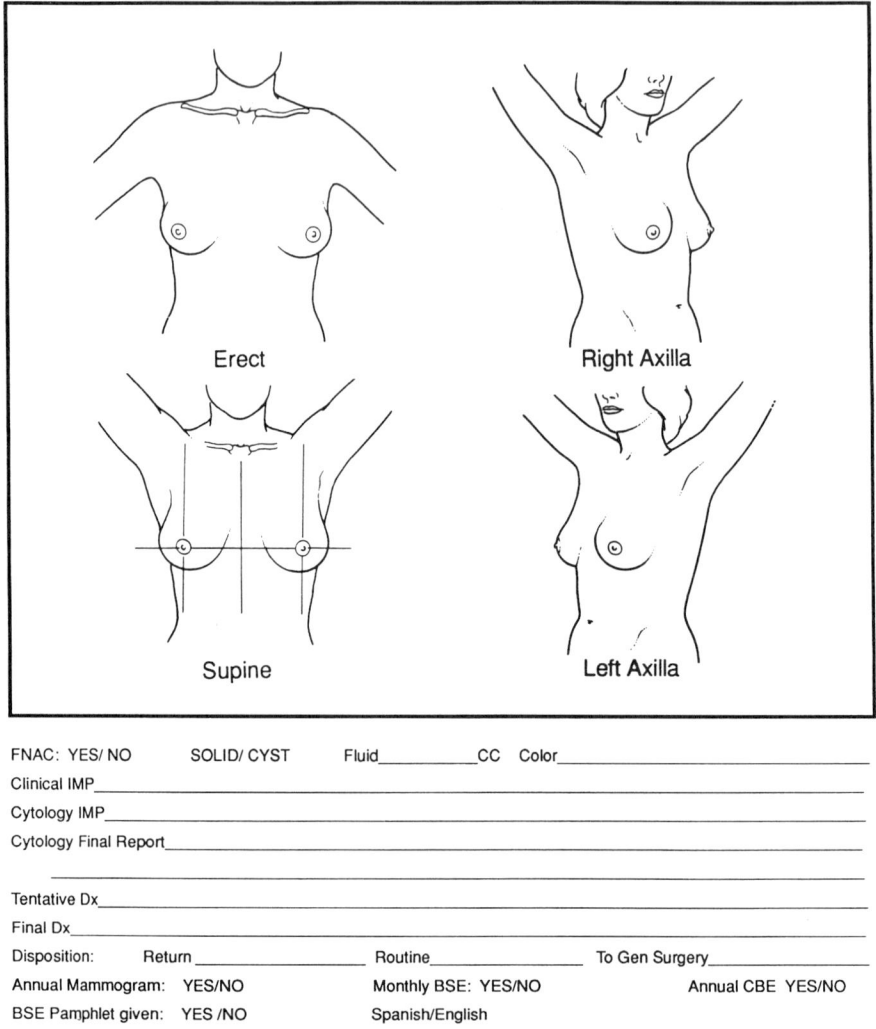

FNAC: YES/ NO   SOLID/ CYST   Fluid_____CC   Color_____

Clinical IMP_____

Cytology IMP_____

Cytology Final Report_____

_____

Tentative Dx_____

Final Dx_____

Disposition: Return _____   Routine_____   To Gen Surgery_____

Annual Mammogram: YES/NO   Monthly BSE: YES/NO   Annual CBE YES/NO

BSE Pamphlet given: YES /NO   Spanish/English

BSE Video shown: YES/ NO   Spanish/English

_____ M.D

LAC/USC Medical Center   *signed*
Womens Hospital
County of Los Angeles   Breast Diagnostic Center   Department of Health Services

Figure A.4. Initial Evaluation, page 2.

and she facilitates access to the LACUSCMC health care system and allied
resources.

SCREENING MAMMOGRAPHY

Screening mammography is offered to all nonpregnant women aged 40 or older
who attend W&CH, and they are encouraged to return for annual routine screening mammography. Currently, screening mammography is being made available
within W&CH by the Department of Radiology on the floor above the BDC. As

County of Los Angeles   LAC/USC Medical Center   Department of Health Services
                                              Womens Hospital
                                          Breast Diagnostic Center

MAMMOGRAPHY REQUISITION/REPORT

Date: _____   Pt. age:_____   Ordered by:_____M.D.
PT Phone:_____   Alternate Phone: _____

☐ **Screening**   ☐ **Diagnostic**

History	Breast Mass	YES / NO	RIGHT/LEFT	Quadrant location
	Nipple Discharge	YES / NO		
	Breast Biopsy	YES / NO		UI | UO
	Breast Surgery	YES / NO	On ERT/OCs YES / NO	
	F Hx Breast CA	YES / NO	Pregnant YES / NO	LI | LO
	Prior Mammography	YES / NO		
	If Yes, where? _____ W.H. LAC E.W. _____			

MAMMOGRAM REPORT: Date:_____

☐ No significant abnormality

  ☐ No significant change since previous mammogram_____

  ☐ Dense fibroglandular parenchyma-bilateral

  ☐ Mammographically benign finding

    ☐ Definable mass

    ☐ Asymmetry and/or architectural distortion

    ☐ Calcifications

    ☐ Developing or new mass/asymmetry

    ☐ Skin thickening and/or retraction   Approximate location of abnormality:

MAMMOGRAPHICALLY SUSPICIOUS FOR CA:

☐ Mass

☐ Calcification

☐ Asymmetry or architectural distortion

☐ Developing or new mass, asymmetry

RECOMMEND: Right   Left

☐ Routine Follow-up

☐ Further mammographic views   Mammographer_____ M.D.

☐ P.E. Correlation

☐ Biopsy/FNA

☐ Repeat in 6 months

          BREAST DIAGNOSTIC CENTER | Name _____ |
             LAC/USC Medical Center | PF# _____ |
                Womens Hospital

Figure A.5.   Mammography Requisition/Report.

soon as the personnel are available, mammography will be expanded to 5 (from 2) days a week and will include on-site diagnostic mammography and ultrasound imaging. The mammography machine will be staffed by a mammography technologist. Basic craniocaudal (CC) and mediolateral oblique (MLO) views are obtained. The films are batch-processed and read by a mammographer later at the Department of Radiology. As soon as the report is read and dictated into the computer system, it is available by fax; a printout of the final verified copy is available several days later.

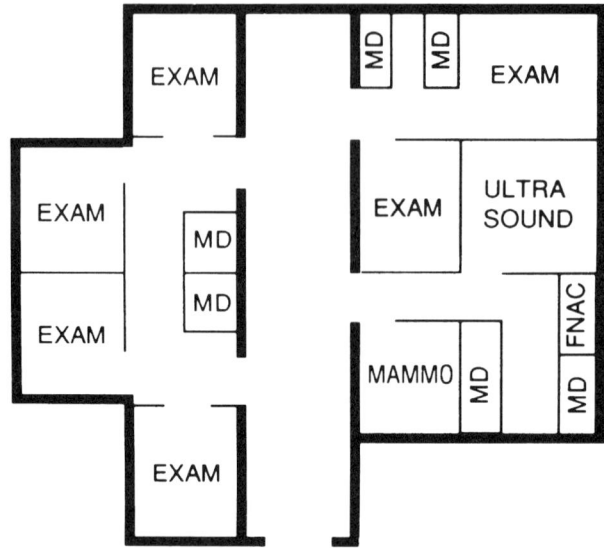

Figure A.6. Floor plan of the Breast Diagnostic Center. MD = Physician desk; FNAC = fine-needle aspiration cyctology slide preparation and viewing.

BDC FNA Reports

As soon as the slides are prepared, within minutes of an FNA, the cytopathologist in the BDC makes a preliminary evaluation and interpretation while the resident physician in charge of the patient views the slides at the same time via a double-headed microscope. The resident physician thus receives valuable on-the-spot instruction on evaluating a cellular specimen and can immediately compare the clinical impression with the preliminary cytologic impression. The resident physician then verbally informs the patient of the preliminary cytologic impression and advises that she will be notified if there is any variance with the final formal interpretation, to be made by the cytopathology division of the department of pathology. However, the preliminary FNA impression allows clinical management to proceed. The final formal reports are available by phone within two working days and are in the computer results system within a week.

State of California Programs

The W&CH participates in the State of California Breast Cancer Early Detection Program (BCEDP) and the State Breast and Cervical Cancer Control Program (BCCCP), both of which provide funding for uninsured or underinsured women of minority ethnic backgrounds. In addition, the BDC participates in the Blue Cross Treatment Fund (BCTF), which also reimburses cancer treatment costs for this patient population.

APPENDIX B: REPORTING SYSTEM*

A. *REPORT ORGANIZATION*

The reporting system should be concise and organized using the following structure. A statement indicating that the present examination has been compared to previous mammograms should be included. If this is not included, it should be assumed that no comparison has been made.

1. A succinct description of the overall breast composition.

   This an overall assessment of the attenuating tissues in the breast to help indicate the relative possibility that a lesion could be hidden by the normal tissues. Generally, this includes fatty, mixed or dense.

   Since mammography cannot detect all breast cancers, physical examination is always a key element of screening. It is important to alert the clinician that in the radiographically dense breast the ability of mammography to detect small cancers is reduced. Although mammography is still useful in these women, the physical examination (which is always important) is increased in importance. The available data do not support the use of mammographic patterns for determining screening frequency (i.e., risk for breast cancer).

   For consistency, this should be included for all patients using the following patterns:

   1) The breast is almost entirely fat.

   2) There are scattered fibroglandular densities that could obscure a lesion on mammography.

   3) The breast tissue is heterogeneously dense. This may lower the sensitivity of mammography.

   4) The breast tissue is extremely dense, which lowers the sensitivity of mammography.

* The source of the material contained in Appendix B is the American College of Radiology. *Breast Imaging Reporting and Data System* (BI-RADS) (2nd ed). Reston, VA, ACR, 1995.

If an implant is present, it should be stated in the report and an implant description code added as appropriate.

2. A clear description of any significant finding. (It is assumed that most significant findings are new.)

    a. Mass

        Size

        Lesion type and modifiers

        Associated calcifications

        Associated findings

        Location

        How changed, if previously present

    b. Calcifications

        Morphology: type of shape and modifiers

        Distribution

        Associated findings

        Location

        How changed, if previously present.

The *clinical location* of the abnormality as extrapolated from the mammographic location (based on the face of a clock).

3. An overall (summary) impression

All final impressions should be complete with each lesion fully categorized and qualified. An indeterminate reading should only be given in the screening setting where additional imaging evaluation is recommended before a final opinion can be rendered.

In the screening situation a suggestion for the next course of action should be given if the study is not conclusive (magnification, ultrasound, etc.).

Interpretation is facilitated by recognizing that most mammograms can be categorized under a few headings. There are listed below and suggested codes are included for computer use.

If a suspicious abnormality is detected, the report should indicate that biopsy should be considered. This is an assessment where the radiologist has sufficient concern that biopsy is warranted unless there are other reasons why the patient and her physician might wish to defer the biopsy.

    a. Assessment is incomplete

    Category 0   Need Additional Imaging Evaluation:

           Finding for which additional imaging evaluation is needed. This is almost always used in a screening situation and should rarely be used after a full imaging workup. A recommendation for additional imaging evaluation includes the use of spot compression, magnification, special mammographic views, ultrasound, etc.

Whenever possible, the present mammogram should be compared to previous studies. The radiologist should use judgment in how vigorously to pursue previous studies.

b. Assessment is complete—*final* categories

Category 1   Negative

There is nothing to comment on. The breasts are symmetrical; and no masses, architectural disturbances or suspicious calcifications are present.

Category 2   Benign finding

This is also a negative mammogram, but the interpreter may wish to describe a finding. Involuting, calcified fibroadenomas, multiple secretory calcifications, fat-containing lesions such as oil cysts, lipomas, galactoceles, and mixed density hamartomas all have characteristic appearances and may be labeled with confidence. The interpreter might wish to describe intramammary lymph nodes, implants, etc. while still concluding that there is no mammographic evidence of malignancy.

Category 3   Probably benign finding: short interval follow-up suggested

A finding placed in this category should have a very high probability of being benign. It is not expected to change over the follow-up interval, but the radiologist would prefer to establish its stability. Data are becoming available that shed light on the efficacy of short-interval follow-up. At the present time, most approaches are intuitive. These will likely undergo future modification as more data accrue as to the validity of an approach, the interval required, and the type of findings that should be followed.

Category 4   Suspicious abnormality: biopsy should be considered

These are lesions that do not have the characteristic morphologies of breast cancer but have a definite probability of being malignant. The radiologist has sufficient concern to urge a biopsy. If possible, the relevant probabilities should be cited so that the patient and her physician can make the decision on the ultimate course of action.

Category 5   Highly suggestive of malignancy: appropriate action should be taken

These lesions have high probability of being cancer.

B. *WORDING THE REPORT*

When available, the present examination should be compared to previous studies, and this should be indicated in the report. Reports should be organized with a brief description of the composition of the breast, any pertinent FINDINGS, followed by the ASSESSMENT with any recommendations. The report should be succinct using terminology from the approved lexicon without embellishment. Note below in the sample reports the definitions and descriptors of the lexicon terms do not appear in the report narrative. Following the impression section of the report, both the assessment category number and the lexicon terminology for the assessment category should be stated. Other aspects of the report data should comply with the ACR Standard on Communication.

1. SAMPLE REPORTS

a. For screening

   The present examination is compared to previous mammograms. The breasts are almost entirely fat. No masses, significant calcifications, or other findings are seen.

   Impression: There is no mammographic evidence of malignancy.

   BI-RADS Category 1: Negative

b. For the patient with a mammographically detected mass

   The breasts are almost entirely fat.

   There is a 7 mm irregular, spiculated mass in the anterior 11:00 region of the right breast.

   Impression: There is a malignant appearing lesion in the right breast.

   BI-RADS Category 5: Highly suggestive of malignancy: appropriate action should be taken.

c. For the patient with a palpable mass when the mammogram is negative

   The breast is extremely dense, which lowers the sensitivity of mammography.

   No masses, significant calcifications, or other abnormalities are visible.

   Impression: There is no mammographic evidence of malignancy, although the dense tissue could obscure a lesion. The decision whether or not to biopsy at this time should be based on the clinical assessment.

   BI-RADS Category 1: Negative

APPENDIX C: BREAST CANCER STAGING*

TNM classification
  T = tumor
  N = node
  M = metastasis

TNM STAGING SYSTEM

Primary Tumor (T)	Definition
TX	Primary tumor cannot be assessed
T0	No evidence of primary tumor
TIS	Carcinoma in situ: intraductal carcinoma lobular carcinoma in situ or Paget's disease of the nipple with no tumor
T1	Tumor ≤2 cm in greatest dimension
T1a	Tumor ≤0.5 cm in greatest dimension
T1b	Tumor >0.5 cm but not >2 cm in greatest dimension
T1c	Tumor >1 cm but not >2 cm in greatest dimension
T2	Tumor >2 cm but not >5 cm in greatest dimension
T3	Tumor >5 cm in greatest dimension
T4	Tumor of any size with direct extension to the chest wall or skin
T4a	Extension to chest wall
T4b	Edema (including peu d'orange) or ulceration of the skin of the breast, or satellite skin nodules confined to the same breast
T4c	Both T4a and T4b
T4d	Inflammatory carcinoma

*The source of the material contained in Appendix C is the American Joint Committee on Cancer. *AJCC Cancer Staging Manual* (5th ed). Philadelphia, Lippincott-Raven, 1997.

Regional Lymph Nodes (N)

NX	Regional lymph nodes cannot be assessed (e.g., previously removed)
N0	No regional lymph node metastasis
N1	Metastasis to movable ipsilateral axillary lymph node(s)
N2	Metastasis to ipsilateral axillary lymph node(s) fixed to one another or to other structures
N3	Metastasis to ipsilateral internal mammary lymph node(s)

Pathologic Classification (PN)

pNX	Regional lymph nodes cannot be assessed (e.g., previously removed or not removed for pathologic study)
pN0	No regional lymph node metastasis
pN1	Metastasis to movable ipsilateral axillary lymph node(s)
pN1a	Only micrometastasis (<0.2 cm)
pN1b	Metastasis to lymph node(s) >0.2 cm
pN1bi	Metastasis in 1–3 lymph nodes, >0.2 cm but not >2 cm in greatest dimension
pN1bii	Metastasis to 4 or more lymph nodes, >0.2 cm but not >2 cm in greatest dimension
pN1biii	Extension of tumor beyond the capsule of a lymph node metastasis, <2 cm in greatest dimension
pN1biv	Metastasis to a lymph node ≥ 2 cm in greatest dimension
pN2	Metastasis to ipsilateral axillary lymph nodes that are fixed to one another or to other structures
pN3	Metastasis to ipsilateral internal mammary lymph node(s)

Distant Metastasis (M)

MX	Presence of distant metastasis cannot be assessed
M0	No distant metastasis
M1	Distant metastasis (includes metastasis to ipsilateral supraclavicular lymph node(s)

STAGE GROUPING

Stage 0	Tis, N0, M0
Stage I	T1, N0, M0
	T1, N1, M0
Stage IIA	T0, N1, M0
	T2, N0, M0
Stage IIB	T2, N1, M0
	T3, N0, M0

Stage IIIA	T0, N2, M0
	T1, N2, M0
	T2, N2, M0
	T3, N1, M0
	T3, N2, M0

Stage IIIB	T4, any N, M0
	Any T, N3, M0

Stage IV	Any T, any N, M1

APPENDIX D: GLOSSARY OF ABBREVIATIONS AND SIGNS

A	Used in chemotherapy for Adriamycin (doxorubicin)
AC	Multidrug chemotherapy: doxorubicin (Adriamycin)/cyclo-phosphamide
APN	Advanced preparation nurse
AxLN	Axillary lymph node(s)
AxLND	Axillary lymph node dissection (removal of levels I and II as part of breast-conserving therapy)
BCDDP	Breast Cancer Detection Demonstration Project
BCT	Breast-conserving therapy
BDC	Breast Diagnostic Center, Women's and Children's Hospital, LAC + USC Medical Center, Los Angeles, California
BI-RADS	Breast imaging reporting and data system
BRCA1	Human breast cancer gene number one (the first identified)
BRCA2	Human breast cancer gene number two (the second identified)
BSE	Breast self-examination
CBE	Clinical breast examination
CC	Craniocaudal (views on mammography) [not to be confused with cc = chief complaint]
CDP	Complete (complex) decongestive physiotherapy
CMF	Polychemotherapy: cyclophosphamide/methotrexate/5-fluo-rouracil
DCIS	Ductal carcinoma in situ
DNA	Deoxyribonucleic acid
EBCTCG	Early Breast Cancer Trialists' Collaborative Group
EIC	Extensive intraductal component
ER	Estrogen receptor
	ER^+ = estrogen receptor positive
	ER^- = estrogen receptor negative
ERT	Estrogen replacement therapy
FAC	Polychemotherapy: 5-fluorouracil/doxorubicin (Adriamycin)/cyclophosphamide

FCC	Fibrocystic change
FNA	Fine-needle aspiration, including "needle alone" (without negative pressure/suction)
5-FU	5-Fluorouracil
HRM	Halsted radical mastectomy
HRT	Hormone replacement therapy (estrogen and progestin)
Hx	History
IDC	Invasive ductal carcinoma
IV	Intravenous
LAC	Los Angeles County
LAC + USC	Los Angeles County plus University of Southern California Medical Center, Los Angeles, California
LCIS	Lobular carcinoma in situ
LMP	Last menstrual period (date of onset)
MLO	Mediolateral oblique (view on mammography)
MRI	Magnetic resonance imaging
MRM	Modified radical mastectomy
NCI	National Cancer Institute (Bethesda, MD)
NDBB	Needle-directed breast biopsy
NIH	National Institutes of Health (Bethesda, MD)
NSABP	National Surgical Adjuvant Breast and Bowel Project
OC	Oral contraceptive
OCT	Oral contraceptive therapy
OSBx	Open surgical biopsy
Pap	Papanicolaou stain for test smears obtained from the uterine cervix for detection of premalignant or malignant cytology
PCP	Primary care physician
PET	Positron emission tomography (scan)
PR	Progesterone receptor
	PR^+ = progesterone receptor positive
	PR^- = progesterone receptor negative
QOL	Quality of life
RNA	Ribonucleic acid
RT	Radiation therapy (used with breast-conserving therapy)
Rx	Treatment or therapy
SEER	Surveillance, Epidemiology, and End Results (NCI)
STAT	Immediately
Tam, Tamox	Used in chemotherapy to indicate tamoxifen
TCNB	Tissue core-needle biopsy
TDLU	Terminal duct lobular unit
TNM	Staging system for breast cancer: T = tumor size, N = nodal status (number), M = presence of metastasis
UOQ	Upper outer quadrant of the breast
US	Ultrasonography
USC	University of Southern California

USC/NBC   University of Southern California/Norris Breast Center, Norris
                   Comprehensive Cancer Center, Los Angeles, California
USC/NCCC   University of Southern California/Norris Comprehensive
                   Cancer Center, Los Angeles
W&CH   Women's and Children's Hospital at LAC + USC Medical
                   Center, Los Angeles

>   more than
<   less than
%   percent
cc   cubic centimeters
cm   centimeters
mg   milligrams
mm   millimeters

Appendix E: Glossary of Definitions of Terms as Used in This Text*

acini (plural): Small sac-like structures, particularly those of glandular nature (function), singular = **acinus**

anecdotal: Not published. Based on descriptions of unmatched individual cases rather than on controlled studies. A short account of a happening (e.g., a single case report).

anechoic: Without internal echoes (ultrasonography).

apoptosis: Fragmentation of a cell into membrane-bound particles that are then eliminated by phagocytosis (e.g., physiologic planned cyclic cell death).

areola: Circular pigmented (dark) area of the skin surrounding the base of the nipple.

axillary lymph node levels (I, II, III): Level I is lateral to the insertion of the pectoralis minor muscle; level II is under the insertion of the pectoralis minor muscle; level III is medial to the insertion of the pectoralis minor muscle.

baseline mammogram: Term originally used for an initial mammogram usually obtained several years before the age for which routine periodic mammography was recommended. This screening concept has been abandoned. Current mammography guidelines begin with routine (usually annual) mammograms.

benign: Characteristic of doing little or no harm; not malignant.

benignity: Condition of being benign (i.e., not malignant).

biopsy: Removal and examination, usually microscopic, of tissue from the living body, performed to establish a precise diagnosis. In the BDC this term is

---

* Adapted from *Dorland's Illustrated Medical Dictionary* (28th ed), Philadelphia, Saunders, 1994; or from *Webster's New World College Dictionary* (3rd ed), New York, Macmillan Simon & Schuster, 1996.

restricted to "tissue" sampling and is *not* used for cellular (cytology) sampling. The term implies histology. In our patient population it is presumed that biopsy entails a surgical incision (of the breast) with anesthesia and a visible scar.

circumareolar: Around the border of the areola (at the pigmented–normal skin junction). Synonym = *periareolar*.

cosmesis: Preservation, restoration, or bestowing of bodily beauty.

cure: Successful treatment of disease; for cancer, the therapeutic result of having no evidence of recurrence (local or metastatic) (i.e., for the remainder of one's life).

desmoplastic: Characterized by or causing the growth of fibrous tissue.

diagnostic mammography: Film screen breast imaging of symptomatic patient beginning with the craniocaudal (CC) and mediolateral oblique (MLO) views; then additional views and techniques (e.g., spot compression or magnification) as indicated.

diagnostic triad: Utilization of clinical breast examination (and breast-oriented history), mammography, and fine-needle aspiration for evaluation of a dominant breast mass. Synonyms = *triple assessment, triple diagnosis, triple test*.

diffuse: Spread out or dispersed; not concentrated.

discohesion: Properly = dyshesion. By common medical usage: lack of cohesion of cells in their normal architectural histologic pattern. Colloquially: *falling-apart pattern*.

dominant breast mass: Three-dimensional distinct mass that is different from the remainder of the breast tissue and the tissue of the other breast.

down-staging: Use of chemotherapy to "shrink" cancers to a smaller size, which reduces the stage (e.g., stage III to stage II) and thereby makes them eligible for breast-conserving therapy or allows surgical resection of previously "inoperable" cancers.

ductogram: Mammographic procedure of injecting contrast medium into a single duct opening on the nipple to visualize an intraductal lesion (e.g., an intraductal papilloma). Synonym = *galactogram*.

dyshesion: Loss of intercellular cohesion, a characteristic of malignancy, as determined by aspiration biopsy; disordered cell appearance. Colloquially, *discohesion*. Adj. = **dyshesive**

dysplasia: Variation in the size, shape, and structure (architecture) of adult cells, with implied premalignant potential and suggestion of malignant transformation (e.g., dysplasia of the squamous epithelial cells of the uterine cervix). The term dysplasia has been inappropriately used (usually to connote extreme mammographic density) when describing mammographic and cytologic findings.

dystrophic: Characterized by dystrophy. Used in mammography to describe certain calcifications.

dystrophy: Any disorder arising from defective or faulty nutrition or physiology.

echogenicity: Ultrasonographic pattern of reflections (echoes) of ultrasound waves (e.g., those produced within a solid mass). Adj. = **echogenic**.

edge shadows: On ultrasound scans, posterior shadows (dark) at the periphery of the mass with loss of signals (echoes) beyond the edge.

elicited: Drawn forth or evoked. Provoked, stimulated (in contrast to spontaneous). Used with normal physiologic nipple discharge.

enucleation: Removal of an organ, tumor, or another body in such a way that it comes out clean and whole, like a nut from its shell. A procedure to remove a mass (e.g., fibroadenoma) by blunt and sharp dissection without removing adherent surrounding tissue.

excise: To remove by cutting out or away.

excision: Removal (of a tumor, organ) by cutting.

excisional biopsy: Biopsy of an entire lesion, including a significant margin of contiguous normal-appearing tissue. Alternately = **excision biopsy**. Often used colloquially as synonymous with open surgical biopsy or lumpectomy.

fibromyxoid: Primitive connective tissue cells and stroma resembling mesenchyme. Myxoid tissue is loose connective tissue rich in mucopolysaccharides. The fibroblasts within the tissue are small and stellate in shape.

fine needle: 22-Gauge (or smaller) needle.

fine-needle aspiration: Technique used to diagnosis (and drain) a cyst or to obtain a cellular sample from a solid mass for cytologic interpretation (in contrast to tissue biopsy for histology).

frond: Leafy-looking (e.g., fern-like) projection.

galactogram: Alternate term for ductogram.

heterogeneous: Consisting or composed of dissimilar elements or ingredients; not having a uniform quality throughout. Noun = **heterogeneity**.

hyperechoic: On ultrasound scans, increased echogenicity compared to that of normal breast parenchyma. Characteristic of the anterior and posterior borders of a cyst.

hypoechoic: On ultrasound scans, decreased echogenicity compared to that of normal breast parenchyma. Characteristic of a solid breast neoplasm.

indeterminate: Used in cytology, histology, and imaging reports to qualify the impression of a lesion that does not have clearly defined characteristics typical of a benign or malignant lesion. Sometimes used colloquially in the same sense as *borderline*.

infiltrating: Penetrating the interstices (spaces or gaps) of a tissue. Used in oncology as a synonym for invasive.

invasive: Tending to infiltrate and actively destroy surrounding tissue. Used in oncology as synonymous with *infiltrating*.

inversion: Of the nipple: inward turning of the nipple upon itself. Nipple usually "comes out" with compression of the areola (see *retraction*). Often bilateral, usually begins during puberty.

involved lymph node: Metastatic cancer growing within a lymph node. Colloquial = "positive," in contrast to a "negative" (clear) lymph node.

irradiation: Application of ionizing radiation for therapeutic purposes (radiation therapy).

lesion: Any pathologic or traumatic discontinuity of tissue or loss of function of a part. Commonly used to denote an abnormal physical (or mammographic) finding including a lump or mass.

localize: Make local; limited or confined to a particular place, area, or locality; to concentrate in one area, especially of the body.

lump: Solid mass of no special shape; a swelling or protuberance. The imprecise definition of lump has led to the precise description of a "dominant breast mass."

lumpectomy: Synonymous with excision biopsy as per the NSABP protocol; also partial mastectomy and segmental mastectomy, which is the term commonly used in Europe, particularly in Italy.

lumpy: Diffuse nodular texture of the breast by palpation, common in most women of reproductive age. "Lumpy bumpy" texture is usually bilateral, more prominent in the upper outer quadrants.

macrocyst: Palpable cyst.

malignant: Virulent with the potential of becoming progressively worse and ultimately causing death (i.e., an anaplastic tumor with invasion that is capable of metastasis).

mass: Lump or body made up of cohering particles. A general term for an accumulation of cells or cohesive tissue. Used in this text for a three-dimensional distinct mass. Often loosely used in the medical literature for a "lump" or "tumor." Confusion as to the definition of "mass" has led to the precise term of "dominant breast mass."

mastalgia: Pain in the mammary gland. The preferred term in this text. Synonym = *mastodynia* (commonly used in Europe).

mastodynia: Pain in the breast. Synonym = *mastalgia*.

medical oncologist: Internal medicine physician specializing in chemotherapy.

mesenchyme (mesenchyma): Meshwork of embryonic connective tissue in the mesoderm from which are formed the connective tissues of the body, blood vessels, and lymphatic vessels.

metastatic: Spreading (of a cancer) from its primary location in the body to another, unrelated location.

microcyst: Nonpalpable cyst.

microdochectomy: Excision of a segment of a single duct, usually below the nipple and through a small circumareolar incision, for spontaneous pathologic nipple discharge.

multiplicity: Quality or state of being manifold, various, numerous. In breast disease, generally accepted as a sign of benignity because two or three cancers hardly ever arise simultaneously. Used in breast imaging as a strong indication of the benign nature of multiple mammographically similar lesions (e.g., cysts or fibroadenomas).

negative: By common medical usage this indicates the absence of a pathologic condition. Patients frequently assume that this term indicates that they are free of disease (e.g., cancer). [The editor prefers to avoid this term because it can lead to lack of appropriate action by the health care provider and false reassurance to the patient, as in a "negative" mammogram.]

neoplasm: Any new and abnormal growth; specifically a new growth of tissue in which the growth is uncontrolled and progressive. Synonym = *tumor*.

nipple–areolar complex: Anatomic term for the entire nipple, areola, and underlying structures as a unit.

nodule: Small knot or irregular rounded lump. **nodular** (adj) **nodularity** (noun).

nondiagnostic: Used in cytology reports when no (or rare) benign ductal epithelial cells are present, such as an FNA smear showing blood, adipose tissue, and stroma.

oncologist: Physician who specializes in tumors, usually cancer.

open surgical biopsy: Often used colloquially as synonymous with excisional biopsy, although technically other types of biopsy would also be included.

parenchyma: Functional (glandular) tissue of an organ or lesion.

pass: Used by cytopathologist to indicate a separate (skin-to-skin) FNA (e.g., "make four passes"). Not to be confused with the thrusts of the needle up and down within the mass. Often used as a synonym for *puncture*.

paucicellular: Few cells present (e.g., on an FNA smear).

periareolar: Circumareolar.

pneumocystogram: Mammographic procedure of injecting air into a cyst after the fluid has been removed to visualize the inner surface of the cyst for signs of an intracystic neoplasm.

polyclonal: Derived from different cell types.

positive: By common medical usage, an adverse pathologic condition, meaning malignantly involved, when applied to a disease process, as in positive nodes, positive margins. [The editor prefers to avoid the use of this emotionally ambiguous term as it is frequently misinterpreted by the patient to mean "good."]

posterior acoustic shadow: On ultrasound scans, a shadow (dark) below the entire mass. Characteristic of a solid mass.

posterior enhancement: On ultrasound scans, increased echoes (white) below a mass. Characteristic of a cyst.

progesterone: Steroid hormone active in preparing the uterus for reception and development of a fertilized ovum and the mammary glands for milk secretion. **progestational** (adj.).

progestin: Colloquially used for synthetic progestational agents.

progestogen: Any substance possessing progestational activity (i.e., natural or synthetic).

puncture: Act of perforating or piercing. Commonly used in Europe as a synonym for fine-needle aspiration. Often used by U.S. cytopathologists to indicate a separate insertion of the needle through the skin (e.g., "four punctures should be made") usually with a separate set of slides for each puncture. Often used as a synonym for *pass*.

retraction: Of the nipple: a secondary change, often of recent onset, caused by contraction of the supporting tissue so the nipple is permanently drawn back. The nipple does not "come out" with pressure on the areola. It can be a secondary sign of breast cancer.

screening mammography: Periodic mammography (CC and MLO views) of asymptomatic women.

second opinion: Evaluation and recommendation for management of a patient by another physician or group of health care providers after the initial physician's diagnosis and treatment plan. It has become routine practice in many urban locations. However, nothing guarantees that the second opinion is any more "correct" than the initial opinion. Optimally, in the case of breast cancer, the second opinion is rendered by an interdisciplinary treatment planning team in a comprehensive cancer center.

spiculated: Having a sharp, needle-like body mammographically characteristic of margins (borders) of invasive ductal carcinoma. "Spiculated" is the BI-RADS' preferred terminology, rather than the previously used "stellate."

Staff: Designates full-time physician faculty of the Department of Obstetrics and Gynecology, University of Southern California Medical School.

stellate: Shaped like a star, arranged in a rosette. Previously used to describe the characteristic appearance of invasive ductal carcinoma seen on a mammogram. "Spiculated" is now the BI-RADS' preferred terminology.

stroma: Supporting (connective) tissue or matrix of an organ or lesion.

subcuticular: Below the surface of the skin (e.g., sutures placed in the dermis) so no sutures are visible when the skin is closed.

synchronous: Happening at the same time; simultaneous; occurring together.

thickening: Thickened part of something. *Thickened* = made or being thick or thicker, as in dimension, density, consistency, articulation.

triple assessment: Diagnostic triad.

triple diagnosis: Diagnostic triad.

triple test: Diagnostic triad.

tumor: Neoplasm.

INDEX